2

D0216369

*Normality Does Not
Equal Mental Health*

Also from Steven James Bartlett

The Pathology of Man: A Study of Human Evil

Reflexivity: A Source Book in Self-Reference

When You Don't Know Where to Turn: A Self-Diagnosing
Guide to Counseling and Therapy

Self-Reference: Reflections on Reflexivity (co-edited with Peter Suber)

Conceptual Therapy: An Introduction to Framework-Relative Epistemology

Metalogic of Reference: A Study in the Foundations of Possibility

VALIDITY: A Learning Game Approach to Mathematical Logic

As editor of these books by Paul Alexander Bartlett:
Voices from the Past – A Quintet of Novels

Sappho's Journal

Christ's Journal

Leonardo da Vinci's Journal

Shakespeare's Journal

Lincoln's Journal

Normality Does Not Equal Mental Health

The Need to Look Elsewhere for Standards of Good Psychological Health

Steven James Bartlett

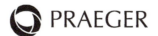

PRAEGER

AN IMPRINT OF ABC-CLIO, LLC
Santa Barbara, California • Denver, Colorado • Oxford, England

Copyright 2011 by Steven James Bartlett

All rights reserved. No part of this publication may be reproduced, stored in a retrieval system, or transmitted, in any form or by any means, electronic, mechanical, photocopying, recording, or otherwise, except for the inclusion of brief quotations in a review, without prior permission in writing from the publisher.

Library of Congress Cataloging-in-Publication Data

Bartlett, Steven J.
  Normality does not equal mental health : the need to look elsewhere for standards of good psychological health / Steven James Bartlett.
    p. cm.
  Includes bibliographical references and index.
    ISBN 978–0–313–39931–2 (hard copy : alk. paper)— ISBN 978–0–313–39932–9 (ebook)
  1. Mental health. 2. Psychology, Pathological. 3. Creative ability. I. Title.
RA790.5.B345   2011
362.2—dc22   2011015147

ISBN: 978–0–313–39931–2
EISBN: 978–0–313–39932–9

15 14 13 12 11   1 2 3 4 5

This book is also available on the World Wide Web as an eBook.
Visit www.abc-clio.com for details.

Praeger
An Imprint of ABC-CLIO, LLC

ABC-CLIO, LLC
130 Cremona Drive, P.O. Box 1911
Santa Barbara, California 93116-1911

This book is printed on acid-free paper ∞

Manufactured in the United States of America

*Dedicated to those who are willing to see things differently,
who may therefore lead the way to better people.*

Einstein was once asked, "What can we do to get a better world?"
He replied, "You have to have better people."
—Quoted in Wynne-Tyson (1985/1989, p. 422)

Contents

Preface

"Normal is good, abnormal is bad" is an unquestioned refrain of conventional wisdom in such varied areas as child-raising, elementary and higher education, peer-reviewed publications, the evaluative judgments of society, and understanding the psychology of creative individuals—and, when translated and clothed in slightly more sophisticated attire, it is the basis for much of the diagnostic framework of contemporary psychiatry and clinical psychology. The general equation of psychological normality with good mental health, and of psychological abnormality with mental illness, together express an uncritical bias that favors what is humanly typical and socially and politically desirable. This equation has had far-reaching consequences, consequences that affect humanity and human culture far beyond the diagnostic confines of psychiatry and clinical psychology.

To examine this issue and certain of its major and sometimes wide-ranging ramifications is the central purpose of this book. Its rationale is to pick up the discussion where two psychologist-authors, Abraham Maslow and Thomas Szasz, left off: Maslow directed attention to the characteristics of "self-actualizing" people in an effort to delineate ways in which they exemplify a better and higher degree of mental health than is to be found among the typical, psychologically average population. Maslow was a pioneer in recognizing the need to raise the criteria used to define positive psychological health from conventionally applied standards to a higher level.

Szasz approached human psychology from a different perspective. He opposed the diagnostic labeling of contemporary psychiatry and clinical psychology because their conception of "mental disorders," in his view, expresses the not-so-hidden agenda to force people to conform to social and political interests. Szasz's criticism of *DSM*-inspired labeling led him to characterize its alleged "mental disorders" as so much ideologically motivated "mythology."

In their challenges to contemporary psychology and psychiatry, neither Maslow nor Szasz apparently thought to question whether the widespread presumption—that psychological normality should be used as a standard, a baseline, for good mental health—is *deserved*. *Normality Does Not Equal Mental Health* is the first book to do this.

To that end, the book moves beyond Maslow and Szasz by seeking to show, first, that psychologically normality cannot serve as a justifiable standard in terms of which to distinguish good from dysfunctional mental health; second, that today's "mental disorders" are not so much a matter of "myth" but of conceptual and empirical error; and, third, that we are in need of revised and revitalized concepts of mental health and the treatment of human psychological problems, both of which the book formulates.

Where Maslow intuitively pointed to positive characteristics of "highly developed" people, the book's purpose is to show why it is *necessary* to look elsewhere, beyond psychological normality, for acceptable standards of positive mental health—because if we fail to do this, we mistakenly base our conception of good psychological health on the model offered by the inherently limiting and often destructive psychology of normality.

Where Szasz saw "mythological thinking" in the creation of today's rapidly inflating lexicon of mental disorders, the book's purpose is to show that the majority of claims concerning such "mental disorders" involve fundamental conceptual errors and a disregard for scientific standards of validity. This is not a matter of directing attention to vested social and clinical interests expressed in the language of myth but of showing such claims to be *wrong* because, first, they conflict with scientific standards of evidence and conceptual coherence, and second, and more importantly, they are *misguided* in holding up as a standard of good mental health what we should by now know to be frequently dysfunctional and indeed pathogenic.

The unexamined presumption of psychological normality as a desirable standard of good mental health has infiltrated a wide variety of contexts, including the psychology of definition in psychiatric nosology (i.e., the definition of 'mental disorders' in the *DSM*), the psychology of higher education, the psychology of creativity, the psychology that impairs human cultural development, the psychology of peer review, and the internally limiting psychology of mediocrity, which has been studied almost not at all. The book shows how the equation of psychological normality with good mental health goes wrong in the real world and how it does this is a wide variety of contexts. In place of that unsatisfactory standard, the book offers a constructive, positive conception of good mental health and outlines how psychotherapy can be redirected to foster it.

Acknowledgments

One of the few advantages of growing older is the privilege of looking as far back as a short human lifespan permits. And looking back, I can't help but see a strong thread of iconoclasm that stitches together the fabric of reflections begun more than four decades ago. As I suspect the reader already knows, iconoclasm isn't generally encouraged by our teachers and mentors, but in this respect I've been lucky in my life that a number of original thinkers, people who did not resist a fresh look at ingrained patterns of thinking, gave me their personal and professional encouragement.

As it is now routine good taste to make clear at this point: none of these people should be held responsible for what each may inadvertently have done as a result of his generosity. Even so, I want to thank the following individualists for their guidance and for the breadth of their perception and compass of their minds: *Melvin Calvin*, Nobel Laureate in chemistry of the University of California at Berkeley, for his warm encouragement in connection with my search for new antibiotics; *Thomas N. Fast* for his generous guidance and free run of the microbiology lab at the University of Santa Clara; *William Altus*, of the University of California, Santa Barbara, for his insightful direction as my interests in pathology grew to include psychiatric pathology; and *Robert M. Hutchins*, founder and director of the Center for the Study of Democratic Institutions, for having been persuaded that through my writing I would contribute to what, in the introductory volume of the *Great Books of the Western World*, he called "The Great Conversation." His scope of perception, intellectual sharpness, generous humanity and spirit, and statesmanship in the nearly forgotten meaning of the word I miss very much. I am also indebted to *Gabriel Marcel* for making it possible for me to study with Paul Ricoeur at the Université de Paris; to *Paul Ricoeur*, whose wide span of interest and scholarly knowledge, along with his intellectual fearlessness and creative capacity, made it possible to turn what is so often an intellectually humdrum dissertation experience into the development of a method and approach that I continue to develop; and to *C. F. von Weizsäcker*, director of the Max-Planck-Institut in Starnberg, Germany, for his support of research that underlies a few of the chapters in this book.

These men had one admirable quality in common: They were sufficiently at home in a noncompartmentalized openness to free inquiry not to be intimidated by it. They were sufficiently secure, both personally and intellectually, not to be threatened by critical thinking and the iconoclasm that is its natural result.

I also wish to thank *Thomas Maloney*, clinical psychologist in Clayton, Missouri, who became a true colleague and good friend. I owe much to him, and now to his memory, for his willingness to provide me with a practicum as his cotherapist.

I want to express my appreciation to *Debbie Carvalko*, Praeger's senior acquisitions editor in psychology and health, and to Praeger's editorial board for their intellectual openness and interest in fresh ideas and new directions of inquiry that challenge the status quo, qualities that are highly valued but increasing rarities among publishers at a time of conservatism and conformity.

Most especially I'm grateful to the significant people in my personal life: to my wife, *Karen Bartlett*, for her love, friendship, and faithful encouragement over the years; to my mother, *Elizabeth Bartlett*, poet; and to my father, *Paul Alexander Bartlett*, novelist-artist. In this less than the best of possible worlds, no one could possibly have had parents who offered a more culturally rich upbringing in which the values of intellectual courage and honesty, independence of mind, and compassion were foremost.

A Note on Conventions

In the course of this book we'll encounter a variety of natural human psychological propensities to believe without adequate justification. One of these is to mistake words for the things we believe they represent. For example, we can be lulled into believing that because we have a name for a psychological disorder such a disorder must exist. To avoid misplaced belief it is essential to distinguish two fundamentally different uses of language.

To do this I use a convention drawn from semiotics, or the theory of signs, to make clear when so-called "autonymous" or "indirect reference" is made to a word, phrase, or other symbol and to distinguish this from its ordinary use. This convention reminds us to be aware when reference is made only to words themselves as opposed to what they mean or what we believe they designate.

When reference is made to a word, phrase, or symbol itself, single quotes (also called inverted commas) are placed around it; they're also used to set off a quote within a quote. Double quotes are reserved for direct quotations and to draw attention to words employed in an important way, or words used in an odd, exaggerated, or illogical fashion that stretches their usual meaning. To illustrate this practice: 'five' contains four letters, in contrast to Einstein's wise maxim, "to keep doing the same things unsuccessfully is insanity."

Whenever feasible I've used gender-neutral language in this book. In infrequent passages where it would be repetitive to the point of ridiculousness to use 'he or she' and its variants, I've followed the equitable convention proposed by Charles Murray (2003, p. xiv) to use the author's own sex as the choice of third-person singular pronouns.

Chapter endnotes have been kept to a minimum; most provide explanatory details.

Introduction

> The range of what we think and do is limited by what we fail to notice.
> And because we fail to notice *that* we fail to notice there is little we can
> do to change until we notice how failing to notice shapes our thoughts
> and deeds.
>
> —Goleman (1985, p. 24)

"I like to believe _____" is a phrase that has often caught my ear in discussions with others. It's been a long time since I've been able pass over the phase in innocence. Now I flinch when I hear it. During the past four decades the focus of much of my research has been the psychology of belief; from this experience the deeply rooted connection between what we *like* and what we *believe* has impressed itself on me. The beliefs we embrace, as I see again and again, express what we *prefer to think*. History unfortunately makes it all too clear that what we like to believe all too often turns out simply to be wrong.

If we chose, we could make this very human disposition a focus of study. We would then examine the psychology underpinning our often passionate commitments to beliefs, ideas, principles, paradigms, and all the other ingredients that make up the approaches, methods, and theories which, in one way or another, we *like* better than others and to which we give our allegiance and defend with sometimes confounding hardihood even when confronted by contrary evidence (and sometimes especially then!).

For better or worse, we are emotionally defined organisms whose choices as to what to believe and what not to are motivated in large measure by a relatively simple psychology of reinforcement, security, and comfort. Conventional thinking *is* the way average people think, not because the majority just *happens* to think that way but because conformity with convention gratifies many people in terms of reinforcement, security, and comfort.

Unfortunately, what we like to think, what we prefer to believe, can be false, misleading, and at times harmful precisely because we resist putting our ideological preferences into question. It is now common practice to refer to "belief *systems*," and this is appropriate since beliefs are built on beliefs, layer upon layer, in interdependent, integrated ways that form systems that possess a dynamic of their own—resistant to change, chameleonlike so as to accommodate to varying environments of fact and fashion, and structured so as to protect and defend those systems, much as the human immune system is organized to withstand and fight back when challenged by a pathogen.

The fortitude and obduracy of systems of belief are their strength but also their downfall. Conservative thinking—adherence to and defense of conventions that are dominant at any particular time—therefore automatically brings with it a limited field of vision and a self-chosen myopia. If any blame can be laid for periods of slowed, nonexistent, or retrograde intellectual and scientific development, for periods of uncreative, sluggish, and at times imperceptible growth, that blame can be placed both on the natural human unwillingness to call into question beliefs that apparently have served well enough in the past and on the deeply entrenched disinclination to step outside of the preferred category set. Individuals who are willing to do these things tend to be few, and they should expect to meet correspondingly deeply rooted resistance, which of course indeed they have throughout the past.

As a consequence of the psychology of belief, when we look at the history of science we see that its most basic concepts and presuppositions are often the least examined. They form the basis for all else in scientific thought, so that in their very mental activity scientists make habitual use of them. This results in it being all the more intellectually difficult and challenging to place them in the light of day. Since they serve as the fundamental, core conceptual vocabulary of scientific thought, they resist critical examination, because for a scientist to do this, he or she believes, often incorrectly, that those very concepts and presuppositions must be used.

It can be hard intellectual work to find ways of stepping back or out of the habitual reference frame, and if necessary to develop new concepts and flexible ways of thinking that make it possible to render basic concepts and presuppositions explicit enough so they can be thought about without being themselves used in the process.

Unfortunately, when efforts like this are made, practitioners of a discipline very naturally often feel that one must step into an altogether different discipline—into "philosophy" or "metatheory"—which is then judged to comprise a separate area of study, one that can safely and conveniently be ignored by the scientist when his or her paradigm, tools of thinking, and habitual approach are made objects of explicit critical evaluation. This reaction has led to an unnecessary and undesirable compartmentalization of science and a divorce of science from "foundational questions" that are held at arm's length and encapsulated as alien—as just so much pure theory entirely divorced from practice.

As a result, the critical examination of the conceptual foundations of science is often disconnected from science and considered to be a distinct discipline, so that responsibility is transferred to philosophy of science or perhaps to epistemology studied within cognitive science. This has served both as an excuse for scientists to shift the responsibility for their conceptual clarity to others and as a source of encouragement for philosophers of science and epistemologists to take on such metathinking without the requirement of firsthand competency in science.

Such a separation of a discipline from an examination of its basic beliefs and concepts is ill-conceived and, indeed, limitative and destructive. If critical examination of the plans for a bridge or for space shuttle construction were divorced from actual bridge and shuttle engineering, bridges would much more frequently collapse and space shuttles disastrously fail. It is long past due that we should make the self-reflective critique of a science an integral and integrated part of scientific activity and part of the responsibility of any science for its own development.

This is not a book about philosophy of science or about epistemology, which is often assigned these tasks of reflective criticism. Like epistemology, much of the book's focus is on extremely basic questions, and its goals are similar: to improve our understanding, to make clear what it is that we actually understand and can know, and in this process to correct and avoid conceptual confusions.

But the approach used here is not epistemological but rather thoroughly psychological. In some of the chapters, my purpose is to challenge conventional thinking in psychiatry and clinical psychology, and to this end I've intentionally resisted the tendency to "philosophize" about psychology from an external standpoint disconnected from psychological study. I do not approach a critique of basic concepts and presuppositions of clinical psychology and psychiatry from outside but situate the discussion and the evidence provided from *within*, applying the observational framework and tools of psychology from inside. And so in some of the chapters I am interested in the psychological basis of much that psychiatrists and clinical psychologists think and do. This reflexive or self-referential use of psychology is natural for human beings to engage in, since we are ourselves reflective organisms, capable of self-awareness and self-criticism. At the same time, such a reflexive, critical turn of psychological thought back upon itself is what psychologically focused self-criticism, if it existed, would set as its subject matter and goal.

In other chapters, I also use the standpoint of clinical psychology and psychiatry to understand aspects of the present human situation, and in these chapters, where there is no intent to engage in presuppositional criticism, still we will push against the confines of established convention.

In both ways it is my conviction that we cannot become aware of our limitations unless we make the boundaries of our beliefs and thinking explicit, and to do this we must of course exceed those boundaries and step beyond what the past has allowed.

This book is about our usually unexamined, underlying, and indeed profoundly rooted psychology. A wide range of interconnected purposes will concern us. They include:

- A radical standing on its head of the view that psychological normality is equivalent to mental health, and therefore good;
- A revision of our understanding of mental health in a way that changes both our conception of mental disorders and, correlatively and perhaps surprisingly, also our understanding of the psychology of creativity;
- A discussion of seldom-recognized psychological problems brought about by two intertwined phenomena: (1) an epidemic of work and materialism that has led to an incapacitating mental disability of values and resulting widespread cultural impoverishment and (2) the associated collapse of a genuinely higher education that has led to demoralization among university faculty who are profoundly committed to that rapidly vanishing ideal;
- A long-avoided examination of the psychology of peer review and editorial bias;
- A detailed study of the psychology of mediocrity, which acts as a powerfully limiting force that hinders individual and group development; and
- The formulation of revised and revitalized concepts of mental health and the treatment of human psychological problems.

In the coming chapters we will discover, often at the very heart of each of the above issues, strongly entrenched commitments to the dominant and unquestioned belief that psychological normality must serve as a gold standard for good mental health. Contemporary psychiatry and clinical psychology base their conception of mental health on the baseline standard of psychological normality. This supposition has come to be accepted uncritically, has become habitual and fundamental to current clinical theory and practice, and lies at the core of the psychiatric classification system of the *DSM*, which has become today's diagnostic authority.

This is the first book to question the equation of psychological normality and mental health. In the chapters ahead, I propose to weigh the evidence and, using strict logic and compelling analysis, to challenge the current paradigm of mental health theorists and practitioners. It will be my intention to show how the presumed standard of normality has come to play a basic role in a surprisingly wide diversity of contexts. The broad and yet focused compass of the study seeks to make evident how this unquestioned presumption has come to permeate contemporary consciousness, often in unrecognized and well-disguised ways.

Throughout this book, as readers can immediately foresee, a variety of toes—that is to say, *beliefs*—will inevitably get stepped on. But I try to do this in as gentle and understanding a way possible, but also with directness and without equivocation, inviting readers to share in the intellectual adventure of sampling directions in psychology that may be new to them.

In writing this book it has been my sustained conviction that little good comes from shielding ourselves from critical thinking, and even less comes from adherence to beliefs simply because we *like* them, beliefs that we defend in the name of political or disciplinary correctness. Iconoclasm need not be felt as a threat: it can be freeing, indeed intellectually a source of playfulness and pleasure as we become unstuck from conventional categories and from social, political, and professional attitudes that serve mainly to narrow our field of vision while giving us a bad case of near-sightedness.

There is an underlying, unifying thread in the discussions that follow, and that is a willingness to examine a group of important psychological problems and subjects from a psychological perspective. This kind of self-referential approach from within psychology is unconventional and likely to be new to readers. It is intended to encourage—and indeed it presupposes—a certain intellectual flexibility and openness.

PART I

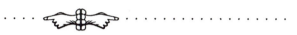

Normality and Mental Health

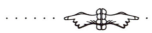

Questioning the Standard of Normality: Steps to a More Effective Understanding of Mental Health

[Y]ou ... talk about the truth, which turns out to be nothing but what you like to believe.
                                        —George Bernard Shaw (1934, p. 182)

Psychological normality has remained one of the last as well as one of the most central unexamined presuppositions of current psychiatry and clinical psychology. With few exceptions in the literature, psychological normality has served as an unquestioned standard of mental health while the same standard has been used to equate deviations from normality with mental illness. This opening chapter reviews some of the most compelling reasons to question that understanding of mental health and of the psychological problems that many people experience and outlines an alternative theoretical and therapeutic framework that offers promise.

To continue thinking unchallenged is, ninety-nine times out of a hundred, our practical substitute for knowing....
                                        —William James (1904/1958, p. 69)

Presuppositions held uncritically can powerfully impede the growth of any branch of learning. Because of the tenacious and obstructive nature of unexamined assumptions, it has often been an intellectually, politically, and sometimes religiously difficult project to place the prevailing beliefs of the day in question before the dispassionate eye of reason. Intrepid souls who have insisted on doing this have often been harshly rewarded for their pains, for unexamined assumptions are often closely tied to vested disciplinary interests, while attempts to question those assumptions are apt to run aground on the shoals of what is perceived to be counterintuitive, in conflict with establishment belief, and therefore seen literally to be "para-doxical."

One of the central assumptions of both the practice and theory of traditional psychiatry and clinical psychology is almost never discussed in the literature, and even more seldom is it questioned. Let us agree to step back to get an unobstructed view of this core assumption by means of a short, fictitious allegory, pretending for a few moments that we are visiting an alien planet populated by a humanoid life form. We on the visiting team are professional psychologists; our observations are described in the following report to be sent back home:

> We see that the planet's population has well-defined psychological characteristics that include a long history of very frequent wars, genocides, revolutions, and acts of terrorism. In all of these deadly quarrels the vast majority of the population has been enthusiastic to participate and can be aroused to engage in mass killing with little needed explanation or justification from their leaders. We find that violent conflicts bring the majority diverse forms of emotional gratification and stimulation. But we also find that there is sometimes a very small minority, averaging less than 1 percent of the adult population, who possess a strong aversion to harming or killing others.
>
> During infrequent periods of peace, as well as during periods of chronic deadly conflict, the majority's overwhelming preference in entertainment is to watch, read, and hear stories in which the plot revolves around violence and murder and to watch athletic contests that are violent. Our psychological testing, moreover, has shown that the majority will—without compunction and under no duress—inflict severe suffering and death on their unknown fellows merely if instructed to do this by those they consider to be authorities. The population is never at a loss to fill the ranks of its military, police, prison guards, or public executioners. If left unsupervised, their military, police, and prison personnel exhibit a pronounced tendency quickly to become violently and maliciously abusive toward their designated enemies or prisoners.
>
> We also find that the inhabitants of the planet take their beliefs with extreme seriousness, so much so that violent outbreaks of prejudice and hatred are a daily occurrence. More than this, we find that, again, the majority of the population receives emotional gratification from inflicting suffering and death on those whom they see as significantly different from themselves, whether because of distinguishable physical features, behavior, or beliefs. Their emotional responses to such signs of difference—expressed in the form of disrespect, ridicule, hatred, and persecution—give the majority satisfaction, and this helps to perpetuate the cycle.
>
> Theirs is a beautiful planet with a rich variety of many forms of life. However, the humanoid population proliferates without any thought to

ecological balance or intelligent judgment concerning the optimal population that the planet is capable of supporting and refuses to think about curtailing its population growth—in fact this topic is taboo in public discussion. As a result, the steadily encroaching humanoid population is extinguishing many thousands of irreplaceable species each year and is responsible for the largest species extinction in their world's geological history. At the same time, the uncontrolled population explosion is causing rapid climate change, which we can see will predictably accelerate and lead to worldwide suffering, famine, refugee migrations, resulting deadly conflicts, desertification and deforestation, the spread of toxic waste, further species extinctions, and a domino effect of these and related catastrophic yet avoidable consequences.

Two psychological characteristics stand out for us in observing this population: First, the majority express strong disapproval, offense, or denial if any of the above observations are brought to their attention. They are very proud of their various national groups and of their social, political, and religious institutions, and exhibit pronounced signs of narcissistic injury if their own psychologists (for they also have them) or our own team members share the foregoing observations with them.

Second, they are also deeply and rigidly committed to a conception of mental health based upon what they judge to be "psychologically normal." The majority are, by definition, psychologically normal, for by this they understand what is statistically average and hence the norm; those who deviate from psychological normality are considered aberrant, and for the aberrant their psychologists have developed a voluminous and detailed taxonomy to label specialized variations of deviation from psychological normality. Those who are so labeled are invalidated and stigmatized by their societies and tend to become social outcasts or involuntary inmates in mental institutions.

It is compellingly obvious to all of our team members that what the inhabitants understand by "psychological normality" is synonymous with the psychological description we have given above—of a form of life that, despite evident signs of intelligence, receives important and addictive emotional and cognitive gratifications from the many ways in which they choose to cause one another, as well as other forms of life, harm, suffering, and death. From our vantage point, their psychology of mental health and disease is a paradigm case of tragic irony, for it is founded on their central and misplaced use of the standard set by their own psychological normality, which has embedded within it the destructive emotional and cognitive predispositions we have already characterized. From our standpoint, we cannot judge their psychological normality to be other than pathological, for the normal, average psychology that characterizes the majority of their population results in harm that is unmistakable throughout the planet and observable in their private domestic lives, in bullying and mass killings in their schools, in their abuse-prone system of justice, in their social, religious, and political conflicts, and even in their preferred kinds of entertainment.

We initially believed that it would be possible to share our conclusions constructively with their psychologists, who at least have been able to recognize what, to us, are unmistakable pathological characteristics of the general population. However, when we have pointed out that their psychology is based on a dysfunctional standard, on a yardstick for mental health that implicitly legitimates planet-wide pathological affective and behavioral patterns, their psychologists take the same sort of narcissistic offense as does their own lay population when observations are expressed that they don't like.

As a result of our visit and the observations our team has made, as behavioral scientists we conclude that the majority, as well as the planet's own psychologists, are on a self-defeating, self-destructive path, heading in a direction about which we cannot be optimistic. Their own idealized conception of mental health, based as it is on a standard imbued with pathology, shows no promise for development unless an altogether different standard of mental health becomes evident and persuasive to the population. For this, their psychologists would need—again paradoxically for them—to study their own very small minorities that are to be found within the overall population, specialized groups that appear to be free from the pathologies of normality that characterize the majority.

FROM THE "BANALITY OF EVIL" TO THE "EVIL OF BANALITY"

The foregoing observations of another planet would be distressing indeed if they were applied to our own human world without a pacifying sugar-coated translation. Were the foregoing psychological observations to be published about the human species, we should anticipate that many people, even many behavioral scientists, would take offense or choose denial, preferring to relegate to silence what they do not want to believe. And yet, despite our predictable response to views that we find unpalatable, there has been some progress in the direction of reaching an honest human psychological self-understanding.

One of the first steps was taken when the meaning of the phrase 'the banality of evil' underwent a quiet change from the time that Hannah Arendt used it as a subtitle for her well-known book *Eichmann in Jerusalem* (Arendt, 1964). Most readers may not know that, surprisingly, Arendt used the phrase only once in her book, and only at its end, employing the phrase without discussion, definition, or explanation. Readers acquired a sense of the meaning of the phrase from context, but the meaning they derived in this way was not what Arendt herself appears to have had in mind.

Years later, more than two and a half decades after Arendt died, her colleague Jerome Kohn collected together some of her essays and published them under the title *Responsibility and Judgment* (Arendt, 2003). In one of her essays, Arendt made clear what the phrase was intended by her to mean—namely, the inability of many people to think:

> Some years ago, reporting the trial of Eichmann in Jerusalem, I spoke of the "banality of evil" and meant with this *no theory or doctrine* but something quite factual, the phenomenon of evil deeds, committed on gigantic scale, which could not be traced to any particularity of wickedness, pathology, or ideological conviction in the doer, whose only personal distinction was perhaps an extraordinary shallowness. However monstrous the deeds were, the doer was neither monstrous nor demonic, and the only specific characteristic one could detect in his past as well as in his behavior during the trial and the preceding police examination was something entirely negative: it was not stupidity but *a curious, quite authentic inability to think.* (Arendt, 2003, p. 159, italics added)

The equation of "banality of evil" with "a curious, quite authentic inability to think" is far from what most readers today associate with the banality of evil. Certainly most people are unaware that any sort of incapacity to think was involved in Arendt's view.

The phrase "banality of evil" has instead come to name, contrary to Arendt's stated intent, precisely the *theory or doctrine* according to which many people who perpetrate monstrous acts of atrocity are recognized to be psychologically normal; indeed, much of the factual reporting in *Eichmann in Jerusalem* bears this out. Once Arendt's thesis has been formulated in this way, it is plausible to find that thesis residing implicitly in the passage quoted above, when Arendt refers to "evil deeds . . . which could not be traced to any . . . pathology."

The "banality of evil" has evolved into the doctrine which claims that many people who perpetrate evil are generally not psychopathological but rather are psychologically normal. Studies that have appeared since Arendt died, such as Browning's *Ordinary Men: Reserve Police Battalion 101 and the Final Solution in Poland* (Browning, 1992) and Zillmer, Harrower, Ritzler, and Archer's *The Quest for the Nazi Personality: A Psychological Investigation of Nazi War Criminals* (Zillmer et al., 1995), have succeeded in bringing together strong evidence for the banality of evil understood in this sense.

Arendt's focus was a specialized population, the Nazi leaders, in which she found abundant evidence of human evil. She, and now others since she wrote, have in different ways supported the contention that many of the Nazi leaders, as well as Nazi soldiers and functionaries, were by and large psychologically normal people. However, Arendt did not undertake a much expanded analysis, not of special groups of war criminals, but of the population at large, in order to study in the psychologically normal majority the prevalence of highly destructive pathologies.

There is a very considerable difference, one which cannot be overemphasized, between finding that a specialized group of people who have committed atrocities are psychological normal, and finding, as our fictitious visiting team found on an alien planet, that the majority consisting of the psychologically normal have a predisposition to inflict harm and suffering on others in a way that can be characterized as pathological. There is clearly a very large difference in the range of application of these two divergent claims. The "banality of evil" has a very limited range of application; "the evil of banality," in contrast, includes most of the human population. In the latter, more inclusive framework, Arendt's work is historically significant, but it does not support the stronger and more embracing thesis. That more encompassing thesis may appropriately be called "*the evil of banality*," for such a thesis would locate the source of much of human psychiatric pathology in the psychological make-up of the psychologically normal person (see Bartlett, 2005, p. 315, and Bartlett, 2008).

I don't intend in this chapter to attempt to support this thesis, for to do this would require a book-length study, which now exists (Bartlett, 2005). Here, as introduction to what follows and for readers unfamiliar with that study, it may be helpful to summarize briefly its approach and some of its conclusions, since it is on this foundation that I want to raise the question here whether psychological normality should continue to be used to define mental health. I do not of course presume that readers should be persuaded by the conclusions that are merely summarized here, for the relevant evidence cannot be presented in a single chapter. Nonetheless some explanation of why I have chosen to go strongly against the prevailing current should be given. Certainly readers have a right to a brief explanation of an author's previously argued position when the author builds upon his or her past research.

Throughout its development, the science of pathology has accepted without question a homocentric bias that reserves the application of the clinical-diagnostic label 'pathogen' to nonhuman agents, such as disease-producing bacteria, viruses, or more recently discovered prions. But the concept of pathogenicity does not of itself dictate an exclusionary application to other-than-human forms of life. In *The Pathology of Man* (Bartlett, 2005), I argued the case expressed by the title, identifying and seeking to explain in psychological terms pathologies for which the human species, and by inclusion the psychologically normal human majority, are responsible. There are unfortunately many such pathologies. They include a varied and psychologically rewarding palette of emotional and cognitive gratifications provided by vicarious or direct participation in violence and hatred; by ideological rigidity and absolutism, obedience to perceived authority, prejudice and persecution, sheer self-defeating stupidity and low levels of moral development, and their many sequelae in genocides, terrorism, and wars; by school, domestic, social, and political bullying; by publicly approved imprisonment, torture, and executions; by an unconstrained proliferation of the human population to its own detriment and the detriment of many other forms of life, the unquestioned placement of human interests above those of all other life forms on the planet, the enforced subservience of nonhuman life to human wishes and convenience; and by the resulting devastation of global biodiversity. (On the psychology of human ecological destructiveness, see Bartlett, 2006.) The list of human pathologies does not end here.

Central to human pathology is human resistance to an awareness of it. "Denial" would be an understatement, for the forces that stand in the way of humankind's reflective consciousness of the psychological and ecological malignancy of the species are incredibly strong, tenacious, and self-preserving.

As a result of human recalcitrance to acknowledge our own pathology, in the history of behavioral science, and in particular in the history of psychology and psychiatry, almost no effort has been made to gain an understanding of human pathology that has its roots in *normal*—as opposed to abnormal—*psychology*. Primarily among psychiatrists there have been a few notable exceptions, including Menninger, Fromm, Peck, Milton Erickson, and others whose observations are discussed in Bartlett (2005), all of whom have had the courage to recognize the pathological constitution of the ordinary person who so often is a willing participant in inflicting suffering, death, and destruction. But despite the work of these few researchers, psychology and psychiatry have doggedly reserved the term 'pathology' exclusively for application to individuals and groups judged to be abnormal, that is, whose psychology deviates from the norm. This, as Bartlett (2005) attempts to show, is short-sightedness in the extreme.

My purpose in giving this preliminary overview is to center our attention on the important role that the standard of normality has played in traditional psychopathology. Psychological normality has served as the fundamental arbiter in the diagnostic judgments that psychiatry and clinical psychology have made when identifying psychiatric pathology. Nosologies of mental disorders have traditionally given center stage to psychological normality as a core criterion of mental health, in relation to which deviations from such psychological normality are judged to constitute psychiatric illness. A vaguely formulated, idealized conception of the "psychologically normal person" has been incorporated into diagnostic judgment. It has usually taken the form of a loosely understood, amalgamated construct formed from the statistical average in a society's

population in conjunction with the psychological and behavioral characteristics which that society judges to be typically acceptable. For as long
as psychiatry and psychology have sought to be scientific, various alternative constructs of this kind have been proposed and equated with the emotional and cognitive constitution of the "mentally healthy person." Such a
"psychologically normal" and hence "mentally healthy" person is believed
to exemplify the traditionally accepted signs of psychological health, such
as the abilities to care for oneself and for others, to be comparatively happy
or contented, to maintain stable and productive human relationships, and
to find satisfaction in work or creative activity.

We need to make a terminological digression at this point: Over the years,
psychology and psychiatry have found themselves mired in a confusing
multiplicity of definitions of the term 'normality', which I cannot discuss
at length here but which nonetheless should be mentioned since these
many definitions form an implicit historical backdrop for our discussion.
These definitions include normality considered as the statistical average
(among the earliest in the last century to focus upon this were Hacker,
1945 and Redlich, 1952); normality as adjustment (Wile, 1940); normality
as optimal functioning (applied to physical health, e.g., by Hacker, 1945);
normality linked to social desirability and conformity (e.g., Reider, 1950;
Szasz, 1970/1997; Bolton, 2008); normality as personality integration
(e.g., Hacker, 1945); normality as the expression of stage of evolution
(e.g., Millon, 1989; Wakefield, 1992); and normality defined in terms of
multiple factors, which in different combinations include those previously
mentioned, along with mental efficiency; diverse utopian ideals; the
pragmatic distinction between normality and mental illness, defined as
what clinicians treat; individual adaptive strength; integrity of personal
meaning; and so forth (representative examples include Jones, 1942;
Sabshin, 1967; Offer & Sabshin, 1966/1974, 1984, 1989; Buck, 1992;
Wood et al., 2007; Bolton, 2008).

   Since we cannot venture into this historical jungle of often conflicting
conceptions of normality, I ask readers to accept, for our purposes here,
a much simplified, intentionally fuzzy, and hence flexible understanding
of the phrase 'psychological normality'. What I will mean by 'psychological normality' is the set of *typical* and *socially approved* characteristics of
affective, cognitive, and behavioral functioning, a set of characteristics
derived from the reference group consisting of the majority in a society's
population and relative to which clinicians understand "deviations from

normality" and hence "mental disorder." I use the term 'normality' in its commonly accepted meaning of 'customary' and 'typical', and 'norm' in its ordinary meaning of 'an authoritative standard'. Finally, I distinguish the term 'normality' from terms like 'normative' and 'normativity', which suggest stipulative and usually ethical injunctions.

With these preliminary comments behind us, let's continue the main discussion.

THE DISPOSITIONAL PATHOLOGY OF PSYCHOLOGICAL NORMALITY

I've used the phrase 'the evil of banality' to place the doctrine that we've come to associate with Arendt in deliberate contrast with the more encompassing claim that psychologically normal people are predisposed, when the situation is right, to inflict harm on others and often on themselves in the process. In this chapter, when I speak of "predispositions" or "propensities" what I mean is that, with the exception of many criminals, bullies, and other people who have already behaved violently or abusively, the majority of psychologically normal people are "*sleepers*"—that is, they are dispositionally inclined, when the situation is right, to aggression and destructiveness. Their patterns of thought and behavior are to be understood dispositionally, that is, in the conditional sense that, if an adequately provoking situation arises, then the behavior that results will tend to be malignant: they have a pathogenic willingness to inflict harm, which remains latent until an appropriate situation arises. Such a situation may, for example, come in the form of war, ideological conflict, unrestricted power over others (as in an inadequately supervised prison), narcissistic injury, or in many other ways. Such "adequately provoking situations" unfortunately, as we know, arise with great frequency and prevalence.

Various psychiatrists, psychologists, ethologists, sociologists, anthropologists, and historians have recognized this dispositional propensity or predisposition of psychologically normal people to manifest aggressiveness and destructiveness. Among them, Freud, Jung, Menninger, Fromm, and Peck have emphasized this; quantitative historians Quincy Wright, Sorokin, Rashevsky, and Richardson came to the same conclusion, as have ethologists Lorenz and Eibl-Eibesfeldt as well (see Bartlett, 2005, Part II). It is both legitimate and appropriate for us to apply the term 'pathology' to this deeply rooted human predisposition.

Should we come to recognize that "psychological normality" is inherently pathogenic, that is, predisposing the majority of typical, normal people to harm others and often themselves as well, then it would seem that we come up short, without reliable bearings in terms of which to orient diagnostic study—without, in other words, possessing an agreed upon, objective standard of reference in terms of which to identify human pathology and to understand what constitutes good mental health.

Hannah Arendt's concept of "the banality of evil," as it has come to be understood, rests upon an unquestioned acceptance of psychological normality as a standard of mental health. We may quickly see that this is the case: implicit acceptance of this standard has understandably led researchers who are sympathetic with Arendt's view and who wish to build upon it to wonder how "psychologically normal people," who *should* be mentally healthy *by definition*, could possibly perpetrate such appalling, terrible acts of atrocity as we routinely see when human beings engage in violent conflicts, genocides, terrorism, or torture. The very fact that our adherence to the standard of psychological normality, intended to identify *the mentally healthy*, would lead to a state of such surprise and perplexity over what causes human evil should alert us that something in our theoretical orientation is fundamentally wrong.

What is wrong is misplaced emphasis. Psychological normality, far from comprising a reliable base from which to judge psychopathology, is essentially pathogenic and can serve as no useful standard for mentally healthy functioning. The very fact that only a tiny minority in any population will resist authority and refuse to kill others in wars that they are enlisted to fight—usually without adequate proof from their leaders that such wars are just or necessary—should tell us that average, majoritarian, psychologically normal people cause great harm. If the long human history of wars, genocides, deadly quarrels, imprisonment, torture, and executions is not enough, and if we need controlled experiments to reach the same conclusion, the now amply reproduced Milgram experiment (Milgram, 1974) and Zimbardo's prison experiment (for a retrospective analysis and update, see Zimbardo, 2007) show how the majority of psychologically normal people do and will, in fact, behave.

If our intent is to understand the psychology of people who resist inflicting suffering and death upon others, then we should look not to psychological normality as a standard of mental health but decisively in another direction: we should feel a need to understand the psychology of those who *resist* perpetrating harm, who are capable of thinking critically for themselves (which, we are reminded, was Arendt's original concern), and who have a level of moral and intellectual development that, in a comparative sense, "immunizes" them from participation in human pathology. (For the groundwork for such a study, see Bartlett, 2005, Chapter 12,

"The Psychology of Those Who Refuse to Participate in Mass Murder" and "Those Who Actively Resist.")

Arendt's conception of the banality of evil has not led us to question the central role in psychiatry and clinical psychology of the standard of normality, with reference to which psychopathologies are identified and judged to be disorders that are deviations from normality. However, were we, on the contrary, to recognize *the evil of banality*, we would already be halfway toward realizing the purpose of this volume, namely to challenge the appropriateness, usefulness, and effectiveness of employing what is merely normal as an arbiter of what is *desirable* in mental health.

PSYCHOLOGICAL NORMALITY IS NOT MENTAL HEALTH

The standard of health advocated by the yardstick of normality has become so habitual, so deeply ingrained in our mental health nosologies and therapeutic outlook that to question it can seem not only counterintuitive but to court the ridiculous and extreme. Certainly a statement becomes true the more it is repeated and never contradicted. And the standard of mental health that equates psychological normality with healthy mental functioning has remained unquestioned for a very long time.

One of the first to equate normality with sanity, and deviations from normality with mental illness, was Benjamin Rush (1746–1813), dean of the Medical School at the University of Pennsylvania and physician general of the Continental Army; his portrait is on the seal of the American Psychiatric Association. Dr. Rush defined sanity and insanity in the following terms: "Sanity—aptitude to judge things like other men, and regular habits, etc. Insanity a departure from this" (quoted in Szasz, 1970/ 1997, p. 141). For Dr. Rush, social conformity is synonymous with mental health, and social nonconformity with mental illness. In the two intervening centuries since Dr. Rush made his diagnostic pronouncements the standard of mental health set by conformity with the psychological norms of everyday society has remained exempt from serious challenge by mainstream psychiatry and clinical psychology.

Has the standard we have created by placing psychological normality on a pedestal become so imperious, so solidly embedded as an undeniable premise of modern psychiatric diagnosis, that as psychologists and psychiatrists we are incapable of thinking without it? Even if we should be persuaded that normal psychology can be correlated with pathological predispositions to prejudice, hatred, violence, and insensitivity to the suffering of others when they are dehumanized, conjoined with emotional gratification when those we see as our adversaries are harmed—even if we should be persuaded that normal, average people can readily be persuaded to become puppets of destruction, what would be accomplished by recognizing that pathology lies so close to home, and is not confined, as we would more comfortably prefer, to the smaller population of those whom we now label as mentally aberrant? This is an important question to which we shall return a little later.

Thomas Szasz has repeatedly emphasized that the labeling of persons as mentally healthy or as diseased is crucial to psychiatric practice. Psychiatric labeling is in and of itself an "act of social validation and invalidation" (Szasz, 1970/1997, p. 267). Psychiatric labeling sanctions society to set the limits on an individual's acceptability to his or her community. It sets the boundaries within which people are expected to conform in their attitudes toward others and themselves through their behavior, their preferences, and how they think and feel. Although this should hardly need to be said, it is important to express the following as explicitly as possible: *When we make the standard of mental health synonymous with psychological normality, we automatically validate normal psychology and invalidate deviations from it.* It makes good sense to do this as long as the standard of mental health we accept is not synonymous with a psychological predisposition to cause harm. At a theoretically fundamental level, theories of disease recognize that identifying a condition as a pathology means that we recognize that it causes *harm*—principally to the afflicted person or to others to whom he or she relates, or to both (for a detailed analysis see Bartlett, 2005, Part I). As in the extraterrestrial allegory with which I began this chapter, it is a tragic irony when what we embrace as mental health coincides with a propensity to cause harm. To use psychological normality as an arbiter of good mental health is to import pathology in our efforts to differentiate health as opposed to disease.

This point of view is, to be sure, a hard pill to swallow. It was hard enough to be faced with the banality of evil—to be forced by evidence to acknowledge that terrible atrocities are often committed by psychologically normal individuals. It has taken a great deal of carefully marshaled evidence to convince us that this is the case, and yet we do still, almost in a reflex arc, continue to look for reassuring signs of "abnormal psychology" in perpetrators of brutal criminal acts.

Now, to be faced with a need to accept the preponderance of evidence for the evil of banality—evidence that establishes that psychologically normal people are predisposed to harm others and often themselves in the process—this is considerably more taxing, and few scholars and researchers in behavioral science have been willing to consider the human species in this light. So that the skeptical reader may see that this understanding of human psychological normality is not as far-fetched as it might at first seem, here are a few examples of mental health professionals who in the past have reached similar conclusions:

Psychiatrist Milton Erickson wrote:

> It is time that society—particularly its psychologists and psychiatrists—takes a realistic view of the nature of undesirable and destructive human behavior and the extent to which, under stress or without stress, the individual, the group or an entire society can be led to enact it.... [N]o effort is made to investigate scientifically the extremes to which the normal, the good, the average, or the intellectual person or group will go if given the opportunity. ... (Erickson, 1968, p. 278)

> [N]ormal and average human beings can be manipulated into inhumane behavior. ... [T]he need is great to study the normal man from this aspect rather than continue to regard such behavior either as incomprehensible or as evidence that the person involved is somehow aberrant, abnormal and atypical. ... (p. 279)

In a parallel way, psychiatrist K. R. Eissler (1960), in a case study of soldiers judged to be "psychologically average," came to this conclusion: "In spite of a general consensus by the whole community that they are to be regarded as prototypes of normality, the psychiatrist finds himself professionally obliged to view these very men as specimens of significant psychopathology" (p. 69). Eissler went on to explain: "The general result pointed to a negative rather than a positive statement, namely, the fact that [a soldier's] efficiency is possible in spite of psychopathology and that quite possibly even that which is arbitrarily called *normality is a special instance of psychopathology*. If so, what the specific nature of that psychopathology is has escaped our knowledge" (p. 71, italics added). His paper concludes by saying: "Thus this paper may be taken as an attempt at trying out the operational value of the concept of *the psychopathology of normality*" (p. 94, italics added).

Also dating back to the 1960s, Daniel Offer and Melvin Sabshin's book, *Normality: Theoretical and Clinical Concepts of Mental Health* (1966/1974), questioned the assumption that psychological normality is free of pathology:

> [I]t is possible that the major impetus of this approach will be the redefinition of the borders of pathology to include a much wider range of phenomena heretofore omitted. It is also possible, of course, that out of such developments ... new ideas going beyond the broadened definition of pathology will develop. Whatever the new direction, it is clear that much more attention will be paid to the normal part of the spectrum than has been in the past. (p. 9)

[A] person who labels himself "normal" and is also labeled "normal" by others is far from being free from psychopathology, and indeed may be quite neurotic. (p. 33)

Psychologist Arthur G. Miller, reflecting on what we've learned from the obedience experiments, proposed what he called the "normality thesis": "The basic argument is that people who would not ordinarily be described as unusual, deviant, sick, mentally ill, or pathological are capable of committing acts of unrestrained violence and evil" (Miller, 1986, p. 184).

My point in citing behavioral scientists like Erickson, Eissler, Offer, Sabshin, and Miller is to ask that we reflect on the justification and desirability of making "mental health" and "psychological normality" synonymous. That they are not is a matter that is not hard to decide empirically, merely by reviewing human history, although we recognize that a willingness to be persuaded by the dismal facts about normal human propensities is still not common among behavioral scientists or the general public.

POSITIVE ILLUSION AND RESISTANCE TO THE PATHOLOGY OF NORMALITY

As far back in time as recorded history permits us to look we find evidence that people have sought to make the difficulties of life more acceptable and emotionally satisfying through recourse to the illusions of myth, the hopes of religion, and the security of systems of social ethics. Despite the evidence provided by history of the human need for such beliefs, for a long time traditional psychology embraced the view that to be mentally healthy a person should be realistic, "in touch with reality," that is, among other qualities, to be nondelusional about one's place in the world and about what one can realistically expect from life. But in the past few decades, the pendulum has swung the other way, affirming that "positive illusions" play a central role in a healthy, satisfying life. Indeed, the propensity to hold positive illusions has now become tantamount to being psychologically normal and hence mentally healthy. "A substantial amount of research testifies to the prevalence of illusion in normal human cognition" (Taylor & Brown, 1988, p. 193). "[T]he healthy mind is a self-deceptive one" (Taylor, 1989, p. xi). "[D]eparture from reality is not harmful, on the contrary. This finding allows us to presume that greater misperceptions of reality are not associated with maladjustment. . . . [I]nflated self-deception is not synonymous with poor adaptation" (Gana, Alaphilippe, & Bailly, 2004, p. 63).

In this trend, three general types of illusion have occupied researchers: distortions of reality that enhance self-esteem, illusions that support and maintain the conviction of personal efficacy, and distortions of reality that encourage optimism toward the future. All of these have been linked to psychological normality and hence to what contemporary psychiatry and psychology believe constitutes mental health: "These three illusions, as we have called them, appear to *foster traditional criteria of mental health*, including the ability to care about the self and others, the ability to be happy or contented, and the ability to engage in productive and creative work" (Taylor & Brown, 1988, p. 204, italics added).

This recent reversal, from asserting the central role of realism and "reality testing" in the mentally healthy person to emphasizing the importance of positive illusion, has explicitly linked self-delusion with psychological normality while retaining psychological normality as the standard of mental health. Some researchers have, however, acknowledged that positive illusions can be harmful and destructive, as when an individual's positive illusion that his or her set of beliefs is superior to those of others results in prejudice, persecution, and violence: "Faith in the inherent goodness of one's beliefs and actions may lead a person to trample on the rights and values of others; centuries of atrocities committed in the name of religious and political values bear witness to the liabilities of such faith" (Taylor & Brown, 1988, p. 204). These authors go on to acknowledge that "[t]he preceding argument is not meant to suggest that positive illusions are without liabilities. Indeed, there may be many" (p. 204).

With even a modest awareness of history and of the current world situation we should be prepared to acknowledge that there are in fact a very great many such liabilities that come from a predilection to engage in illusional thinking, liabilities that pose threats to our species' and to our world's well-being. They should make us hesitant to associate the average, psychologically normal person's propensity to engage in illusion—a propensity exercised throughout human history and now recognized in social psychological research—with genuine mental health.

The social psychology of positive illusion has generally focused on individual psychology. But what is true on an individual level is also in this case true on a collective level. Stubbornly entrenched, collective positive illusions that magnify group self-esteem and the conviction of the group's effective control and that promote a collective delusional optimism about the future are not only counterproductive but serve as obstacles if we are realistically and responsibly to face and solve the problems for which our species is responsible. To take only one example, which has become "politically hot" even to mention: There are now some 300,000 human babies born into the world *each day*. This means that each week, 2 million come into the world, adding to the world's human burden that must ideally be fed, housed, educated, and enabled to lead healthy and meaningful lives. Many will subsist in the world's rapidly growing slums of 830 million people today, expected by the United Nation's division UN Habitat over the next two decades to swell to 2 billion—enough people living in slums to populate present-day China one-and-a-half times over. Despite Al Gore's admirable efforts to educate the public and its political leaders about the need to take concrete, significant steps to avert climate catastrophe, his book (Gore, 2006) contains only two pages that refer to the burgeoning human population, while in the section of his book devoted to "what you can personally do to help solve the climate crisis" (pp. 305–321), the suggestion "have few or no children" is conspicuously *not* included. Systematic avoidance in discussing the overwhelming need for intelligent human population management is the expression of positive illusion gone awry.[1]

The potential ecological disaster that has begun to intrude on our consciousness needs to be seen realistically, not through the rose-tinted lenses of collective positive illusion and optimistic denial. And yet, even to suggest this is to tilt against windmills. It is important that we recognize—again realistically—how fundamentally important positive illusion is to our species, to its homocentric bias, and to its preference for optimism toward the future even when this is based on illusion. And we need to recognize what is central in our conception of mental health and psychiatric pathology, that psychological normality has achieved its unquestioned status as the standard of mental health without adequate study, justification, or evidence.

WHERE WE MIGHT GO FROM HERE

If we were to accept the main points raised in the foregoing discussion, it would be hard *not* to feel that the deck is stacked against the suggestion that we look beyond psychological normality for an appropriate mental health standard. The prevalence of human pathology, of human denial of that pathology, and of the unrelenting force of human illusion together would seem to make the challenge such a proposal faces close to insurmountable.

Earlier in this chapter, I raised the question, "What would be accomplished by recognizing that pathology lies so close to home, and is not confined, as we would prefer, to the smaller population of those whom we now label as mentally aberrant?" Let me now try to respond to that question. Two principal purposes would be realized by acknowledging the pathology of normality: First, we would no longer remain in a state of denial concerning normal psychology. We would see it as it is, recognizing its so often realized potential for aggression and destructiveness—to cause harm, which is, after all, the central meaning of pathogenicity. Second, we should be motivated to redefine mental health in a way that does not import into our understanding of the functioning of the mentally healthy person the very psychological constitution that has, in so many ways, caused people, their families, their societies, their nations, and other forms of life such a great deal of harm.

Critics of such a proposal will be quick to ask, "Just how then do you propose to understand mental health and psychiatric disorder if the standard of psychological normality is discarded?" This is a fair question, and in the space available here I'll try to sketch how it might be answered. But before proceeding, after the grim tone of the foregoing discussion, it may help our mood to inject some humor—humor which at the same time isn't altogether tongue-in-cheek:

Psychiatrist Louis E. Bisch many years ago thought rather poorly of the psychologically average. To say this is to probably to overstate his affection for normality, for he wrote: "The great, great majority of the people who make a nation, who make a world, are normal . . . even if it be a low normal, just about missing moronity or falling upon the bottom levels of adolescence" (Bisch, 1936, p. 17). He bravely defended his antipathy toward normality: "What this country needs is not more normals—not even the exceptionally fine ones—but more neurotics; neurotics who are glad of it; neurotics who have the courage to stress their individuality and sensitiveness and make it outstanding and telling" (p. 28).

Bisch was not afraid of political incorrectness; he boldly claimed: "to be normal is nothing to brag about! When I study normals and compare them with neurotics I wonder sometimes whether to be normal is not something to be ashamed about" (p. 32). We might be reminded of the definition of 'abnormal' given by Ambrose Bierce—"Not conforming to standard. In matters of thought and conduct, to be independent is to be abnormal, to be abnormal is to be detested" (Bierce, 1946/1989, p. 189)—and his definition of 'mad'—"Affected with a high degree of intellectual independence; not conforming to standards of thought, speech and action derived by the conformants from study of themselves; at odds with the majority; in short, unusual" (p. 300).

Bisch saw in neurotics a collection of potentially affirmative traits that tend not to be found in the average, psychologically normal person. "What [well-meaning persons] do not realize is that the child who later becomes neurotic is different, consequently does not fit in, because he has been born with potentials for development that are greater than, and unlike, the average. Remember he is not neurotic at birth, only supercharged and hypersensitive. His neurotic reactions appear only later" (p. 45). To be a neurotic in this sense is, he felt, something of a privilege (p. 180). If his humorous yet serious book were taken to heart, some of the unproductive stigma, shame, and alienation associated with neuroticism might be lifted. And would this be such a bad thing?

However, to turn from this lighter thought, there are, as I see the situation we face, two main directions in which mental health theory might develop. For both there are good grounds to believe that they are therapeutically promising. Both avoid the misplaced emphasis traditionally invested in psychological normality as a standard of mental health, and both are more realistic as well as accurate in their understanding of human psychological problems. If we were, if only for the purposes of a thought experiment here, to suspend reliance upon psychological normality as a standard for mental health, the following are two potential directions for future development that open to psychiatry and clinical psychology. They are not mutually exclusive but complementary; they can be employed fruitfully together.

The first seeks to understand mental health in terms of special, smaller populations that exhibit signs of healthy, benign—nonpathogenic— mental functioning, that is, in terms of identifiable marks of good mental health that can be distinguished and freed from the context of pressure to conform to the majoritarian larger population. I cannot develop this suggestion in detail here, but instead offer a few examples by way of illustration. If we accept that the human propensity to engage in deadly quarrels, manifested so often throughout human history, is far from being an expression of good mental health, we might do well to consider a special group whose psychology has been little studied: the population of conscientious objectors. It would be potentially enlightening to study their degree of moral development and their capacity for autonomous thought and behavior as contrasted with the general population. Instead of relying upon the general population's normal psychology as a criterion of mental health, we could learn how individuals function on a psychological level who are able to resist the pressures of authority, who are able to think critically for themselves (à la Arendt), and who have the courage to respect and act upon their own sense of individual autonomy. Such a person would share in important ways characteristics identified by Maslow (1970, 1971) in his paradigm of a "self-actualizing individual," which offers a seldom-to-be-found, detailed model of positive mental health that avoids reliance upon a standard of psychological normality.

The suggestion that we establish one viable locus for good mental health in the psychological constitution of conscientious objectors will surely strike some readers as unexpected and perhaps tug at the boundaries of credibility. And yet I wonder if the surprise or incredulity they may experience may not be a reflective aftertaste of contact with the counterintuitive, which, given the history of psychiatry and clinical psychology, is an altogether understandable and even predictable reaction. It has become so habitual to equate psychological normality with good mental health that to question the equation and then look to a special group, such as conscientious objectors, for defining signs of good mental health can indeed run counter to prevailing beliefs and hence feel paradoxical.

There are without question other conceivably appropriate loci in terms of which to understand good mental health and by means of which we should be able to broaden our conception of beneficial, well-functioning psychology. To mention a few other examples, one could study the psychology of those who have developed compassion to a high degree (e.g., Buddhist and yoga practitioners, as in Walsh & Shapiro, 1983), of those who have highly developed aesthetic sensibility (e.g., artists, sculptors, and poets, as we'll discuss in Chapter 3; see also Bartlett, 2009), and of those who have cultivated impressive cognitive abilities of concentration, discipline, synthesis, and creative thought (original thinkers in such fields as mathematics, music, philosophy, natural science, etc., as in Simonton, 1994 and Andreasen, 2005). From an integrated study of such special groups of people selected because they exemplify fully functional, healthy, benign cognitive and emotional abilities, we should be able to integrate into a clear and cohering whole what genuine mental health means and then make use of what we have learned to establish a set of enlightened and effective criteria of healthy psychological functioning.

As should be clear, the resulting conception of mental health would not coincide with "psychological normality," nor would we make recourse to a standard of psychological normality to define mental health.

A second approach, which again can be employed in conjunction with the first, involves a return to an individualized, human-centered, nonregimented, nontaxonomic understanding of psychological problems—dispensing with technically structured algorithmic catalogs of constructed diagnostic codes. Such an approach was proposed by psychiatrist J. H. van den Berg. He developed an approach to clinical psychiatry that he called phenomenological psychiatry (van den Berg, 1955, 1972, 1980; de Konig, 1982). It avoids standard psychiatric classification and diagnostic pigeonholing and instead seeks to help individuals through nonjudgmental support of the patient by the therapist, support that is situated from a phenomenological standpoint that recognizes the reality and legitimacy of the patient's own experience.

From this perspective, a therapist helps patients less through *intervention* and more through *collaborative understanding* (my way of putting this, not van den Berg's). Van den Berg observed in many of his patients that their inability to live effectively and at peace with themselves was at the root of their psychiatric problems. Psychiatric treatment can be effective, he found, when the therapist helps the patient to improve the degree to which he or she is able to accommodate, without inner conflict, to his or her own personal needs, interests, and values as these are expressed in the individual's "life-world," the patient's world of experience. Therapeutic self-acceptance does not necessarily adjust the patient to the needs and expectations of prevailing society, but it does often help the patient adjust to himself or herself so as to establish a healthy congruity and integrity. Although van den Berg did not formulate his approach in these terms, one can describe his approach as seeking to help people find appropriate, to them acceptable, ways to adapt to their experienced environments.

what if that environment is hostile?

Recognizing that van den Berg's European-phenomenological approach has not been in keeping with prevailing American clinical tastes, it may be worth mentioning in passing that Alfred Adler offered a related perspective that considers many psychological difficulties to be expressions of "problems of living" (see, e.g., Adler, 1924 and the collection of his work in Ansbacher & Ansbacher, 1956). Adlerians understand that they are treating an individual's discouragement in life rather than forms of mental "sickness." Adlerian therapy uses encouragement tailored to the individual's self-understanding and view of the world. Like van den Berg, Adler did not pathologize human problems as varieties of mental illness, but rather observed that such problems comprise challenging emotional and behavioral difficulties in life, blocking people in their efforts to realize themselves. Many of the problems that Adlerian therapists seek to treat are therefore considered by them to be characteristic, naturally occurring problems of living, problems that are part of life. Adler and his followers have endorsed an approach to therapy that seeks, somewhat like van den Berg's, to understand and help the patient in essential relation to his or her perceived total environment.[2]

As with the first approach suggested above, which derives an understanding of mental health from a study of special groups, it is important to note that van den Berg's and Adler's conceptions of mental health do not rely upon the application of a standard of psychological normality.

Both ways of understanding mental health that I've outlined in this section reject the technical classification mechanism of psychopathological diagnosis; both approaches turn away from traditional psychiatric diagnostic criteria that derive their meaning from deviations from psychological normality and a constructed nosology of mental disorders. Instead, one approach seeks to understand healthy mental functioning through a study of specialized groups chosen both because their members do not

cause harm and because they posses identifiable abilities to function especially well. The second approach seeks to help people on an individualized
basis to reach an improved level of self-understanding, self-acceptance,
and integration within the framework of their perception of their environments and to learn to function effectively in their own terms. Neither
approach aims to proselytize or inculcate in patients the behavioral goals
and cognitive values of majority society; they do not aim to adjust patients
to conform with what is perceived to be psychologically normal. Neither
approach leads to a stigmatization of "deviations from normality," since
deviation from psychological normality is no longer an indication of mental illness. Individuals who are seen to be in need of therapy are not identified due to their deviation from normality and the fact that their
symptoms satisfy conditions specified by diagnostic algorithms that are
themselves based on the benchmark of normality. The people who need
and may profit from therapy are rather those who experience impairments
which, most especially from their own points of view, are harmful and
undesirable.

In summary, both approaches are open to a recognition that psychiatric
pathology afflicts psychologically normal populations that include the
majority of people. Neither approach seeks, implicitly or explicitly, to
import into diagnostic classifications or into the practice of therapy an
endorsement that psychological normality is a core criterion of mental
health. One approach establishes a locus of psychiatric health in individuals who function exceptionally well and nonpathogenically in one or
more aspects of their cognitive, affective, or behavioral lives. The other
seeks to help patients develop a foundation for their own effective functioning from within, without social indoctrination or socializing goals.

TOWARD A MORE EFFECTIVE UNDERSTANDING
OF MENTAL HEALTH

To give up the exclusionist standard of normality in psychiatry and
clinical psychology is no small thing. To develop and apply an alternative
theory of mental health and of psychological pathology that does without
such a standard requires the majority of clinicians to revise their understanding of pathology, mental health, and therapy. We should need
to look in a different direction from the one in which we are accustomed
to look.

From the standpoint of current psychiatric diagnosis-centered thought,
if we were to try to define its presupposed concept of "mental health"—
which is seldom attempted—we'd get something like this: Mental health
explicitly presupposes psychological normality, and implicitly it calls for

an *absence of perceptible mental dysfunction* (as in Offer & Sabshin, 1989, pp. 405–17). And yet mental health, like physical health, is a good deal more than a state of not having a disease: genuinely good health is not just not having anything manifestly wrong with you. Positive physical health derives much of its meaning from the *optimal* functioning of the body— as exemplified and most fully attained by those who are in *excellent* physical condition, and who epitomize a *realizable ideal*. The concept of 'excellence' here is important for it emphasizes the need to have a clear appreciation of the high end of the spectrum, and not just the mean. *Excellence* connotes distinction of quality, superiority of merit, worth, development, or attainment; it is what the ancient Greeks had in mind when they spoke of *aretē*: its central meaning was excellence as evidenced in an individual's ability to reach the highest level of performance in any arena of human capacity. *Optimal* is a derivative and subordinate concept, and yet one which relies upon a grasp of what excellence consists in. 'Optimal functioning', as I propose to use this phrase here, has a more relative meaning that seeks to take into account the limitations of the individual, which may not permit him or her to achieve true excellence. An individual functions at an optimal level—for him or for her—when he or she functions as well as possible given individual limitations. In contrast, an individual functions at a level of excellence when, in comparison with others, the level of attainment reached is truly superior. It will be important later on that we recognize this distinction between 'optimal' and 'excellent'.

Although we are not accustomed to thinking in these terms, what would it be to be in excellent (or optimal) psychological condition? The customary equation of mental health with psychological normality, perhaps coupled with not having any noticeable mental problem, fails to tell us anything significant about excellent (or optimal) psychological functioning.

Modern psychiatry and clinical psychology, although putatively proposing to help people reach a state of genuine mental health, have developed no clear understanding of excellent mental health, with few exceptions. One exception is provided by research concerning the nature of human intelligence. Intellectual intelligence, understood as a measurable degree of excellence in cognitive functioning, has been studied with more success and specificity than has more comprehensive psychological functioning.

In the evolution of our knowledge of human intellectual intelligence perhaps the most significant development has come about as a result of the widened range of abilities that we have come to recognize to express forms of intelligence. We've learned that there are many forms of cognitive intelligence—verbal, spatial, quantitative, comprehension ability, memory, imagination, ability to think critically, and so forth. This multifactorial—or as Guilford (1967, p. 467) preferred to call it, multidimensional—understanding of intelligence has given us a richer and more detailed explanation of what it is to be intellectually intelligent. In studying the varieties of intellectual intelligence, we have looked not simply at normal functioning but at their expression in individuals *who possess those abilities to a superior degree*. In this way, we have derived a sense of what excellence means in connection with verbal ability, spatial relations skills, calculation, memory, and any of the other cognitive skills that together create a composite description of outstanding cognitive functioning. Excellence is a realizable, nonfictitious ideal; it is a construct created through the study of individuals who manifest certain skills to the highest degree.

We have not yet reached a similar, widely accepted, composite understanding of identifiable, special "abilities" or other characteristics which, when taken together, would tell us what excellence in *psychological health* means. A few psychologists and psychiatrists have sought to focus study on highly developed people who exemplify excellence in psychological health: Fromm emphasized the "autonomous person"; Rogers, the "fully functioning person"; Jung, the "individuated person"; and, with the greatest descriptive detail, Maslow identified a large group of psychological characteristics possessed by "self-actualizing" individuals, who are "psychologically healthy, psychologically 'superior' people" (Maslow, 1971, p. 6; cf. also Maslow, 1964, 1970).

A level of excellence in psychological health is clearly a broad and inclusive concept, embracing qualities of person, dispositions, and a range of skills, including such intellectual abilities as we have already mentioned. A few efforts have been made to distinguish and study on their own certain of the extra-intellectual "abilities" that would play a central role in a more comprehensive account of excellent psychological functioning as envisioned here. There are, for example, *social abilities* that are often desirable in healthy social interaction. Nearly a century ago, E. L. Thorndike (1920) proposed that there is a special kind of "social intelligence" distinct from intellectual intelligence, which he characterized as "the ability to understand and manage people" (p. 275). A few years later, Charles E. Spearman (1927) noted that some people have the ability to create within themselves a vicarious experience of the thoughts and feelings of others by analogy with their own experience; Spearman, too, recognized that this ability is the expression of a variety of intelligence. Others, including Bruner and Tagiuri (1954), Taft (1956), and Eysenck (1998/1999), have emphasized skills that can be subsumed under the same heading of social intelligence. (For a more detailed discussion see Bartlett, 2005, pp. 278ff.)

Complementing such social abilities, and overlapping with them, are *emotional skills* that are involved in accurately perceiving one's own emotions and those of others. Salovey and Mayer (1990), Gardner (1983/1993 and 1993), and Goleman (1995) have grouped such skills under the heading of "emotional intelligence."

A third variety of nonintellectual intelligence is *moral intelligence*, which had not previously been studied and which I have characterized in terms of a set of specific dispositions and skills. They include a psychological aversion to participation in behavior that harms others, a fully functioning capacity for empathy, a well-developed sensibility that is expressed in normative weighing tied to aversion that a morally intelligent person feels when confronted by typical human aggression and destructiveness, and a strong moral conviction that bridges skills in moral reasoning with commitment to act accordingly. (For a more detailed elaboration of the concept of moral intelligence, see Bartlett, 2005, pp. 277–80 and passim.)

These are a few examples of skills and dispositions that shed light on how excellence in psychological functioning can be understood—without recourse to the inappropriate standard of normality. There is clearly a need, although it is not often acknowledged, to identify the essential factors of outstanding psychological health. Were we to acquire such an understanding of psychological health by studying specialized expressions of mental health, we should be able to bring together a composite understanding of what genuine mental health means. We need to learn what it is for both cognitive or intellectual skills and the nonintellectual skills mentioned here to be realized in individuals to a degree that expresses excellence of individual development or attainment. This would enable us to formulate a *realizable ideal*, a standard, a set of criteria that tells us what genuine mental health entails. *We should then appreciate that mental health is a good deal more than conformity with psychological normality, and a great deal more than absence of mental illness.*

Such an approach would extend and build upon the way in which human intellectual intelligence has to date been successfully studied, namely by consolidating multiple factors that represent different forms of cognitive intelligence. The current emphasis of psychiatry and clinical psychology has unfortunately been on identifying and distinguishing mental disorders rather than understanding mental health. To reach an effective and clear understanding of mental health, we need to be able to consolidate what we now know, and have yet to learn, about the best in human beings when they think, feel, and behave to a fully developed degree.

MENTAL HEALTH AS EXCEPTION TO THE RULE

The phrase 'psychological normality' has attained the secondhand status of habitual stock expressions "tossed," as Clifton Fadiman has said, "on the scrapheap of popular misuse."[3] 'Psychological normality' is a phrase so widely used and intuitively comfortable as to have become second nature in current thinking. It is hard to loosen the grip we have on it, and it on us.

In this chapter I've argued two general claims: First, the notion of psychological normality, far from throwing light on the nature of mental health, has become a habitual way of referring at one and the same time to psychological characteristics which are socially approved and which are generally invariant across a broad population.[4] Second, and more importantly, the concept of psychological normality has come to function wrongly and inadequately as a standard of mental health. The justification for this second claim rests on several more specific observations:

(a) *Typical* and *socially approved* characteristics of affective, cognitive, and behavioral functioning very frequently are pathogenic, as we've noted earlier.

(b) Genuine mental health therefore needs to be understood in the context of a range of nonpathological emotional, cognitive, and behavioral characteristics and abilities. To formulate criteria of *excellence of functioning* with respect to these abilities requires that we study and develop a clearer understanding of what it is to be a highly developed person from the standpoint of psychological health.

(c) Clinical practice, if it is to avoid the imposition of an inappropriate standard of psychological normality, must center its attention on helping individuals to *optimize* their own mental health within the context of highly individual life situations.

And, finally, as a corollary to (c):

(d) The idea of normality is the result of a selective process of averaging, thereby suppressing an awareness of individual variation by choosing to ignore it through abstraction and generalization. A well-developed concept of mental health, on the contrary, requires compatibility with the significant variation to be found in real individuals, whose psychological functioning cannot adequately be understood in terms of a generalized rule or norm but rather requires a clinician's awareness of their uniqueness as persons who have unique life situations and sources of personal meaning. It follows from the perspective of the individual that there is no one

univocally defined way for all individuals to be psychologically healthy
but many individual paths to mental health. Depending upon the individual, his or her circumstances, and his or her sources of meaning in
life, certain abilities, dispositions, and qualities of person will be essential to that person's optimal functioning and others less so.

To recognize the truth of the above propositions is not to embrace a
vague multiculturalist generality incapable of practical, individual application. Although mental health as I propose we understand it encompasses a
wide range of individual variability, it is a conception that encourages
therapeutic approaches designed to be sensitive to individual needs and
perceptions. At the same time, and on the most fundamental level, such
a theory of mental health expressly (1) defines and affirms specific criteria
of healthy mental functioning that are nonpathogenic, and which, as a
consequence, (2) has no use for a univocal standard of psychological normality in terms of which mental health is assessed.

The current understanding of mental health does not accomplish these
ends. The one-size-fits-all adherence to the standard of psychological
normality not only bases our understanding of mental health on a dysfunctional and destructive model, but is all too frequently a cause of
shame and stigmatization for those upon whom *DSM* labels are affixed.
Furthermore, stipulating that mental health is synonymous with psychological normality can plausibly cause many individuals—and here I literally mean genuine individuals who are exceptions to the norm—to
become psychologically dysfunctional. This happens because they are
labeled dysfunctional both by clinicians and as a result by their society
and are so treated, and because labeling them as having mental disorders
often creates inner obstacles—of self-disparagement, alienation, isolation,
and a self-fulfilling prophesy of "illness"—obstacles to their effective
functioning as the individuals they are. We'll look in more detail at the
psychology of such individualists, who are often artists, poets, writers, or
sculptors, in Chapter 3, and will return to consider the destructive consequences of diagnostic labeling in Chapter 9.

As I've argued, adherence to the standard of psychological normality is
fundamentally flawed. The identical conclusion—that average, psychologically ordinary people hold rigidly to beliefs and have an emotional
constitution such that, when the situation is right, they will inflict harm
on others and often themselves—has been reached from a variety of disciplinary points of view by many researchers in psychiatry, psychology,
ethology, sociology, anthropology, and history (Bartlett, 2005, Part II).
They have reached mutually reinforcing negative conclusions about the
psychology of normal people. None of these researchers, however, has

yet advised that we should replace psychological normality as a standard for mental health, although this conclusion has been staring us in the face for a long time.

A PRELIMINARY CONCLUSION

There are three compelling reasons why psychological normality should not be equated with psychological health: the factual disposition of the psychologically normal person to feel, think, and behave in such harmful—that is, pathogenic—ways as have been outlined here; the strong recalcitrance of the psychologically normal population to pay attention to, much less acknowledge and then make intelligent choices based on, the evidence of their own harmful predispositions; and the deeply rooted willfulness with which psychologically normal people embrace illusions about themselves, others, and the future.

It would take us a meaningful step forward should we be willing to replace our defective, dysfunctional standard of mental health with a new understanding of what mentally healthy functioning involves. Genuine mental health might then be understood as involving, to mention some of the main factors, general cognitive, social-emotional, and moral intelligence that incorporates compassion, aversion to violence, moral conviction, unwillingness automatically and uncritically to obey authority, self-discipline, and the ability to think and make choices autonomously. All of these make up important ingredients essential to mental health. It follows from this understanding that mentally healthy individuals are fundamentally exceptions to the rule. Most of our human population continues to have an inherently dysfunctional set of emotional and behavioral dispositions. A standard of mental health that assumes psychological normality to be a central criterion of mentally healthy functioning is fundamentally mistaken, hence misguided, and does not serve the constructive interests of our as well as other species.

In summary, in this chapter I've proposed: (1) the criteria which we use to define mental health should promote thought, feeling, and conduct that do not result in harm; (2) these criteria should take into account excellence of functioning derived from a study of special groups whose members excel in certain mentally healthy respects; and (3) on an individualized level, these criteria should be applied by clinicians in a manner so as to promote the individual client's or patient's optimal functioning. The standard of psychological normality does not fulfill these requirements. What we should wish to adopt as a standard of mental health is *the exception to the rule* in the sense developed here, the exception to what is and has been the human norm. The normal has failed us as a species, and rather miserably.

To continue to employ the standard of normality is not only a mistake, it fosters the continuation of our species' destructive propensity.

NOTES

1. Population biologist Paul Ehrlich recently made the observation: "Even though virtually every environmental and social problem nationally and globally is exacerbated today by continued population growth, the topic of human numbers is absent not only from policy discussions in the United States but also largely from public discourse" (Ehrlich & Ehrlich, 2008, p. 207).

2. It is interesting to note that this, too, was the conception of beneficial therapy proposed by one of psychiatry's most outspoken critics: "[t]he possibility of helping the client accept his existing inclinations with greater equanimity, to help him value his own authentic selfhood more than his society's judgment of it." (Szasz, 1970/1997, p. 172).

3. An expression used by Fadiman in the course of an oral presentation at the Center for the Study of Democratic Institutions in Santa Barbara during the academic year 1969–70.

4. In the literature there has sometimes been an unfortunate confusion and unconscious blending together of two distinct concepts: normality, on the one hand, versus normativity, on the other. The statistical average, what is typical in a population, is clearly very different from an endorsement of values, which expresses normative preferences. This problem permeates some discussions, confusing the issue (as we find, for example, in Freides, 1960). This confusion probably has its base in the fact that the traditional standard of psychological normality has functioned as a norm in both ordinary senses of that word: as a standard it selects what is typical in a population as a basis for judgment, and then to this it *adds* an *evaluative preference* for what is thereby identified as typical or normal. These two senses need to be disengaged from one another since we can obviously refer to average characteristics of a population without valuing those characteristics.

2

The Psychology of Definition in Psychiatric Nosology

Contemporary psychiatry has sought to adhere to an essentially *medical* conception of pathology in its definition of mental disorders. This chapter looks closely at the psychology that underlies the largely successful attempt of psychiatry to persuade us that the medical paradigm validly applies to psychological conditions judged to be harmful and disabling. The psychiatric conception of pathology—that is, medical psychopathology— is, however, not the only way in which psychological pathology can be understood. Later chapters discuss psychological pathology that is not conceptualized along medical lines. But in this chapter we'll look specifically at psychiatric pathology, pathology as it is understood from a medical standpoint.

Underlying the formulation and endorsement of psychiatric nosologies is the little-studied *psychology of definition of mental disorders*, comprising both the psychology of nosologists who seek to define and classify mental disorders as well as the related psychology of supporting clinicians, institutions, drug companies, and the larger society. The psychologically normal predispositions that come into play are seldom recognized and are responsible, as we shall see, not only for certain flawed judgments embedded in current psychiatric nosology but also for the way mental disorder definitions are frequently misconstrued by clinicians and by the wider society. By recognizing this fundamentally normal psychology we gain a clarified understanding of the nature of definition in psychiatric nosology and see that mental illness and the majority of mental disorders are frequently not what we allow ourselves to believe.

This is but one instance in which our uncritical acceptance of and submission to psychologically normal limitations lead us astray. We shall meet a variety of others in future chapters.

[N]o problems of knowledge are less settled than those of definition, and
no subject is more in need of a fresh approach.
                                                            —Abelson (1967, p. 314)

[B]y the content of their field, psychiatrists are the least well equipped to
confront the issue of defining [the fundamental concept of] normality.
                                                            —Murphy (1979, p. 414)

[T]here ends up being, so far as I can see, no stable reality or concept of
mental disorder; it breaks up into many, quite different kinds. . . . I would
have settled for one clear proposal as to what mental disorder really is, but
couldn't find one.
                                                            —Bolton (2008, p. viii)

These three quotes, spanning four decades, represent a few of many similar comments which have been made in the literature and which highlight
the conceptual confusion and lack of theoretical integration that we continue to face in psychiatry and clinical psychology. This state of disorder
in our concepts and how we apply them has evidently been brought about
in large measure by the rapid increase in the number and theoretical complexity of approaches to psychological therapy. The greatly expanded
range of choice offered by the diversity of theories and methods of
psychotherapeutic treatment can be nothing short of overwhelming, especially in the context of widespread disagreement as to how practitioners
should go about making intelligent, justifiable decisions given the many
alternatives and their possible combinations.[1] On the most elemental
level, conceptual confusion in current psychiatric nosology has come
about due to the great variety of distinct, overlapping, and sometimes
incompatible definitions that have been proposed for such central terms
as 'normality', 'mental disorder', and 'mental health'.

In addition to these sources of theoretical complexity, ambiguity, and
resulting turmoil, there is a hidden dimension that has been responsible
for a substantial amount of avoidable confusion, a dimension that has been
universally neglected throughout the literature. That hidden dimension
concerns *the psychology of definition in psychiatric nosology*. By this I mean the
psychological predispositions that lead nosologists as well as many others
in the mental health profession to lose control over self-critical, deliberate,
intelligent understanding of what they are doing when they define concepts
central to psychiatric or psychological diagnosis and treatment.

The phrase 'the psychology of definition' may suggest several hypotheses:
(1) that we mistakenly consider the process of definition to be simple,

straightforward, and well-understood; (2) that definition brings into play psychological propensities of which most of us tend not to be aware; and (3) that these psychological propensities, if clearly and self-consciously understood, would help us to control them and thereby gain a significant measure of conceptual clarity and theoretical integration, in the process lessening much of the conceptual turmoil that encumbers current psychiatry and clinical psychology. The purpose of this chapter is to show that these three hypotheses are true specifically in the context of definitions of mental disorders.

THE NEED FOR A PSYCHOLOGY OF DEFINITION

Controversies from the careless employment of terms ought to be impossible, and they can be prevented mainly through the agency of Definition. Well-defined words, clearly understood and intelligently expressed meanings, are a sort of panacea for the thinker; and, in proportion as we approach the ideal here or recede from it, we may expect accuracy and progress in thought or deterioration and confusion.

—Davidson (1885, p. 2)

It is a psychological fact that the human mind thinks, and thinks among other things about logical matters including definitions; and the adequate investigation of this must be both psychological and logical.

—Robinson (1950/1962, p. 14)

A great proportion of essential human affairs rests on definition. How much an insurance company will pay for a particular property or medical claim depends on definitions set forth in one's insurance policy or contract. How much a court may provide in settlement of a lawsuit or how many years it may sentence a person to prison equally depend on definitions. How votes are to be counted in an election similarly rests on definitions. What percentage of a forest can be logged may depend on the definition of 'old growth'. And, of course, definitions of 'mental disorders' determine how patients or clients are diagnosed and treated, to what degree they may ultimately be stigmatized by diagnostic labeling, whether a person can be involuntarily confined to a mental institution, and whether the perpetrator of a crime will be judged mentally incompetent to stand trial. The majority of debates over pressing human interests and ideologies have definitions at their core.

Definitions are of many kinds. Some stipulate that a word or phrase is to have a certain meaning, as we often encounter in legal documents and in mathematics. Some definitions state that a word has a certain customary meaning, as we find in dictionaries, which offer definitions through

synonyms. Some definitions offer an informative analysis or explanation
(e.g., "DNA is composed of any of various nucleic acids that serve as the
molecular basis of heredity, are localized in cell nuclei, and are constructed
of a double helix (etc.)."). Many definitions mix together claims that have to
do with wholly different contexts, as we often find in definitions that are
advanced with the desire to persuade others to accept them. (Defining at
what stage and under what conditions a human embryo is to have the legal
rights of personhood is a good example, blending ethical, religious, scientific, and legal definitions.)

The remainder of this chapter focuses on the particular kind of definition that is found in psychiatric nosologies and on how such definitions
are interpreted and understood by mental health professionals, drug
companies, social and legal institutions, and the surrounding society.
As we shall see, even the specialized variety of definition that we find in
psychiatric nosology performs varied functions, which bring about mis-
conceptions and distortions to which the human psychology of definition
is vulnerable.

THE PURPOSES OF DEFINITION IN PSYCHIATRIC NOSOLOGIES

The definition and classification of mental disorders has today become
synonymous in the United States and increasingly in many other countries with the American Psychiatric Association's series of *Diagnostic and
Statistical Manuals of Mental Disorders*, but the *DSM* is only the small, currently perceived promontory of a sprawling historical mainland of competing psychiatric nosologies. Karl Menninger, Martin Mayman, and
Paul Pruyser (1963, pp. 419–89) give a concise yet detailed digest of many
of the psychiatric nosologies formulated over the past two millennia, from
primitive diagnostic classifications to those offered by the ancient Greeks
and Romans and subsequently supplemented and repeatedly modified
during the Middle Ages, Renaissance, and in the centuries since. Their
introductory comment places the swinging pendulum of fashion or paradigm revision in perspective: "From simple beginnings there have been
eras of tremendous expansion, with the inclusion of many [disease]
entities, and—as now—eras of return to greater simplicity." (p. 419). This
was more than four decades ago; since that time, the *DSM*, published
since 1952, has undergone revisions that have expanded the number of
diagnostic definitions from 106 mental disorders identified in the 128
pages of the first edition to 368 disorders defined in the 943 pages of the
2000 edition, *DSM-IV-TR.* —This has certainly not been the "return to
greater simplicity" envisioned by Menninger, Mayman, and Pruyser!

During its long history, psychiatric nosology has in varying degrees been committed to several definite and broadly inclusive purposes: to define mental illness and its specific forms; to describe manifestations of mental illness so they can be identified in a reliable, uniform way despite subjective differences of practitioners; to arrive at insight into the nature and causes of mental disorders; and to organize these definitions, descriptions, and explanations in a systematically integrated and comprehensive taxonomy. In this chapter, we'll be concerned in particular with the first three of these purposes, which concern definition, its descriptive elaboration, and etiology.

Historically, the role of definition in the formulation of psychiatric nosologies has had several concrete purposes intended to support and contribute to the realization of the broader purposes just mentioned. Definitions of pivotal diagnostic concepts are intended to allow mental health practitioners to communicate efficiently and effectively with one another—so that they, as a group, achieve an adequate degree of consensus about what they are referring to in a manner that is as clear, unambiguous, and specific as possible. However, such definitions are not intended to be mere conceptual creations unanchored in reality but are intended to refer to actual symptoms[2] and known causes of individual, distinct forms of real mental illness. In the latter sense, diagnostic definitions may throw explanatory light on how and why individual forms of mental illness arise. Further, in an additional capacity, definitions of mental disorders are intended to function as coordinative rules, today often expressed in the form of diagnostic algorithms, in terms of which practitioners can reliably link an identified disease with a specified symptomatology, family and patient medical history, the course of a disorder, its likely outcome, and so on.

Diagnostic definitions are formulated, then, for the primary purposes of efficient, effective, clear identification of real "disease entities"; beyond these purposes, they serve others that are less immediately evident, among them that the definitions propounded be judged to be *authoritative* and that they, as a result, be *persuasive*. Diagnostic definitions are implicitly intended to establish authority and credibility.

Definitions, as we've noted, come in many forms, and so far we've mentioned a few of these. They have names: There is *stipulative definition*, for specifying how important terms are to be understood, either by equivalence with synonymous terms (word-word definitions), or by reference to things (word-thing); both of these are called *nominal definitions*. Then there are word-thing definitions that have empirical content that may be true or false, and may, as we've already seen in the example of DNA, offer an informative analysis or explanation, called *real definitions*.[3] Further, as we've noted in connection with diagnostic algorithms, there are so-called *coordinative definitions* that establish relationships between the terms of a theory and the phenomena the theory is intended to be about (e.g., Reichenbach, 1965, Chap. IV). And then there are what we might call the "meta-purposes" of definition, that is, to serve the function of *authoritative persuasion*.

With this short summary of the types of definition encountered in psychiatric nosologies, we turn to consider the psychology that underlies their formulation and implementation.

STIPULATIVE DEFINITIONS AS SOURCES OF AUTHORITY

Humpty Dumpty was adamant in claiming that the meanings of words *were* the meanings that he chose that they *should* mean. This is stipulative definition in a nutshell. It differs from the lexical variety of definition that we find in dictionaries; that variety describes how people have used a word or phrase in the past, which is the history of word use. Definitions are stipulative when they decree how a word *is to be used* from now on, which is the future. Stipulative definitions can be laid down for purely formal purposes, as is done in mathematics and in a formal system of logic, or they can be propounded for practical purposes, as we find in law. Stipulative definition is also found in psychiatric nosology, as one main variety of psychiatric definition; there is another we shall discuss in the next section. In both law and psychiatric nosology, stipulative definitions serve an intended role as *arbiters* of endorsed or acceptable future usage and practice. Those who formulate such definitions consider themselves and want others to consider them to be credible authorities whose judgment in these matters should be respected and followed in the future. When the definitions they advocate are widely accepted, their authority and credibility increase; a self-reinforcing cycle is established that lends further authority and credibility to their future stipulative definitions and revisions of past definitions. As further stipulations are made and these are accepted, the degree of recognized authority continues to increase.

In other words, stipulative definitions of this kind are inherently *legislative*: they are not statements that are true or false, but are *rules of usage* that are recommended or urged. Stipulatively defined terms, when they are accepted, become a group-endorsed, socially correct vocabulary in terms of which both the future usage of those terms and practice in accordance with their definitions are to adhere.

To call for *proof* of stipulative definitions is inappropriate because, as we have noted, such definitions are not statements of fact that can be shown to be true or false. The stipulative definitions found in psychiatric nosologies are often misinterpreted to consist of statements that are true about the world, but in fact they are legislated *choices* that are true or false statements in appearance only; in actuality they are announcements or decrees made by the recognized authorities of the time that certain sets of rules should be accepted. To wish to "prove the stipulative definitions of a nosology" is to misuse the word 'proof': One cannot prove that rules, which are agreed-upon conventions, are true of the world. One cannot prove that the Celsius temperature scale or the metric system is "true." Rules cannot be true or false; they can only be accepted or rejected—useful in connection with a certain set of purposes or not useful. What is at issue when we consider the definitions set forth in a nosology are the choices made by those who enact the stipulative definitions of the nosology, coupled with the choices made by those who accept and then implement those definitions. The history of psychiatric nosologies is a history of how such choices have changed over time.

In nonscientific language the meaning of most words is ambiguous, since most ordinary, nontechnical words can be used in different senses. In science, ambiguity and resulting vagueness tend to be undesirable, and for this reason stipulative definition can serve an important function, ensuring that colleagues in a discipline are all talking about the same thing when they use the same word. From the standpoint of psychiatric diagnosis, it is desirable that mental health practitioners reach mutually supporting, consistent evaluations of patients, and here agreed-upon stipulative definitions are important; such agreement is what we mean when we refer to the "reliability" of diagnosis.

When the number of specialized kinds of disease or disorder that are named and classified by a nosology increases or decreases, when the stipulated definitions of those forms of illness shift and frequent revisions are made, we need to be alert to the active role of stipulation. The psychology that characterizes human legislative activity is an expression of the psychology of persuasion, recognized in those whom we accept as experts when they seek the power of authority and credibility. The psychology of persuasion, on which rhetoric in its traditional meaning rests, is therefore at the core of the formulation and acceptance of definitions of mental disorders in psychiatric nosologies. As we shall see, stipulative definitions of this kind frequently lead to inappropriate and indeed fallacious inferences concerning the nature of what is defined, contributing to the conceptual confusion we have remarked on. This, too, is a psychological matter.

REAL DEFINITION AND REIFICATION

Writers from Epictetus on have noted that what a person thinks is real is usually more important than what is real, which is just another way of saying that a person's construction of events will psychologically channelize his processes.

—Sechrest (1977, p. 234)

Real definition plays a major role in science. Real definition is part of the process of obtaining and expressing new knowledge of things. It has a long history from the time of the ancient Greeks to the present. Real definition was understood by Aristotle to be a statement of the essence of a thing, and two millennia later this remains the goal of natural and behavioral science. Real definition seeks to express important facts about an object of reference, from which other true propositions about that object can be deduced or otherwise related. Einstein's definition of 'simultaneity' or psychiatry's definition of 'mental disorder' alike intend to fulfill this purpose. Unlike stipulative definition, real definition is believed to communicate not merely conventionally agreed-upon meaning but real information about things. In other words, real definitions are believed to be *empirically descriptive* and hence to be true or false.

Real definition, then, by virtue of its intended purpose, purports to be about what is real, contrary to a definition that is a pure conceptual construct and has the status of a fiction. We recognize that the definition of 'unicorn' is not a real definition, nor are the definitions of 'point' and 'line' in Euclidean geometry. Real definitions implicitly or explicitly assert real existence and hence imply existential propositions.

It is sometimes difficult to know whether a definition refers to what is real or fictitious. Here psychology comes decidedly into play. British mathematician and philosopher Alfred North Whitehead (1925) described what he called "the fallacy of misplaced concreteness," the error of believing that what is only abstract exists physically. Whitehead's name for this conceptual mistake may be more descriptive than the more commonly used name 'reification', derived from the Latin *facere*, meaning "to make," and *res*, meaning "thing," which when both are brought together means "converting something that is purely an idea into an object believed to exist." Both 'misplaced concreteness' and 'reification' are names for the fallacy of believing that a construct, a purely hypothetical idea, refers to a real physical entity.

Misplacing concreteness or reifying are not mere parlor-game fallacies of logic but are fundamental to the psychologically normal human constitution. The propensity to believe that many of the things we define must be real expresses one of a variety of forms of "conceptual pathology" that I have studied elsewhere (Bartlett 1971; 1975; 1976; 1982; 1983; 2005, Part III). The human disposition to reify has often been expressed in the history of science: In physics, appeal was made to the concepts of a luminiferous aether and of phlogiston in order to provide for a substantive, real medium in space that could carry light waves and for the "fiery substance" released during combustion. In medicine, similar reifications were made through the concept of bodily humors, miasma, and vital force or by stethoscope inventor René-Théophile-Hyacinth Laënnec's (1982, MS. 2186 [III]) *principe vital*. And of course reification is pervasive in ideologies and religions (the nation is partially reified in its flag, gods and goddesses are reified by systems of religion and mythology, etc.). It is practically impossible for most people to *refrain* from believing that what appears to be a real definition or description actually refers to things that exist.

The tendency to reify is deeply engrained in the human psychologically normal propensity to engage in what I have elsewhere called "projective misconstructions." Expressed in compressed form, a projective misconstruction occurs when we believe that that to which we refer is independent of the very conditions that render such reference possible (Bartlett 1971; 1975; 1976; 1982; 1983; 2005, Part II). For our purposes here, this is a theoretically abstract way of saying several simple things at once: when we formulate definitions that we misconstrue to be real definitions, we are often led to build on these, making further statements that we take to be true, when in fact on a very basic level we do not know what we're actually referring to and talking about, and yet nonetheless insist that we do and that what we're talking about is real. To engage in projective misconstruction in the context of our present discussion is to be caught by the delusional power of definition, that is, to believe that our seemingly real definitions refer to empirical realities. In psychiatric nosology, this takes the form of believing that what is authoritatively defined as a "mental disorder" corresponds to "a distinct and real disease entity."

Once a purported illness has been defined, a *psychological shift* to reification often takes place: after a nosologist has stipulated a disease definition, it is a psychologically normal tendency to transform the definition, without giving this shift reflective thought, into a judgment that a corresponding object, a "real disease entity," exists with the defined properties. Definitions that purport to be real definitions carry with them, often in disguise, existential propositions that claim that what has been defined is empirically real. A name is given to a disease, its symptomatology is described, and then a leap of misplaced concreteness frequently takes place that results in an unquestioned acceptance that a "disease entity" exists: a "mental illness" or "mental disorder." Let us look at this psychological shift in greater detail.

DEFINING MENTAL DISORDERS INTO EXISTENCE

> Like the personifications of the religions, these [disease] entities offer certain advantages as transition stages for untrained reasoning, but from the scientific point of view they are unacceptable.
> —German physician and bacteriologist Ferdinand Hueppe (1852–1938)
> (quoted by Faber, 1923/1930, pp. 191–92)

As we have seen, stipulative or legislative definition can be a great aid to effective, efficient communication. It also has its disadvantages, for many legislative definitions are easily mistaken for real definitions, which, unlike stipulative, legislative definitions, can, as we've noted, refer to empirical realities and communicate information about the world. All definitions of course communicate information, but only some definitions formulate empirical claims to knowledge, which can be true or false. We've seen that stipulative definitions are not true or false but rather express an authoritative request or insistence that they be adopted. Stipulative definitions in a nosology express judgments that certain choices should be made—most especially choices that specify which medical conditions we should consider harmful or disabling and how those conditions are to be understood in terms of sets of symptoms, family and patient history, the course of a disease, its prognosis, and other factors. In short, some definitions that appear to be real definitions are only that in disguise, camouflaging the fact that they express evaluative choices in favor of the shared allegiance of an expert group that wishes to persuade others to adopt the same choices. But beyond such misleading definitions, there are other disease definitions that successfully function as genuinely real definitions: They combine stipulation with empirical description and indicate how observable symptoms are associated with underlying physiological pathology, often recognized or confirmed by laboratory tests, as is common in physical medicine.

The history of both psychiatry and physical medicine attests to the frequency of change in the choices expressed by nosologies: In recent decades within psychiatry, we've witnessed a succession of modifications, reclassifications, indecision, and controversy in diagnostic choices concerning, for example, homosexuality, mathematics disorder, masochistic personality disorder, caffeine intoxication, posttraumatic stress disorder, nightmare disorder, perileuteal phase dysphoric disorder (a.k.a. PMS), depression, intermittent explosive disorder, pathological gambling, alcoholism, learning disorders, kleptomania, attention deficit disorder, sibling relational problem, autism, conduct disorders, and eating disorders—and the list could of course be lengthened. Some diagnostic judgments about "disorders" thought to be real are now considered to be dead wrong, for instance, masturbation and female orgasm.

In physical medicine, perhaps more extravagant and outrageous in hindsight, we have seen diseases come and go, as in the case of physician Samuel Cartwright's (1851) discovery of *drapetomania* (the disease causing slaves to want to abscond) and *dysæsthesia æthiopsis* (the disease causing slaves to destroy property); or going back a little further in time, of physician Benjamin Rush's 1792 discovery of *Negritude*, "the disease of being black" (Reznek, 1987, pp. 17–18). When, with the clarity that looking back permits us, such putative "diseases" are recognized to have been disguised evaluations that promoted the social or political correctness of the times, we can see that these seemingly real definitions of disease were actually definitions that aimed to persuade. As Robinson (1950/1962), whose work was not concerned with psychiatric matters, asked in one of the few books wholly devoted to cataloguing varieties of definition,

> What is the value of persuasive definition? The habit of evaluating things is presumably ineradicable from human nature, and certainly desirable. The habit of trying to get other persons to share our own valuations is equally ineradicable and equally legitimate. What is hard to decide is whether persuasive definition is a desirable way of trying to change people's opinions. The argument against it is that it involves error and perhaps also deceit. The only persons who are influenced by a persuasive definition, it may be said, are those who do not realize its true nature, but take it to be what every real definition professes to be, a description of the objective nature of things. A persuasive definition, it may be urged, is at best a mistake and at worst a lie, because it consists in getting someone to alter his valuations under the false impression that he is not altering his valuations but correcting his knowledge of the facts. (pp. 169–70)

Robinson notes: "This ... form of real definition is a moral or evaluative appeal misrepresented as a statement of fact, and gaining force from its pseudo-scientific character. The general pattern of this [is] ... exhortation and appeal and moral judgement masquerading as science" (p. 167).

However, we would be thrown off course if we were to accept that persuasive definitions are, as Robinson suggests, of themselves error-inducing and deceit-causing. It is not the definitions themselves that are responsible but the psychologically normal propensity that willingly, and indeed often willfully, *insists* that our conceptual constructs correspond to physical realities.

THE DYSFUNCTIONAL NATURE OF THE PSYCHOLOGY OF DEFINITION

We have seen how stipulative definitions that appear to be or are mistaken to be real definitions often lead to existence claims. Again, it is important to stress that the fault for this mistake is not simply attributable to clumsy or inarticulate language but rests with psychological propensities that are normal, pervasive, and expressed in many aspects of life—in politics, religion, mythology, literature, and the history of many disciplines. It is certainly not a mistake confined to the way we construe definitions in psychiatric nosology. We use words to point, and it is psychologically normal to succumb to the belief that that to which they point is *real*. What J. R. R. Tolkien called in a nonfiction essay the *reality consistency* of literature (mentioning the New Testament as an example) touches precisely on the psychological facility we have of endowing with imagined, projected reality whatever is portrayed sufficiently well in words to create in us a sense of its "inner consistency of reality" (Tolkien, 1965, p. 47).

Legislative definitions—especially when they are enacted by panels of experts in which the full faith of a profession is invested and when they are set forth in a well-developed, detailed, descriptive system of disease classification—can easily exercise a powerfully persuasive influence over its professional audience and, in a psychological domino effect, also over the general public. This is especially true if that audience and the public are psychologically predisposed to engage in "projective misconstructions"—specifically if they are predisposed to misplace concreteness and reify the diseases stipulatively defined by the authorized nosology. This is, to be sure, most likely to happen when many of the stipulatively defined diseases are not known to have organic origins and are instead understood primarily in terms of sets of symptoms. We shall look more carefully into this aspect of psychiatric disease definition later.

When normal human psychology supports and indeed promotes the delusional reification of stipulated definitions it becomes dysfunctional, for to equate what is purely a construct and hence fictitious with what is real is delusion, while to recognize delusion is to acknowledge that cognitive failure has occurred. In the context of psychiatric nosology, when stipulated definitions of "mental disorders" inappropriately lead to their reification as real "disease entities," nosology similarly becomes dysfunctional.

We need to take this statement out of the abstract framework of nosology and to place it within the framework of the people who are directly and indirectly affected—psychiatrists, clinical psychologists, social workers, their patients or clients, pharmaceutical and insurance companies, the courts, the political system, and the wider society. When we do this and find our feet firmly planted on the ground, it is hard to avoid the strong impression that group delusion must be at work when definitions are constructed by panels of experts, then are agreed upon and ratified, then are given official endorsement as diagnostic *rules* by today's psychiatric community (recall once again that rules are not true or false), and then are misconstrued by psychiatrists themselves, and subsequently by much of the rest of society, as "true statements" about *real diseases.*

Is this, however, what actually happens? Are all "mental disorders" that are stipulatively defined by contemporary psychiatric nosology no more than theoretical fictions? Does the concept of "mental illness" lose medical meaning as "real disease" because of the propensity of human projective psychology to reify? Surely, it is natural to think, not in all cases. At this point, we need to make explicit what the stipulative definitions of today's psychiatric nosology in fact refer to.

CHOICES IN THE INTERPRETATION AND RECOGNITION OF DISEASE: PHYSICAL PATHOLOGY AND MENTAL DISORDER

In matters of definition there is no right or wrong.
—Hardin (1982, p. 138)

Stipulative definitions and the lexical definitions that we find in dictionaries are not dictated by reality, but, as we've noted, they express conventions: the stipulative variety lay down conventions that are intended to serve an author's or a group's purposes in the future; the lexical variety describes conventions that language use in the past has followed. Definitions of either kind reflect choices that could have been made otherwise if human purposes had been different. Empirical reality does not prescribe the definitions human beings have chosen for their words that we find in dictionaries, nor do facts determine what we recognize as disease. Farmers judge that the blight that attacks corn or potatoes is most certainly disease, yet

> if man wished to cultivate parasites (rather than potatoes or corn) there would be no "blight," but simply the necessary foddering of the parasite-crop.... Outside of the significances that man voluntarily attaches to certain conditions, *there are no illnesses in nature....* The fracture of a septuagenarian's femur has, within the world of nature, no more significance than the snapping of an autumn leaf from its twig: and the invasion of a human organism by cholera-germs carries with it no more the stamp of "illness" than does the souring of milk by other forms of bacteria.... [I]f some plant-species in which man had no interest (a desert grass, let us say) were to be attacked by a fungus or parasite, we should speak not of a disease, but merely of the competition between two species. The medical enterprise is from its inception value-loaded; it is not simply an applied biology, but a biology applied in accordance with the dictates of social interest. (Sedgwick, 1973, pp. 30, 31)

There are, however, levels of choice. The medical definition of disease does not involve the degree of freedom that we often see in the stipulative definitions of mathematics or law or that we recognize in the dictionary definition of a word where a choice is recorded, indicating that someone, at a certain time, chose to associate the sound or symbol of a word with a certain meaning. Historically, the prototypical medical definition of disease has been derived from physical medicine, which claims that the presence of disease is made evident through its symptomatology (as noted earlier, here taken to include both the symptoms the patient is capable of reporting as well as the signs observed by the treating physician). We are reminded that a *symptom* is a physical or psychological phenomenon that is believed to arise from or accompany a presumed disease and to constitute an indication of it.[4] The prototypical medical understanding of disease claims that symptoms are the consequence of underlying pathology and that the main goal of medical treatment is to detect and eliminate that pathology.

The medical theory of disease distinguishes various types of organic disease ranging from disease caused by an infectious agent to environmental disease, nutritional disease, metabolic disease, autoimmune disease, genetically based disease, and so on. (cf. Bartlett, 2005, Chapter 1). A specific and clear schematic concept of physical disease is expressed by the Systematized Nomenclature of Pathology (SNOP), which seeks to standardize nomenclature for diagnostic pathologists and to assist pathologists in classifying laboratory specimens. SNOP defines a physical disease in terms of four fields: the part of the body affected ("topography"), structural changes that result from the disease ("morphology"), the cause of the disorder ("etiology"), and functional manifestations ("function"). For each field, a four-digit code is assigned, the first digit designating the section of the field and the subsequent digits specifying subdivisions (College of American Pathologists Committee on Nomenclature and Classification of Disease, 1965). The Systematized Nomenclature of Medicine (SNOMED) is similarly organized, being an extension of the SNOP. SNOMED uses the four fields of the SNOP plus three additional fields consisting of a disease classification field, a procedure field for administrative records, and an occupation field for occupational record keeping (College of American Pathologists Committee on Nomenclature and Classification of Disease, 1979).

There is a significant—literally, a *substantive*—difference between such an evidence-based, physical definition of disease and the definition of 'mental disorder' or 'mental illness'. Psychiatric nosologies throughout history have been influenced by their love affair with the model offered by physical disease, but the definitions of physical disease and mental disorder have in general diverged very considerably.

If we were to take the medical model of physical disease as an ideal standard in defining disease, then several criteria of definition follow. In order for a medical definition of an individual disease to go beyond stipulative definition, it would need to accomplish all four of the following things: (1) the definition must identify a disorder that is judged to result in disability or harm either to individuals themselves who are afflicted with that malady, to their society, or to both; (2) it integrates the description of the disease within a systematic framework of classification of other known diseases; (3) it specifies conditions under which the disease is observable by enumerating physical, behavioral, cognitive, and affective symptoms and signs that serve as indications to the physician and to the patient of the presence of the disease; and (4) the definition describes the separately specifiable conditions, states, or physiological pathology known to give rise to the characteristic symptomatology of that disease.[5] Emphasis must be placed on the phrase "separately specifiable," for it is here that a medical definition of physical disease is anchored in what we might, if it were not such a mouthful, call "extrasymptomatological reality."

In other words, we must have these *two* different contexts of reference— stipulative definition plus empirical confirmation of pathology—in order for a defined disorder or disease, whether in psychiatry or in physical medicine, to have more than symptomatological status. Unless a mental disorder is to be equated with a set of symptoms, condition 4 must be satisfied. However, as we shall soon see, the great majority of mental disorders in fact *have* been identified and reduced only to sets of symptoms (commonly supplemented by individual and family history and by assessment of the course of the purported disorder and of its likely outcome).

THE PSYCHOLOGY OF SYMPTOM CLUSTERING

A disease without physical findings is an anomaly.
—Stempsey (1999, p. 190)

Symptom-complexes cannot pass for diseases.
—Hungarian neurologist Eugen Jendrassik (1829–1891) (quoted by Faber, 1923/1930, p. 183)

A "syndrome" is a group of symptoms that occur together and are used to identify a state or condition judged to be medically undesirable. Nearly all purported "mental disorders" are syndromes, that is, their definitions are symptom-based and fail to meet the last condition (4) above. The term 'syndrome' is at the core of the definition of 'mental disorders' that we find relatively unchanged in the *DSM-III-R* (1987), *DSM-IV* (1994), and *DSM-IV-R* (2000):[6]

> [E]ach of the mental disorders is conceptualized as a clinically significant behavioral or psychological *syndrome* or pattern that occurs in an individual and that is associated with present distress (e.g. a painful symptom) or disability (i.e. an impairment in one or more important areas of functioning) or with a significantly increased risk of suffering death, pain, disability, or an important loss of freedom.... Whatever its original cause, it *must* currently be considered a manifestation of a behavioral, psychological, or biological dysfunction in the individual. (American Psychiatric Association, 1994, p. xxii, italics added)

This is intellectually honest language that places the word 'syndrome' alongside its nontechnical synonym 'pattern', for the perception of patterns plays an important role in the definition of disease. Before 1980, when *DSM-III* was published, "syndromes" were implicitly regarded as being "proper sets," that is, they were generally understood in terms of well-defined symptom sets, each symptom of which was necessary, and all symptoms taken together were sufficient, to determine the presence of the disorder in question. Since then, a tolerance for less well-defined, "fuzzy" syndromes has developed so that often no set of symptoms is jointly sufficient to define a particular disorder. We now typically find psychiatric disorders defined in terms of multiple symptoms, a specified minimum number of which must be satisfied in order for a patient to be considered correspondingly "disordered."

There are several recognized problems with such a symptom-based approach to defining mental illness: one is that the same symptoms are frequently found in patients who are judged to have different disorders, another is that a patient may have a mixture of symptoms that are considered to belong to several different disorders, still another is that a single patient may have symptomatology that satisfies the definitions of two or more mental disorders (so-called "comorbidity"), and still another is that two patients with the same diagnosis may have different sets of symptoms ("heterogeneity"). These problems, which together we'll call "problems of diagnostic haze," when coupled with the psychology of pattern recognition that we'll look at in a moment, make symptom-based definitions of mental disorders inherently prone to uncertainty about the status of a syndrome as a disease or disorder in itself. This naturally leads to doubt whether the diagnostic criteria stipulated by a definition of a mental disorder refer to distinct "disease entities" and whether such definitions themselves are well formulated.

Fever and depression are examples: A fever can be a symptom of an illness, but is not itself a distinct disease, for fevers may accompany many diseases. Similarly, depression can be associated with various psychiatric conditions—some 60 percent of general psychiatric patients show symptoms of depression, more than 40 percent of those diagnosed with anxiety disorders, and 30 to 70 percent of those judged to have a personality disorder (Beutler & Malik, 2002, p. 257). The incidence of depressive symptoms is, in other words, not neatly delimited, and this fact leads to suspicion that depression is not a specific "disease entity," not a specifiable "real mental disorder" in its own right, but a human psychological state that has "a nonspecific etiology, an irregular course, and no specific treatment" (p. 265). Depression, in this sense, is like the nonspecific symptom of physical pain; the "emotional pain" of depression can accompany many psychological conditions. It was therefore natural for Beutler and Malik to conclude: "If this is true of the most frequently diagnosed and most problematic of the mental health disorders, by extension one must be concerned about the very nature of the assumptions underlying the *DSM* itself" (p. 265).

It is evident that here, in the recognition and naming of symptom patterns, several human psychological propensities are deeply involved. The sets of symptoms that are grouped into syndromes are commonly and graphically referred to by nosologists as "constellations." Certain elements of the psychology of perception, involving a subject's interests and purposes, underlie the definition of constellations. It is easy to see this in connection with constellations of another sort, the astronomical "objects" we see on a starry night. Pattern recognition plays a leading role in the form that perceived clusters of stars come to take—once we are instructed what to look for—whether Orion, Cassiopeia, or the seven Pleiades. The psychology that is part of this process of clustering has not been studied in connection with the construction of nosologies, but that it plays a leading part is evident.

When as children we played "connect the dots," the game would be time-consuming indeed were it not for the numbering of the dots. The greater the number of dots (in analogy here with symptoms), the greater the number of possible patterns (in analogy with syndromes). To come a little closer to the real world, consider a three-dimensional group of numerous but unnumbered dots, and consider how many different patterns can result from connecting them with straight lines. If arbitrarily curved lines are allowed instead, the number of patterns explodes infinitely. If we bring in the dimension of time, the potential number of patterns quickly becomes dizzying. Although at this point we are on a fairly high level of theoretical abstraction, we should quickly see that, on a specific and concrete level, the clustering of symptoms can occur as a function of many variables, some of which have been the object of discussion and at times contention in the psychiatric literature: namely, to what extent definitions of syndromes are a function, for example, of social, political, religious, moral, and commercial interests (e.g., Laing, 1960; Szasz, 1957/1961 and 1970/1997; Scheff, 1966/1984; Breggin, 1994; Stempsey, 1999; Beutler & Malik, 2002; Sadler, 2002; Schiappa, 2003; Bartlett, 2005, Part I; Cooper, 2005; Sadler, 2005).

With respect to both kinds of constellations, of stars or of symptoms, selective human choice is involved in the patterns we recognize. The clustering that we sometimes say we "discover" and sometimes say we "create" can be understood in terms of selective interest, for nature provides no lines of categorical division, just as the map lines that define counties, states, and nations are not determined by nature but are chosen and legislated. As Stempsey (1999, p. 99) expressed this, "our descriptions of these [symptom] constellations are in an important sense socially constructed. We have a choice as to which clusters of phenomena we see as constituting a disease, and which we choose to interpret as background noise."

As we've noted, by 'symptoms' we include behavior, affective and physical states, and cognitive activity, whether reported by the patient or observed as signs by the clinician. These phenomena are highly individual, related to the individuating context of a patient's life history and ongoing experience. Depending on the criteria by which these phenomena are sorted and placed in symptom clusters, they can be grouped in essentially innumerable ways.[7]

It might be appropriate to single out and name this open-ended human propensity that clusters symptoms in diverse ways. One might be tempted to name it the "Endless Multiplication of Syndromes *Principle*," were it not for the fact that it itself constitutes a syndrome, a collection of characteristic psychologically normal dispositions. And so perhaps we may call it the "Endless Multiplication of Syndromes Syndrome" (EMSS). By naming the EMSS I want to underscore that we need to take seriously that "endless multiplication" is really at issue, for there is, in principle, *nothing*—psychologically or logically—to halt it. We shall see that psychiatry does not, like physical medicine, have available an "empirical brake" that can reign in runaway syndrome multiplication.

The psychology of symptom clustering is also involved in the phenomenon of *diagnostic filtering*. In much the same way as the constellation of Orion leaps out—a clear pattern detaching itself from its starry background—*as soon as you know what to look for*, so do the diagnostic classifications learned by clinicians *define*, in both main senses of this word, how they are likely to perceive their patients' behavior and psychological symptomatology. Human beings cannot make observations outside of a frame of reference that reflects adherence to some group of conceptual commitments, however basic these may be. The conceptual commitments with which a clinician evaluates a patient are generally those that are advocated by the nosology he or she has been taught, and these, in turn, of course can sometimes be further influenced by prevailing nonclinical values such as diagnostic expedience (using *DSM* codes to meet insurance payment criteria, etc.).

Diagnostic filtering extends beyond a clinician's perception of patients: it serves to check or limit the scope of what he or she is able to see or is able *most easily* to see. As Malik and Beutler (2002) expressed this metaphorically, "the very success and widespread use of the *DSM* model of diagnosis may have the unintended side effect of constraining us to work within a less-than-optimal system of diagnosis, a situation analogous to that of expending considerable time and resources in the ascent of a single mountain, while neglecting to explore the possibility that even higher peaks may exist nearby" (pp. 7–8). They concluded: "[T]he longer diagnosis is determined according to the *DSM*, the fewer opportunities there will be for the exploration of alternatives" (p. 9).

PSYCHIATRY'S INFLATIONARY ONTOLOGY

> Those groups of symptoms which are [called "diseases" by my colleagues] are metaphysical abstractions which by no means represent a constant unchangeable morbid condition, and which we cannot be certain of finding in nature. They are factitious entities (entités factices), and all those who study medicine according to this method are ontologists.
> —French physician François-Joseph-Victor Broussias (1772–1838)
> (quoted by Faber, 1930/1978, p. 48)

> Such a view which takes abstract concepts for things, implying their actual existence and at once treating them as entities, is called ontology.... [T]o the ontologist the assumed disease is a dogma; the group once collected, it becomes a concept, an entity.
> —German physician and psychiatrist Carl Reinhold August Wunderlich
> (1815–1877) (quoted by Faber, 1923/1930, pp. 66–67)

As human needs and vested interests change, it is to be expected that so will the choice of symptom sets, for what human beings regard as harmful or disabling behavior, affect, or cognitive function is subject to very considerable change with time. Hence, correspondingly harmful "syndromes" of these phenomena can be expected also to multiply without end, along with, as we shall see, their correspondingly reified "internal dysfunctions." Diagnosable "patterns" will change, sometimes inflating and sometimes contracting in number, but open-ended definitional change in psychiatric nosology is formally assured as well as being guaranteed by the psychologically normal human predisposition to recognize patterns in experience that fit, or conflict, with perceived needs and interests. As long as "mental disorders" are equivalent to *free-floating stipulated syndromes*, uncorrelated with an empirical basis that can be tested and thereby be confirmed or disconfirmed, they will remain on the historically primitive level of mere beliefs subject to the vagaries of changing fashion, changing interests, and values ever in flux.

Henrik Wulff has divided disease into four types: disease defined in terms of symptoms, syndromal disease, anatomically defined disease, and causally defined disease. He has argued that symptom diagnoses are used to describe "the most primitive form of disease entity" (Wulff, 1976, p. 67), with syndromes occupying the next level of scientific development. As an example, he gives chronic diarrhea, which could come from ulcerative colitis (a syndrome), cancer of the colon (an anatomically defined disease), or lactase deficiency (a causally defined disease).

Similarly, J. G. Scadding has described scientific progress in medicine in terms of a "ladder of taxonomic knowledge" (Scadding, 1990, 1996). The first rung of the ladder corresponds to disorders that physicians were able to understand only in terms of symptomatology. This level of medical knowledge is the most elementary and forms a starting point for future needed work. Scadding situates the majority of "psychiatric disorders" on this primitive stage of development. As scientific medicine progresses, the discovery of structural anomalies replaces the rudimentary and informal descriptions of syndromes; this occurred, for example, when the structural knowledge of tubercles replaced exclusive reliance on the syndromal description of tuberculosis. As scientific medicine progresses further, a third rung in the ladder of knowledge is reached when evidence of physical pathophysiology or of disorders of function becomes available. Finally, the top rung of the ladder is reached when medicine comes to understand the etiology of disease, which occurred when the tubercle bacillus, *Mycobacterium tuberculosis*, was discovered to be the origin both for the morbid structure it causes and for a resulting failure of physiological functions.

From this evaluative-historical perspective, medicine advances not when syndromally defined disorders explode in number, as they have in psychiatric nosology during the past several decades, but when etiological explanations are found for diseases that previously had been defined on the elementary syndromal level. As physical medicine has gradually been able to detect identifiable pathology at the root of what were previously described only as free-floating syndromes, it has made significant, solid progress.

In contrast, the history of psychiatric nosologies shows little signs of such progress. Few of the syndromally defined "disorders" in the most recent edition of *DSM* can be associated with an empirically verifiable etiology (e.g., Houts, 2002, p. 44). R. L. Spitzer, who has played a central role in recent *DSM* revisions, estimated that more than 200 of the "disorders" listed in *DSM-III* (it listed 265) would not have been included had the criterion of empirical support from the research literature been applied (Spitzer, 1991; Houts, 2002, p. 53). And since Spitzer published this admission, syndrome multiplication has continued as more than 100 additional alleged "mental disorders" have been added to the *DSM*, nearly all of these also lacking an empirical basis.

The globally influential *International Classification of Diseases (ICD-10)* shows a similar inflationary trend. Where the previous edition, *ICD-9*, contained only 30 categories for mental disorders, the new standalone volume, *ICD-10 Classification of Mental and Behavioural Disorders: Clinical Descriptions and Diagnostic Guidelines*, devotes 100 categories (some still unused) to mental disorders, of which some 90 percent of those listed have no known organic basis.

This recent exuberance for recognizing and naming new syndromal disorders stands in conflict with the precepts of disease theory urged by the most eminent of nosologists of the past two centuries. Emil Kraepelin (1856–1926) understood mental illness in essential connection with associated organic pathology, course, and outcome. When there was an absence of knowledge of the etiology of a purported mental disorder, he fell back upon symptom-based definitions. Kihlstrom (2002), recognizing the importance of Kraepelin's basic medical objective, has urged: "[W]e can honor Kraepelin not by repealing his principles, but by reaffirming them—by moving beyond symptoms and diagnosing mental illness in terms of underlying pathology. For Kraepelin, diagnosis by symptoms was a temporary fallback, to be used only because diagnosis by pathology and etiology was not possible" (p. 297).

THE CONCEPT OF MENTAL ILLNESS IS NO MYTH BUT THE RESULT OF DYSFUNCTIONAL THOUGHT

It is important not to equate the need for an observable physical etiology, for an empirically established origin of stipulated symptom sets, with a simplistic and dogmatic preference for the paradigm offered by physical diagnosis. For it is not simply that a preferred paradigm may be in view, but something a good deal more central: that is, the need for symptom sets to be correlated with a *detectable, underlying disorder or dysfunction*. This is needed, not purely in order to honor Kraepelin's ideal nor to satisfy the antipsychiatrists' complaint against the use of "mental illness" as a "metaphor" or "myth" (Szasz, 1957/1961, 1970/1997), *but in order for the psychology of definition to be nonarbitrary and not merely stipulative*. This is an important fact, and it distinguishes "the myth of mental illness" from "a concept of mental illness that results from psychological misconception." The first is a matter of metaphor or analogy that has gone astray, while the second is a matter of *dysfunctional thinking*. Szasz's anti-mental-disorder position was correct, not for the surface reason that mental illness labeling is mythical or metaphorical but because the human psychology of definition has become dysfunctional, that is, it has resulted in delusional reification of mental illness by means of constructed definitions, stipulated, agreed upon, and ratified by today's psychiatric community, with no confirmable basis in empirical pathology, and then systematically misconstrued by psychiatrists themselves and then by the rest of society as referring to real diseases.

In order for the psychology of definition in psychiatric nosology to rise above the arbitrariness of symptom clustering, it is essential to find a basis for any alleged "mental disorder" in empirically detectable pathology. It should be clear how psychologically easy it is, in relation to whatever may be the dominant social, political, and, indeed, monetary interests at any time, to select forms of behavior and ways of feeling and thinking that are perceived as undesirable, to cluster these into symptom sets, and then deceptively to designate the resulting reified syndromes "mental disorders."

Contemporary psychiatric nosology, as expressed in the *DSM* and the *ICD* (implicitly included in our discussion from now on), has not been blind to the need we are discussing: Although it may take some sympathetic interpretation to see it this way, the *DSM* appears somewhat half-heartedly and dimly to have recognized that, if a stipulated syndrome is to be an indication a "real mental disorder," this requires that an observable inner disorder, a detectable harmful inner dysfunction, a verifiable pathology, actually *exist*. But, unfortunately, in nearly every instance of a purported, *DSM*-classified "mental disorder," this necessary link with reality has gone begging; the failure to establish such a link tends largely to be ignored; and *DSM*-coded syndromes are then taken to name real mental disorders—by clinicians; their patients; medical, legal, and social institutions; and the surrounding society. The endless ramification, combination, and recombination potential, for which the psychology of symptom clustering is responsible when there is no detectable underlying pathology, makes "the reality of mental disorders" a contemporary empty fiction—to paraphrase Robinson—clothing an evaluative appeal in pseudoscientific dress (1950/1962, p. 167). The fiction arises not because the concept of mental disorder is "metaphorical" or a "myth" but because without empirical anchoring definitions of alleged mental illness can only be stipulative, legislated, and promoted with the goal to persuade. Definition within any legitimate nosology must be more than this.

THE PSYCHOLOGY OF RESISTANCE TO IDIOPATHIC DISEASE

> This moral idiopathy, which neither proceeds from nor depends on any other disease, . . . this itch for seeing memorable places . . . is peculiarly English.
>
> —*The New Monthly Magazine* (XXXIX, 1833, p. 129)

As in the quote above, it becomes very easy—often too easy—to label as "idiopathic disease" any phenomenon for which we do not know its cause. A disease is said to be "idiopathic" when, so far as we know, it arises by itself and is not symptomatic or the result of another disease. This is a lexical definition of the word 'idiopathic'; the definition states what a common usage has been in the past. The definition I've given is a paraphrase of the main definition in the *Oxford English Dictionary*; in medical contexts it is often expanded to include a phrase like "arising from an obscure or unknown cause," reflecting another psychologically prevalent predisposition, the need to postulate underlying physical causes, which we'll look at briefly here in the guise of resistance to idiopathic labeling.

Concerning the symptom-based definitions that the *DSM* contains—the majority that do not have a known etiology—could we reasonably say that they are "idiopathic" in nature, insofar as current knowledge is concerned? To suggest, if Dr. Spitzer's estimate, noted a few pages back, is brought up to date, that somewhere in the general neighborhood of 300 of the 368 presently recognized "mental disorders" are "idiopathic clusters of symptoms"—to suggest this would certainly not gladden many psychiatric hearts. And to suggest further, given the shifting sands of fashion, taste, and perceived need, that these syndromes or patterns can and no doubt will in the future be rearranged into varied and alternative clusters, this surely would also not please. There is an unmistakable psychological resistance in taking what one has believed to be a "real disease entity" and downgrading it to the medically shabby level of a mere "idiopathic syndrome" with no fixed identity and an obscure, or merely presumed, cause.

One of the clearest expressions of this resistance can be found in the recently published book by Allan V. Horwitz and Jerome C. Wakefield (2007), which contains a preface by Dr. Spitzer. He tips his hat to critics who "have been suspicious of the very notion of a mental disorder," and goes on, in a revealingly stark, candid, and telling disclosure, to praise Horwitz and Wakefield because they "recognize the *DSM*'s contributions and accept *its assumption* that there are genuine mental disorders in the strict medical sense" (pp. vii–ix, italics added). This is an important admission; indeed it is central to the psychology of definition in psychiatric nosology. For some decades, Dr. Spitzer has been a prominent organizing force as the *DSM* has undergone multiple revisions and updating. If anyone should know what the psychological status is of the claim that mental disorders are genuinely real, it would be Dr. Spitzer. And yet he tells us that this, the very core of a nosology, the very fabric out of which it is stitched, is actually no more and no less than an "*assumption*," which he, presumably, was persuaded to make for reasons rooted in our subject, the psychology of definition. Or was this just a slip of the pen?

That doesn't seem likely. The two authors, Horwitz and Wakefield, also make the same candid admission: "Because of the role that diagnosis has in so many areas of our lives and *the assumption that a diagnosis represents a genuine medical condition*, confusing depressive disorder with normal sadness should not be taken lightly" (p. 22, italics added). Toward the end of their book, they remark: "It is now *generally accepted* that there are genuine medical disorders of the mind" (p. 225, italics added). —Do we then, in vicious circularity, assert the existence of genuine mental disorders *because* they are "generally accepted *assumptions*"? This was the way of the aether, phlogiston, bodily humors, and in psychiatry of Negritude, Homosexuality, and the other phantom pathologies that also for a time gained alleged existence as "genuine medical disorders." Only on the basis of refutable or confirmable *evidence* of an "underlying dysfunction," *can* it make sense to claim that a disease is real.

DO INTERNAL MALFUNCTIONS OR DYSFUNCTIONS UNDERLIE PSYCHIATRIC SYNDROMES?

It isn't my intention to pick on Horwitz and Wakefield, but their book is recent; it is up to date; and it exhibits much of the psychology of definition that this chapter is about; it is therefore instructive to turn to. Any critical observations I express here are directed not so much toward their book as toward the prevailing psychology of contemporary psychiatric nosology. Here are a few sample passages that I suggest we put at arm's length and examine critically:

The authors state: "Because [depressions without cause, so-called *melancholia*] . . . were not proportional reactions to actual events, such conditions were *assumed* to stem from *some sort of internal defect or dysfunction* that required professional attention" (p. 6, italics added). Note here the explicit role of assumption.

They go on to say: "By depressive disorders . . . we mean sadness that is caused by a harmful dysfunction (HD) of *loss response mechanisms. According to the HD definition*, a collection of symptoms indicates a mental disorder only when it meets both of two criteria. The first is dysfunction: something has gone wrong with *some internal mechanism*'s ability to perform one of its biologically designed functions. Second, the dysfunction must be harmful" (p. 17, italics added). Note here that the existence of this "internal mechanism" is again a presumption, thanks to a definition that says it must exist.

Following this claim, the authors accept the following stipulative definition: "Endogenous depressions *by definition* arise in the absence of real loss, *and so are almost always due to internal dysfunctions*" (p. 18, italics added). We need to ask whether it makes sense to claim that endogenous depressions can reasonably be thought to arise as a result of definitional requirements, for this is what the authors seem to be telling us—so that the assumption made by the stipulated definition, that an "internal dysfunction" must be involved, comes, through reification, to be equated with reality. And so it is natural to ask, "What is it about the psychology of psychiatric definition that impels one to believe that behind any syndrome certain 'internal dysfunctions' must exist?"

Not to beat a horse that may already be gasping its last, suffice it to mention that the authors repeatedly refer to "internal dysfunctions" without any confirmable empirical referents whatsoever. The claim is made repeatedly in various forms that depressive conditions are maintained "by *some internal dysfunction* and *thus are likely to be disordered*" (pp. 210; also 20, 22, and passim). This is stipulative insistence that such dysfunctions *exist*, as the authors' preferred definitions would have it.

The *DSM* itself fares no better (nor does the *ICD*). Earlier in this chapter in the section "The Psychology of Symptom Clustering," I quoted the definition of 'mental disorders' found in several editions of the *DSM*. The last sentence in that passage read as follows: "Whatever [the syndrome's] original cause, it *must* currently be considered a manifestation of a behavioral, psychological, or biological *dysfunction* in the individual" (italics added). Why "must" it be considered a manifestation of a *dysfunction*? Have we learned that all (most? any?) symptom sets that we happen to cluster together and judge at any particular time to be harmful and undesirable, are *necessarily* the manifestations of real dysfunctions in the individual? Contrast this barefaced and unjustified assumption of the very thing that is in need of empirical evidence with the way physical medicine confirms, for example, through a patient's blood analysis, that he or she has TB.

We cannot evade the conclusion that it is the psychology of definition as it is deployed in contemporary nosology that is responsible for the misperceived *necessity* that there *exist* a *dysfunction* in the individual patient. Today's nosologists, like many in psychiatry's history, are psychologically induced to claim that corresponding to a definition of a mental disorder—one which has been legislated and enacted by a powerful professional body perceived as a source of authority—is a real disease.

THE PSYCHOLOGY OF DEFINITION AND CLAIMS TO TRUTH

An examination of the psychology of psychiatric definition shows that it is no accident that the majority of definitions of mental disorders, as found today in editions of the *DSM* and the *ICD*, are construed to be true statements. Yet, as we have seen, such definitions are first and foremost prescriptions that aim to persuade others that what is stipulated and legislated should be accepted as diagnostic *rules*, and rules, we are reminded, are never true or false; they are only conventions, some of which have a value, and others of which do not. The definitions of psychiatric nosologies get into trouble when nosologists include descriptive content in their stipulated definitions. It is a psychologically normal characteristic for diagnosticians and other clinicians to construe this descriptive content, which typically enumerates behavioral and psychological symptomatology, as referring to the real world in a true or false manner. But, in fact, this is a psychological deception.

When a mental disorder is stipulatively defined in terms of sets of symptoms, then an individual will be judged to have that putative disorder when he or she exhibits the corresponding set of symptoms. The diagnostic judgment that is involved will be asserted to be "true," and true *by virtue of the definition* with which the patient's symptoms are associated! That judgment is *necessarily true* because it asserts nothing more than a tautology! Here is the way another author expressed much the same point:

> The key issue is this: What is the basis for claiming that when A is broken, the result is C, the observed set of behaviors? For this type of argument to be valid, we would need independent evidence that the hypothetical statement "if A were broken, C would be the expected result" was in fact true. . . . For most of the mental disorders listed in the modern *DSM*s, we

have no such evidence. (Certain organic brain syndromes and substance use problems may be the only exceptions.) The fact is, without such independent evidence for a causal relationship between the broken hypothetical mechanism and the observed behavior, this line of reasoning is tautological, entirely circular (Houts, 2001; Houts & Follette, 1998). (Houts, 2002, p. 43)

But instead of recognizing this fact, the diagnostician believes that he or she has made a statement about the patient's real mental condition and further believes that this statement is verified by virtue of the patient's symptoms. But this is a far cry from what "verification" means in empirical science, for it is not verification at all: We are simply caught in a definitional circle in which we can't lose! There is no way for the diagnostician's application of his or her definition to be disconfirmed.

A basic criterion of the truth or falsity of statements in science is their *falsifiability*. If a scientific proposition cannot, even in principle, be falsified—if *no test* could possibly show that the proposition is false—then we reject the notion that the proposition has a proper place in science. Scientific statements, which can be tested empirically and potentially shown to be false, are contrasted with essentially metaphysical statements, which are held, with great intellectual recalcitrance and fortitude, to be true—no matter what the empirical facts may be.

We have seen how the definitions of mental disorders are thought and believed to entail statements about the real existence of those disorders and even about the existence of unknown yet nevertheless vigorously imagined and propounded dysfunctions that are claimed to be involved in or to underlie them. In what sense are these statements that assert existence falsifiable? It might be tempting to resort to some hoped-for future by saying, "Well, yes, there is a problem here, but maybe these alleged disorders *will* at some future time be shown to come from an underlying empirical pathology." But that won't do: it simply begs the question and legitimates whatever nosological phantoms we happen to feel like postulating.

Could we somehow stretch our imaginations in some Procrustean way so as to conceive how it would be *possible*, today, to falsify these assertions that mental disorders are real, and similarly do this for the conjectured corresponding inner dysfunctions? If your mind works at all like mine, it is too much of a stretch to consider falsifiable that which on the surface looks like an empirical belief but has no basis whatever in evidence in the empirical world.

Our powers of imagination aside, we here face a "conceptual pathology" of the kind alluded to earlier: we seek to refer to what, in principle, we simply cannot successfully refer to in the context of present knowledge, and yet we nonetheless insist that we do, and claim to know what we're talking about. It can be difficult indeed to break through a systematically held, psychologically motivated delusion of this kind, whether it is found in an individual patient or is shared by a professional community of many thousands.

THE NEXT STEP IN REIFICATION

Within the framework of the psychiatric definition of mental disorder, the psychology of "faculties" is making something of a comeback, but in slightly disguised form. In the many centuries since Aristotle distinguished the nutritive, perceptual, and intellectual faculties, numerous other human faculties have been recognized—and then reified into existence—in the form of such "faculties of the soul" as hungering, feeling, knowing, reasoning, judging, perceiving, remembering, and so on.

Each of these "faculties" was presumed to exist as the generating source of the corresponding activity. We may have thought that this old "faculty psychology" had seen its last in nosologies of the nineteenth century, but it is back in vogue to assert the existence of similar "internal mechanisms"—now in order to support the presumed existence of disease entities. This has happened largely, it is reasonable to suggest, because it has not been possible to substantiate with empirical findings the insistent belief that there *simply must be* an identifiable etiology that lies behind today's purely symptom-based psychiatric diagnoses and disorders.

Here is an example of this kind of dysfunctional thinking. To explain the etiology of alleged mental disorders, Cooper (2005) reasons: "Plausibly there are *mental mechanisms* that are not under our conscious control. ... When something goes wrong with such *mechanisms* the behaviours produced might well be involuntary and yet mentally caused" (p. 40, my italics). Kihlstrom (2002) keeps reification company with Cooper. Although he recognizes that diseases in physical medicine are now most often not primarily diagnosed on the basis of symptoms but rather on the basis of laboratory tests that serve to detect ongoing pathology, for psychiatric disorders Kihlstrom believes instead in the existence of underlying "*mental modules* . . . specially *geared* to perform a particular cognitive, emotional, motivational, or behavioral task. . . . [T]he linguist Noam Chomsky has often referred to these modules *as mental organs*" (Kihlstrom, 2002, p. 294; italics added in the first sentence).

In such empirically unfounded claims we see a combination of two of the widespread psychological predispositions that we've described: reification plus tautological verification of the "truth" of stipulative definitions. These psychological predispositions culminate in a view like Kihlstrom's view: "Attention deficit disorder may involve damage to a module that focuses attention, leaving modules that disengage or shift attention intact.... [A]utism results from a specific deficit in a particular mental module, called the *theory-of-mind mechanism*.... [T]he others are an intentionality detector, an eye-direction detector, and a shared attention mechanism" (pp. 295–96). As we have seen, once misplaced concreteness gets started, there is no holding it back! Reified "mechanisms," "modules," and "geared" devices proliferate *ad libitum*!

INTELLIGENT SCIENCE AND STOPGAP DEFINITIONS

> Instead of debating alternative ways of handling information about symptoms, we should be moving beyond symptoms to diagnosis on the basis of underlying pathology.
>
> —Kihlstrom (2002, p. 290)

We have seen how definitions of disease can be very different in physical medicine and in psychiatry. When I have pointed to psychologically based ways in which psychiatric definitions of disease are lacking, this is not due to an unalloyed and exclusionary admiration for the approach that has been successful in physical medicine. What I hope to communicate is the need to understand what the two different approaches to definition yield in terms of our understanding of pathology. Definitions of disease in physical medicine often have lexical, stipulative, and empirical components: unless a totally new disease has been discovered or new knowledge has come to replace old, disease labels tend to be consistent with established, that is, lexical, usage. Yet there is, in addition, agreement among practitioners as to what they will, at least in the foreseeable future, stipulatively understand a given disease label to mean. But most importantly, by virtue of requiring confirmation of a real disease independently of its symptomatology, physical medicine permits statements to be made that are informative, empirically confirmable, and not tautologically true by definition.

The majority of psychiatric definitions of "mental disorders," however, do not meet the scientific standard of falsifiability; although they contain descriptions of symptom clusters, they do not communicate empirical knowledge of pathology but rather an intent to establish consensus agreement to designate those symptom clusters *as if* they were symptoms of an underlying but as yet unknown pathology. As Stempsey (1999, p. 175) observed in connection with physical medicine:

> Mere descriptions of symptoms are ... generally not looked upon as definitive diseases, but merely problems to be further elucidated. However, sometimes symptom diagnoses are seen as definitive. Dermatology offers

many examples. The old joke defines a dermatologist as a doctor who tells you in Latin what you just told him in English. There is a kernel of truth in this. A patient may present with a greasy, scaly red rash, and go away with a diagnosis of seborrheic dermatitis. A patient with an itchy rash might enjoy some psychological comfort (or distress) in having a diagnosis of eczema rather than just a rash. However, this type of symptom diagnosis per se tells virtually nothing about such things as cause and prognosis,*which usually are the point of making diagnoses in the first place.* [italics added]

In this, Stempsey is in agreement with Wulff (1976), who judged, first, that syndromes are only and at best preliminary, tentative, and indeed primitive means of designating possible disease processes; and, second, that syndromes must wait for a satisfactory explanation that may—or may not—be forthcoming through eventual knowledge of etiology. The Centers for Disease Control endorsed this view in connection, for example, with the series of syndrome definitions of AIDS that it has formulated over the years. The CDC called its evolving definitions of AIDS *surveillance definitions*, to emphasize that the intent behind its syndromal definitions has been provisional, to provide a basis for planning and prevention. Tentative surveillance definitions are what we might call "stopgap definitions": they express a medical commitment to shift from a syndromal definition to an empirically based etiological definition as soon as this can be accomplished.

The same degree of conceptual modesty and honesty has been expressed by the American Rheumatism Association when it enacted a new syndrome-based definition of rheumatoid arthritis: The ARA specified seven criteria, stipulating that at least four of these must be satisfied in order for a diagnosis of rheumatoid arthritis to be made. Here is what the ARA nosologists noted about their definition: "Disease criteria which are descriptive reflect our current understanding of these disorders. Elucidation of specific pathogenetic mechanisms may at some point permit classification to be based directly on disease biology. However, these new criteria for RA will necessarily serve to improve understanding, classification, and comparability to patients with rheumatoid arthritis *until other methods of achieving this purpose are available*" (Arnett, Edworthy, Bloch, et al., 1988, p. 323, italics added).

The *ICD* follows a similarly modest and honest wait-and-see approach that is self-avowedly provisional in its comments relating to "mood disorders":

[I]t seems likely that psychiatrists will continue to disagree about the classification of disorders of mood until methods of dividing the clinical syndromes are developed that rely at least in part upon physiological or biochemical measurement, rather than being limited as at present to clinical descriptions of emotions and behaviour. As long as this limitation persists, one of the major choices lies between a comparatively simple classification with only a few degrees of severity, and one with greater details and more subdivisions. (World Health Organization, 1994, p. 13)

Medical definitions of physical disease are not considered complete until their etiology is known. A set of free-floating symptoms that in the future may or may not be found to be associated with a disease does not designate a disease today; at most it has the status of an unanswered question or a hypothesis. A symptom-based definition of alleged disease is simply preliminary, and when no "underlying pathology" is empirically known, such symptom-based definitions need to be taken with a grain of salt. We then need to be alert to the potential for such definitions to be misconstrued as though we know that they refer to "real disease entities," as though we know that these symptoms occur due to a "breakdown," "dysfunction," or "disorder" in the individual, despite having no empirical evidence whatsoever for this.

If psychiatry is to take seriously its status as part of medicine, the profession cannot afford to acquiesce in a psychology that promotes potentially capricious symptom clustering and its empirically unjustified transformation into assumed or asserted reified dysfunctions and correspondingly reified disease entities. *DSM*, instead of being regarded as an authoritative "diagnostic and statistical manual of mental disorders," must be recognized as a provisional listing of forms of behavior and psychological symptoms that may or may not eventually be found to be the result of basic, empirically observed pathology. Seen from this perspective, *DSM* may be thought of as setting before us a highly speculative and substantial research project for the future. For many clinicians it may serve to offer provisional surveillance definitions, but in no way, with the exception of the relatively few organic brain diseases it now includes, should *DSM* be construed as meaning what its title claims.

TO SUMMARIZE

Kraepelin's [nosology] ... arbitrarily set up disease entities in the absence of substantiating empirical data, and subordinated empirical analysis to the practical problems of prognosis.
—Menninger, Mayman, & Pruyser (1963/1967, p. 468)

The most damaging error in the psychology of definition is the confusion of words with things. With respect to psychiatric nosology, there has been abundant and widespread confusion of this sort due to the role played by seven psychological propensities that we've analyzed. To summarize, they are: (1) Nosologists selectively cluster observed symptoms in terms of stipulated patterns that are linked to forms of individual harm and disability, while neglecting to acknowledge the fact that such clustering without empirical reference to confirmable pathology is unscientific and arbitrary. (2) The recognition of such patterns often reflects a psychological dynamic involving various kinds of individual and group-endorsed motivations and interests—social, political, religious, moral, monetary, and so forth. The resulting clustering of allegedly harmful or disabling symptoms then provides a channel for three interrelated forms of delusional projective thinking: (3) Clusters of symptoms are given, so to speak, an "ontological promotion" to the clinically recognized status of syndrome constellations. With no anchor in empirical pathology, (4) these are then construed as necessarily involving internal disorders or dysfunctions that underlie them, and a presumption is made concerning their reified existence. (5) A nonfalsifiable claim is then made that a terminus for this snowballing process *exists* in the form of a reified "disease entity."

The psychological propensity to look for confirmation of the "truth" or "validity" of a nosology's stipulative definitions of disorders is then free to be exercised through (6) the circular, no-lose mechanism of tautological verification. Finally, (7) the diagnostic categories that have been stipulatively established by nosologists are internalized by them and by clinicians who accept and advocate the nosology, resulting in the phenomenon of diagnostic filtering, a predisposition that is then transmitted, spread, and perpetuated by supporting social, pharmaceutical, insurance, political, legal, and other interest groups.

This psychology of definition underpins psychiatric nosology and yet has been virtually ignored for centuries. Stipulative definitions have systematically been misconstrued to be real definitions that are "true" thanks to a psychology of reifying projection and tautological verification that has dominated psychiatric nosology and has remained safely out of sight, implicit, and unquestioned.

Toward the beginning of this chapter, I proposed to show that three hypotheses are true: (1) that we mistakenly consider the process of psychiatric definition in nosology to be simple, straightforward, and well-understood; (2) that such definition brings into play psychological propensities of which most of us are not conscious; and (3) that these psychological propensities, if clearly and self-consciously understood, would help us to control them, gain a significant measure of conceptual clarity and theoretical integration, and in the process lessen much of the conceptual confusion that encumbers current psychiatry and clinical psychology. I have done what I can within the confines of a single chapter to show that the first two hypotheses are true. In connection with the third, I'd like to offer several observations.

We have taken note of a number of serious deficiencies that accompany a symptom-based psychiatric nosology such as the *DSM* or the *ICD*. It may be useful in retrospect to assemble them together: First, as we've seen, purely symptom-based stipulative definitions of psychiatric disorders fail to have a basis in evidence of pathology. Second, due to the related heavy reliance upon a changeable psychology of pattern recognition in clustering symptoms, there is an intrinsic arbitrariness that besets nosology; this makes it easy for stipulative syndrome and disease definitions to shift with prevailing interests, whether these are social, political, medical, monetary, or other interests. Third, symptom-based definitions of mental disorders represent a rudimentary, immature, or at the very least provisional stage of medical knowledge, given that they fail to express knowledge of the origins of disease, the main point of diagnosis. Fourth, symptom-based definitions draw attention to the fact that we are uncertain whether there exists or does not exist an explanatory, originating pathology in the form of an empirically detectable dysfunction or state of disorder. Fifth, such definitions routinely provide a medium in which the psychologically normal human propensity to engage in misplaced concreteness or reification can be enthusiastically exercised without critical oversight. Sixth, symptom-based definitions of mental disorders lead to the interrelated *problems of diagnostic haze* mentioned earlier in this chapter, which result from the lack of distinctness of syndromes and their diagnostic designations and the conceptually untidy tendency of these to overlap. And last, not previously discussed, is the fact that symptom-based definitions of disease fail to be useful in detecting so-called "lanthanic" disease, that is, disease that is present but has not developed sufficiently to be expressed in the form of symptoms (Feinstein, 1967, p. 145; Bartlett, 2005, pp. 40, 68, 179, 284). Lanthanic disease is of course of major diagnostic importance, as we can see from the emphasis placed upon early detection through mammograms, colonoscopies, pap smears, prostate-specific antigen (PSA) and routine blood tests, and other laboratory and imaging procedures.

Given these many drawbacks of symptom-based diagnosis and disease definition, and accepting the fact that at present the majority of alleged psychiatric disorders have no known etiology, it is natural to ask whether a psychiatric nosology as we know it is truly essential to effective clinical practice today.

IS NOSOLOGY ESSENTIAL TO EFFECTIVE
CLINICAL PRACTICE?

There are no diseases, only sick people.

—Old medical aphorism

Earlier we noted how the conceptual commitments embedded in a nosology can lead to *diagnostic filtering*, that is, to perceive, habitually and reflexively, the patterns defined by one's nosology in the symptomatology of one's patients and to be limited by the nosology's diagnostic vocabulary so that, in a Sapir-Whorf-like way, the category set of the nosology determines, or at the very least constrains, one's perception of clinical reality. There is, furthermore, a secondary result of nosology that also is unfortunate, and it applies equally well to physical as to psychiatric medicine. That is the tendency for clinicians to treat diseases instead of individual people, a complaint commonly expressed by the antipsychiatrists. When the focus of treatment is the "disease entity" rather than the afflicted patient, we once again face the human proclivity to reify, for human maladies are never encountered in some metaphysical state of existence independent of individual persons who are sick or injured. If anything, human diseases are abstractions from sick people, and not the other way around. The psychology of definition in psychiatric nosology has the following unintended and unwanted consequence—again, a result of misplaced concreteness: The diagnostic code becomes the object of clinical, social, and reimbursement attention, while the individual person recedes into the background. For many clinicians, the diagnostic label has become more important than the person.

Although the *DSM* has only been around for one lifetime, its spread of influence has been enormous. The *DSM* didn't exist when Tolstoy was alive, but he understood the nature of such power and sway:

> Morally the wielder of power appears to cause the event; physically it is those who submit to the power. But as the moral activity is inconceivable without the physical, the cause of the event is neither in the one nor in the other but in the union of the two.
>
> Or in other words, the conception of a cause is inapplicable to the phenomena we are examining. (Tolstoy, 1869/1952, p. 687)

It is not that the *DSM* in and of itself is the powerful cause of its spreading influence, but that we have participated willingly in allowing its conceptual commitments to influence us deeply and pervasively. As participants in submitting to its persuasive authority we have approved the nosology ratified by its committees, not on the basis of empirical evidence but on *faith*—faith that its stipulative definitions of symptom clusters refer to genuine illnesses named by the nosology; faith that these are the result of unknown but pathologically confirmable mental disorders; and faith that the stipulative definitions of mental disorders in turn designate real disease entities, that is, distinct diseases that are caused by real internal dysfunctions to be found in individual patients. At this time, unless we are referring to organic brain disease, belief in the reality of "mental disorders" defined in this way is clearly a matter of blind and baseless faith, not science.

We need to be persuaded by this conclusion, increasingly hard though it is at a time when the reified nosology of the *DSM* continues to develop rapidly by accretion and the habit of diagnostic compliance establishes more and more reality consistency for us. For readers who are persuaded by this conclusion, what then? Is there effective clinical practice beyond the *DSM*?

To answer this we need to be reminded of the larger clinical world that lies beyond that of the framers and advocates of the *DSM*. To mention but a few of the clinical approaches that eschew nosology, there are behavior therapists who focus on individualized symptom amelioration and who for this reason often do not find classificatory diagnosis useful; clinicians who are psychoanalytically oriented and who wish to put diagnostic labeling behind them; person-oriented therapists, followers of Rogers, Adler, Maslow, Kelly, and others; phenomenologically or existentially oriented clinicians, such as psychiatrist J. H. van den Berg and psychologist Rollo May; to be sure, the antipsychiatrists, including Laing and Szasz; and of course there are others.[8] All of these groups of clinicians have advocated both a "return to the individual" and a recognition that the majority of the problems and suffering that people bring to psychiatrists, clinical psychologists, and other mental health professionals are not, at least insofar as we possess empirical knowledge today, appropriately treated in terms of the paradigm of physical medicine.

Earlier in this chapter, I made a few brief observations concerning psychological resistance to the default label 'idiopathic' when psychiatric syndromes with no known etiology are in view. My purpose in introducing this generic label should be clearer now in retrospect: The term 'idiopathy' heralds from the Greek *idiopatheia*, which breaks down into *idios*, meaning "proper" or "peculiar," and *pathein*, meaning "to suffer." An "idiopathic syndrome" from this etymological point of view would then be something like "a set of symptoms expressing the suffering of an individual." If we want to strain at the halter of medical terminology and insist on using the nomenclature of disorders, an "idiopathic psychiatric disorder" would amount to "the individual symptomatology expressed by a person who is in psychological distress."

Horwitz and Wakefield (2007, p. 115) observed that the *DSM* "gives no criteria for distinguishing symptoms of mental disorders from those that are nondisordered problems in living." The psychology of definition in psychiatric nosology supports this conclusion but regards it as tentative, recognizing that such criteria may yet evolve in the light of future empirical findings, perhaps in neuroscience.[9]

In the meantime, effective clinical treatment for symptoms that express psychological distress has been the focus of the variety of approaches mentioned above, none of which considers psychologically based symptomatology to be more than just that—expressions by an individual who is in need of symptom alleviation, much as a patient in physical pain may need the assistance of a specialist in pain management. For syndromes that have no known etiology, alleviation of symptoms is often the best that can be hoped for. If such syndromes are considered to be truly idiopathic in the individualized sense of the word, then an intellectually honest and scientific conception of psychological distress will avoid diagnostic categorization for all but organically based disorders and diseases for which there is compelling etiological knowledge.

For other forms of psychological distress, harm, and disability, some readers may be willing to lend a new and perhaps somewhat differently attuned ear to a wait-and-see perspective, perhaps similar to the following overall assessment:

Contemporary psychiatric nosology is basically flawed. It has sought to identify and classify increasingly many overlapping and often indistinct varieties of harmful or disabling behavior and psychological response that people have to life. In the process of establishing a nosology, the psychology of which this chapter has described in some detail, psychiatry has imposed a medical frame of reference, usually without empirical justification, upon difficulties that people experience in living. But unless empirically confirmable disorders and diseases are in view, the difficulties that people encounter in living are highly individual in nature and dependent upon context; individual sensitivities; life goals; personal values; age; physical, marital, social, and financial health; and the many other factors that affect, complicate, and individualize life. Unless such difficulties are traceable to organically based pathologies, however much they may cause discouragement and suffering, harm, or disability they are inappropriately treated if they are judged to be medical in nature—not because of a "myth of mental illness" or an inappropriately forced "metaphor" but because *the psychology of definition in psychiatric nosology has for a long time been recognizably dysfunctional, engaging in stipulative definition that has been systematically misconstrued to be real definition and fostering a projective mentality of reification that has no place in modern science.* Such dysfunctional thinking is

characteristic of the common, pervasive, and indeed psychologically normal human propensity to engage in what I earlier termed projective misconstructions. They occur whenever we believe that we can
meaningfully claim to trespass beyond the boundaries of what we can
meaningfully think and assert. What then results are metaphysical fictions, the products of delusional thinking, not science.

To be sure, there are numerous kinds of harmful or disabling psychological and behavioral difficulties that people experience in the course of
their lives. Those that are known to be medical in nature should be appropriately treated. The others, when we lack sufficient knowledge that
shows them to be medically based, should be dealt with outside the medical model as compassionately and honestly as we can. What we have
learned from the psychology of definition in psychiatric nosology is that,
in the absence of knowledge of etiology, a *palliative* approach to alleviate
harm and disability is desirable, while a diagnostic approach, which places
on people mental disorder labels for which there is no empirical basis,
continues to fall victim to a dysfunctional psychology that has dominated
psychiatric nosology for many centuries.

Writing about the APA's first 128-page 1952 edition of the *DSM*, which
we recall listed a mere 106 disorders, Menninger and his co-authors had
this to say: "The carefully prepared booklet has the merit of containing
working definitions of terms and descriptions of syndromes. It is, we are
assured, shortly to be revised—let us hope in the direction of simplifica-
tion" (Menninger et al., 1963/1967, p. 478).

As the *DSM* continues to expand in keeping with the EMSS (the Endless
Multiplication of Syndromes Syndrome), we would do well to remember
Menninger's wise counsel, to simplify in the interest of scientific unifica-
tion. An awareness of the psychology of definition in psychiatric nosology
warns us of the need to embrace Newton's motto, "hypotheses non fingo"
("I do not make hypotheses"), as well as Occam's Razor (to refrain from
multiplying entities beyond necessity)—in short, to accept responsibility
for science that is undertaken intelligently and with intellectual modesty,
admitting into the category of "real disorders" only those that have met
the dispassionate criteria of empirical evidence.

NOTES

1. The recently published book on the nosology of depression by Horwitz and
Wakefield (2007) reflects the present situation: The authors stress the importance

of awareness of the conceptual confusion in current psychiatric nosology and the need to reduce that confusion. They point to "conceptual challenges" that face psychiatry (p. 194) and to the existence of "conceptual problems" that need to be solved (p. 168), express the need for "conceptual analysis" (p. 112), refer to "conceptual errors" (p. 26) that need to be avoided, remark on "the need for greater conceptual clarity" (p. 193), refer to "logical problems" (p. 212) and "semantic confusion" (p. 225) that are involved in diagnostic definition, and so forth. The authors repeatedly direct attention to *conceptual* issues in psychiatric nosology that require attention but instead are disregarded.

2. To avoid repetitive language, I will not always make explicit the conventional distinction between "symptoms" and "signs," the former reported by the patient/client, the latter observed by the psychiatrist/clinical psychologist. When I refer to "symptoms" both are to be understood.

3. For a more comprehensive and detailed inventory and discussion of general types of definition, but without application to psychiatric nosology, see Robinson (1950/1962).

4. As soon as we begin to use the medical concepts and terminology of 'symptoms' and 'syndromes', we admittedly are already biased in terms of our choice of frame of reference. To call a behavior, affect, or cognitive phenomenon a "symptom" is already to presume that it *indicates* something other than itself, that it points toward some pathogenic source. As we shall see, this presumption already expresses certain of the psychological predispositions that typically come into play in psychiatric definition.

5. This medical understanding of physical disease is now well established. In the 1950s René Dubos (1959, p. 183) formulated a "doctrine of specific etiology" that many disease theorists have built on since, according to which disease is understood in terms of four components: a cause (typically a pathogen), a consequent lesion, uniform and unvarying symptoms, and a confirmed expectation that injury to health or death will result.

A comment concerning the first of these components is order. Etiology, the study of the causes of disease, is understandably complex; we need to be wary of a naïve or oversimplified conception of causality, a subject we cannot consider in detail here. In connection with disease, there is usually no "decisive cause" in the genesis of a pathology, which is instead almost always multifactorial, involving the total state of the organism, its susceptibility to illness or injury, its genetic or constitutional predisposition to disease, and other factors. This subject would take us far from our present concerns.

6. Outside of the U.S., the *International Classification of Diseases and Related Health Problems* is widely used. The *ICD-10*, like the *DSM*, defines mental disorders in terms of symptoms: "The term 'disorder' is used throughout the classification, so as to avoid even greater problems inherent in the use of terms such as 'disease' and 'illness'. 'Disorder' is not an exact term, but it is used here to imply the existence of a clinically recognizable set of symptoms or behaviour associated in most cases with distress and with interference with personal functions. Social deviance or conflict alone, *without personal dysfunction*, should not be included in mental disorder as defined here" (World Health Organization, 1994, p. 5, italics added). Note the italicized phrase, which serves the same purpose as the more

obvious assertion of inner dysfunction made by the *DSM* in the quote that follows above in the text.

7. Readers familiar with set theory and number theory will immediately recognize that infinitely many disjoint sets of symptoms can be constructed from the universal set of all symptoms. Hence there is, on a set-theoretical basis alone, no criterion that can "promote" any one symptom set, or any finite number of such sets, to a privileged position of syndromes that are "real" or "most valid." From a strictly formal point of view, this is enough to undermine the claim that "syndromal diseases" are in any sense more than conceptual constructs.

8. In the history of physical medicine, there have been many researchers who have similarly resisted thinking of diseases as objects, who have advocated a focus on the individual patient, among them physicist-physiologist Hermann Helmholtz, Friedrich Gustav Jacob Henle, Emil DuBois-Reymond, Ottomar Rosenbach, Theodor Schwann, Rudolf Virchow, Carl Wunderlich, and others.

9. Already one can see an emerging tendency among neuroscientists to make the central presumption that is questioned in this book: In comparing the brain functioning of "psychological normal" individuals with those who exhibit a specific psychological symptom constellation, differences in brain function are sometimes observed. When such differences are noted, it becomes immediately tempting, again, to *assume* that "dysfunctions" have been identified in the nonnormal patients.

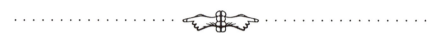

3

The Abnormal Psychology of Creativity and the Pathology of Normality

Psychiatry and clinical psychology face a little-recognized dilemma in understanding and treating creative individuals. On the one hand, it is well established that extremes of mood among the creative are often valued by them, and hence they may resist treatment for what are conventionally diagnosed as affective disorders, and discontinue prescribed medication. On the other hand, it is not well understood that many of the putative disorders ascribed to creative individuals are the result of their justifiable response to widespread but seldom-recognized pathologies found in the normal population. Understanding the interplay between these two horns of the dilemma can help mental health professionals appreciate the need to be especially circumspect and reflective in their diagnostic classification and treatment of mood extremes among creative people.

A significant but as yet not entirely self-conscious change is occurring within psychiatry. While contributors to the rapidly proliferating diagnostic categories of mental illness continue to identify and vote in new disorders for inclusion in perennially updated editions of the *DSM*, other researchers are beginning to question and even erode psychiatry's largely unquestioned belief in the desirability of providing customary treatment for certain routinely classified mental disorders.

This countermovement within psychiatry has branched in different directions; all but one of these have occurred quietly and been given scant attention in the literature. Explicitly critical opposition to the diagnostic pronouncements of the *DSM* has come from several divergent lines of study. The main ones are these: Most widely known has been the skepticism and downright rejection of "mental illness" as a legitimate medical category of disease by Thomas Szasz (e.g., 1957/1961), Thomas Scheff (1966/1984), and others. Less well-known has been a second line of psychiatric thought pioneered by J. H. van den Berg (1955, 1972, 1980), whose "phenomenological psychiatry" avoids standard psychiatric classification and diagnostic pigeonholing and instead seeks to help individuals through nonjudgmental support of the patient by the psychiatrist, support situated from a phenomenological standpoint that recognizes the reality and legitimacy of the patient's own experience. A third line of study by the present author (Bartlett, 2005) is characterized by a reversal of diagnostic classification, turning away from traditional psychiatric diagnostic criteria that derive their meaning in terms of deviations from psychological normality to a distinct variety of socially focused study. Such an approach recognizes that a wide range of psychological pathologies afflict psychologically normal populations that include the majority of people and establishes a locus of psychiatric health in those individuals who are exceptional in their predominant psychology, who do not have the pathologies that afflict the psychologically normal, and who may be at variance with standards of psychological normality.

In this chapter, I bring together the empathic and clinically noncategorizing approach of phenomenological psychiatry with my own studies that have directed attention to the pathology of majority, psychologically normal populations. This integration of these two very distinct approaches offers a new perspective for understanding the psychology of creative individuals. While their difficulties in living have sometimes benefited from careful and penetrating study, they have still failed to be adequately understood by psychiatry, as well as by clinical psychology to the extent that the latter has accepted, wholesale, the diagnostic categories formulated and promulgated by psychiatry.

THE ABNORMAL PSYCHOLOGY OF CREATIVITY

Psychiatry has studied the temperament of creative individuals comparatively little. One of the most detailed studies was published by Kay Redfield Jamison (1993; cf. also Goodwin & Jamison, 1990, Chap. 14; Andreasen, 2005), in which she observed that

> the idea of using formal psychiatric diagnostic criteria in the arts has been anathema, and, in any event, biological psychiatrists have displayed relatively little interest in studying mood disorders in artists, writers, or musicians. Certainly those in the arts have been less than enthusiastic about being seen through a biological or diagnostic grid. Those in the best position to link the two worlds—scholars of creativity—only recently have begun to address the problem. (Jamison, 1993, p. 3)

Adding to the reluctance of psychiatrists to study the psychology of creativity has been the intrinsically fuzzy, amorphous, elusive nature of creativity itself, making it difficult for researchers to know and to pin down exactly what they are referring to. It is a challenge to examine a phenomenon that, by its very character, exists in an area where attempts to define creativity can be limiting, inadequate, or simply mistaken. I therefore make no attempt to define creativity and through a definition delimit it, but will a little later instead refer to some of its psychological roots in observable characteristics of creative individuals.

An understanding of the psychology of the creative has been dominated by the unquestioned application of medical-diagnostic categories that derive their meaning and value relative to a baseline of psychological normality (see Chapter 1). That is, psychopathology has been understood in terms that have equated harmful deviations from psychological normality with pathology. The "harm" involved is either harm to the patient or harm as perceived by his or her surrounding society, or both.[1]

Unfortunately, the situation with respect to creative individuals is not clear cut. The lack of "enthusiasm" on the part of creative individuals toward diagnostic labeling mentioned by Jamison is, as we'll note later, sometimes well warranted by their own experience. There also can be a justifiable resistance by the creative to clinical treatment—despite the overwhelmingly high incidence rate, greatly disproportionate to the baseline normal population, of what clinicians recognize as depression, cyclothymia, manic depression, psychosis, and suicide among many artists, writers, poets, sculptors, composers, mathematicians, and other creative thinkers.

Many creative individuals resist diagnostic labeling and treatment for what seem to them to be compellingly good reasons: First, creative people who are historically aware may justifiably resist mental illness labeling: They may remember that many thousands of people were executed during the Holocaust precisely because the label of mental illness was placed on them, and in the United States many thousands more were involuntarily sterilized due to the same judgment.

Second, from the standpoint of creative individuals, the heights and depths of mood can be valued in and of themselves. What psychiatrists routinely consider to be affective disorders can, for such creative people, be the lifeblood of creativity. We'll consider this perspective below, under the heading of "The Inner Turmoil Thesis."

Third, it is not clear that deep depression, the extreme variations of mood in cyclothymia and manic depression, and even suicide, constitute, for many creative people, unwarranted or undesirable moods or choice. The potentially valuable nature of a life experience that possesses rich emotional intensity and range, as experienced by creative individuals, has, as we will see, led some clinicians to propose a category of "advantageous psychiatric disorders."

Fourth, it has been unappreciated by researchers who are concerned with clinical aspects of creativity that extreme moods experienced by the creative are frequently *situationally induced*, that is, are understandable involuntary responses of creative individuals to their environment. The creative face numerous challenges and suffer considerable ordeals that are unknown to the psychologically normal and that to a meaningful degree are likely to be unintelligible to them. We consider this topic later, where I refer to it as "the situational thesis."

Last, there is an identifiable "constitutional predisposition" shared by many creative artists, writers, poets, composers, and other creative people, that plays a central role in their emotional responses to other people, to the world in which they must work, and to society generally, and this, too, must be taken into account since it forms the basis for their reactions to their life situations.

As we consider each of the above subjects in what follows, to avoid the monotony of a one-phrase-vocabulary, I'll often use the term 'artist' to mean any individual with pronounced creative abilities and temperament, unless the context limits the intended reference.

THE INNER TURMOIL THESIS

Norwegian painter Edvard Munch, who was hospitalized several times for psychiatric illness, remarked: "A German once said to me: 'But if you could rid yourself of many of your troubles.' To which I replied: 'They are part of me and my art. They are indistinguishable from me, and it would destroy my art. I want to keep those sufferings' " (quoted in Stang, 1979, p. 107). Writing about Munch's claim, Jamison (1993, p. 241) noted:

> This is a common concern. Many artists and writers believe that turmoil, suffering, and extremes in emotional experience are integral not only to the human condition but to their abilities as artists. They fear that psychiatric treatment will transform them into normal, well-adjusted, dampened, and bloodless souls—unable, or unmotivated, to write, paint, or compose.

There is no doubt that negative moods and the power of mania can sometimes make positive contributions to creative thought. But such moods do not of course of themselves produce it, or every sufferer from abnormal mood intensity and swings would show signs of creativity. Yet it is typical of anyone who engages in creative work to feel excited, elated, perhaps euphoric or ecstatic, to feel increased self-confidence, the mental efficiency of speed combined with focused concentration, zest, perhaps expansiveness and heightened mental clarity. And, in a parallel fashion, unhappiness, profound sadness, and grief can no less be the inner partners to creative effort, as novelist Herman Melville, who suffered from severe variations of mood, commented: "The intensest light of reason and revelation combined, can not shed such blazonings upon the deeper truths in man, as will sometimes proceed from his own profoundest gloom. Utter darkness is then his light, and cat-like he distinctly sees all objects through a medium which is mere blindness to common vision" (Melville 1852/1995, p. 242).

Melville lived before empirical studies showed that a moderate degree of depression can serve as an aid in reality checking, for perceptions and beliefs while in a depressed state can be more realistic than while in a more normal mood (cf., e.g., Dobson & Franche, 1989; Sackheim, 1983; Taylor & Brown, 1988). In other words, we now know empirically that Melville's poetically expressed observation at times can hold true.

The often beneficial yet potentially destructive peaks and troughs of mood have been called by some psychiatrists "advantageous psychiatric disease" (e.g., Jamison, 1993, p. 235). Yet, from the standpoint of the general theory of disease (cf. Bartlett, 2005, Part I), such a phrase is a contradiction in terms: if a condition qualifies as a "disease," it must be responsible for bringing about harm, rather than advantage or benefit. To call the intense and sometimes destructive moods of artists "advantageous" without substantial qualification is misleading. A more accurate picture requires that we accept the two prongs of a true diagnostic dilemma, for they are incompatibilities that cannot be fused:

> There is a great deal of evidence to suggest that, compared to "normal" individuals, artists, writers, and creative people in general, are both psychologically "sicker"—that is, they score higher on a wide variety of measures of psychopathology—and psychologically healthier (for example, they show quite elevated scores on measures of self-confidence and ego strength). (Jamison, 1993, p. 97 see also note on pp. 300–301, where more than a dozen works supporting this result are cited.)

Despite many avowals by artists of the high worth of melancholy and elation, we need to be reminded that we should take their claims with caution, knowing full well how many creative souls end their lives in misery, impoverished both financially and mentally, often in suicide. For example, Ludwig (1992) found that some 18 percent of poets have committed suicide, while artists have two to three times the rate of mood disorders, psychosis, and suicide as the normal population, and the rate of involuntary hospitalizations of artists, writers, and composers is six to seven times that of normal controls. Similar incidence rates have been borne out by various other studies (e.g., Juda, 1949; Andreasen, 1987 and 2005; Jamison, 1989). It follows that any serious scientific attempt to understand the psychology of creativity must avoid the temptation to romanticize the extremes of creative moods, for they evidently can be associated with very serious and destructive consequences. There is unquestionably a point, for many artists, when the pit of depression or the high pitch of mania can come to interfere with and wreck the very creative spirit that the artist believes these make possible. A point can be reached when many artists recognize, on behalf of themselves and their art, that they must seek clinical treatment. It is important to emphasize this fact and not lose sight of it in the discussion that follows.

WHO IS HARMED? THE ASCRIPTION OF PATHOLOGY

A danger exists from the opposite direction, that of insisting, unilaterally, that society is harmed by those who are identified as "affectively disordered." Who precisely was harmed when Sylvia Plath took her life—as did poets Thomas Lovell Beddoes, John Berryman, Barcroft Boake, Paul Celan, Thomas Chatterton, Hart Crane, John Davidson, Tove Ditlevsen, Sergey Esenin, John Gould Fletcher, Adam Lindsay Gordon, Randall Jarrell, Heinrich von Kleist, Vachel Lindsay, Vladimir Mayakovsky, Cesare Pavese, Anne Sexton, Sara Teasdale, Georg Trakl, and Marina Ivanovna Tsvetayeva, and writers Romain Gary, Ernest Hemingway, William Inge, Malcolm Lowry, Yukio Mishima, Gérard de Nerval, John Kennedy Toole, and Virginia Woolf, and composers Jeremiah Clarke, Peter Warlock, and Bernd Alois Zimmerman, and painters and sculptors Ralph Barton, Francesco Bassano, Franceso Borromini, Edward Dayes, Vincent van Gogh, Arshile Gorky, Benjamin Haydon, Ernst Ludwig Kirchner, Wilhelm Lehmbruck, Jules Pascin, Mark Rothko, Nicolas de Staël, Pietro Testa, and Henry Tilson (from Jamison, 1993, pp. 249, 267–70)? Surely—one can't help but ask—surely not only society, and often, of course, their families, but foremost is it not the creative person who is "harmed" by suicide—and if not by that, then hasn't 'harm' lost its meaning?

Yet it is exactly when the patient denies that his or her condition is experienced as harmful (even should creative life end in suicide), while at the same time society resolutely imposes its standards of "mental correctness," that we come to have Holocaust exterminations of "mental patients" and involuntary sterilization programs in the United States. In *The Pathology of Man* (Bartlett, 2005, Part I), I discuss the main competing theories of disease and advance a general, unified theory of disease. From that standpoint,

I've argued that any judgment to the effect that a condition constitutes a disease—that it qualifies as a genuine pathology—is intrinsically framework-relative. This is not to say that such judgment is subject to relativism, for a disorder that an individual experiences as harmful does this as a matter of self-confirming experienced fact. However, "harm" must be understood contextually: there is harm to the individual—as felt and judged by him or her to constitute harm—and harm as judged by the society in which he or she lives. They do not always coincide. In the case of the creative artist, they often do not. To put the matter rather bleakly: the depression, mania, cyclothymia, and even suicide of the artist will frequently be judged harmful by society but yet at times not by the artist. When the patient and the treating psychiatrist are in disagreement that harm is involved, we are left in a position where it would be ridiculous as well as therapeutically wrong to force the application of diagnostic standards of psychopathology without stopping in our tracks and pausing to reflect. For there are other issues that must be taken into account.

THE SITUATIONAL THESIS

> To bring forth immaterial things, things partaking of spirit, not flesh, we must be jealous of spending time or trouble upon physical demands, since in most men, the soul ages long before the body. Mankind has been no gainer by its drudges.
> —T. E. Lawrence, *The Seven Pillars of Wisdom*

By "the situational thesis" I mean the claim that the alleged "psychopathology" of creative people needs to be understood in the context of their struggle to exist in, cope with, and resist pressures to adapt to, the world of the psychologically normal.

From a phenomenological point of view, an individual's "situation" must be understood in relation to his or her values, sensitivities, and aesthetic and creative skills, as these are expressed in the individual's experience. It is important that we keep clearly in mind that these realities together form a dynamically interrelated group in terms of which the artist's experienced situation in life is defined. We are not able within the span of a chapter to enter into this subject in great detail, but we nonetheless need a framework to understand what is at issue here.

It is a familiar truism that creative people are "more sensitive" than the psychologically normal, but this fails to capture the fact that the experienced world of the creative person can be qualitatively different from normal experience in a variety of ways. First, frequently the artist feels a sense of passionate commitment to his or her art for no *extraneous* reason: for some artists, it is not money or fame that fires the drive to create (though he or she may also want these); the need to create is simply there, for no other reason than itself; it is an intrinsically meaningful and important goal in and of itself. Second, the artist's "sensitivity" may encompass a host of characteristics and skills. The creative person may, for example, be greatly more sensitive to any undesirable disturbance from the physical and human environment: Proust's pronounced sensitivity to noise comes to mind. Yet such "sensitivities" may also be tied to skills: Turner's ability to feel intensely the beauty of a sunset, or Shakespeare's to feel the tragedy of life. These are aesthetic skills, both in terms of the acute responsiveness of an artist to his or her subject and in terms of the ability to communicate that heightened aesthetic response. And last, there is the creative individual's ability to go beyond the bounds of established thought and practice in his or her field of endeavor and to offer new and original insights and approaches.

By *creative sensibility* what I have in mind is the following group of inter-related values, heightened sensitivities and vulnerabilities, and skills in the context of lived experience: (1) passionate commitment to creation as an intrinsically meaningful process and end in itself; (2) sensitivities to the artist's environment that can jeopardize or foster creative work; (3) skills of aesthetic awareness and communication; and (4) the capacity to break free from the confining ruts of the customary and established patterns of thought and practice of the time. These are all sources of meaning in which the creative individual's experience often differs qualitatively from that of the normal population.

There are some truths which, as psychologist George Romanes would nod in assent, do not require supporting statistical studies.[2] One of these is the undeniable truth of the plight of creative individuals in most countries in the world—the still insufficiently appreciated, grueling lives of many poets, independent writers of literary fiction and scholarly nonfiction, painters, sculptors, composers, independent basic scientists and mathematicians, and others. Few parents of modest means are unable to anticipate the challenge their children would face if they decided upon the creative life. Unless they are the rare, lucky exceptions, it will be a serious challenge for the creative to make ends meet and to live, often never fitting in, within an industrialized society whose values displace virtually all else but exclusively materialist interests.

The average person has no idea of the investment purchased by personal sacrifice, toil, long hours of intense concentration, and love poured into an artist's creations. Yet, sustained by an inner need to create, the artist does what he or she must, and yet must somehow try to cope with what is often perceived to be a brutish encompassing society that does not understand artistic sensibility and the care required to bring beauty into the world—and does not wish to. The artist can suffer from a variety of situational depression that has yet to be named and classified by the *DSM*. The painter must deal with tight-fisted opportunist art dealers, galleries that claim half or more of the proceeds from an artist's sales, and consumers of art whose main criterion is whether a painting will match the color of the sofa; the writer must cope with the closed-mindedness and short-sightedness of publishers whose main concerns are word count, page count, printing cost, list price, and market appeal—frequently at the expense of literary or scholarly merit; the composer, sculptor, architect, and poet alike must peddle their wares, often to the deaf ears of publishers, patrons, contracting businesses, and a small and fickle "literary-cultural" market. The potential, and the real, disappointments are legion, the frustrations immense, and the toll on life energies frequently depleting and demoralizing.

Consider the following credo for the living of one's life advocated by novelist Hermann Hesse, who himself experienced wide swings of mood, was hospitalized, and attempted suicide:

> I consider reality to be the thing one need concern oneself about least of all, for it is, tediously enough, always at hand while more beautiful and necessary things demand our attention and care. Reality is that which one must not under any circumstances worship and revere, for it is chance, the refuse of life. And it is in no wise to be changed, this shabby, consistently disappointing reality, except by our denying it and proving in the process that we are stronger than it. (Hesse, 1925/1954, p. 67)

The creative person who has taken the meaning of this passage to heart and bases his or her life on such an outlook is almost guaranteed very substantial hardships. The hardships are likely to be of two different kinds: those experienced in order to "earn a living" and those encountered if and when one is immersed in living a creative existence. Often, in the lives of creative individuals, the first set of hurdles has to be cleared before the artist—rarely—acquires the financial independence to tackle the second. Virginia Woolf described the first set of hurdles in writing about her past life:

> [W]hat still remains with me as a worse infliction ... was the poison of fear and bitterness which those days bred in me. To begin with, always to be doing work that one did not wish to do, and to do it like a slave, flattering and fawning, not always necessarily perhaps, but it seemed necessary and the stakes were too great to run risks; and then the thought of that one

gift which it was death to hide—a small one but dear to the possessor—
perishing and with it myself, my soul—all this became like a rust eating
away the bloom of the spring, destroying the tree at its heart. (Woolf, 1929,
p. 64)

The second group of hurdles will concern us in the next section.

"Situational depression" is a phrase not yet in common use. As most
readers will be aware, clinical psychology and psychiatry often construe
depression in different ways. Biologically focused psychiatrists believe
depression results from biochemical imbalance and should therefore be
treated primarily with medication. Some clinical psychologists urge that
psychotherapy should comprise the main approach; other psychologists
claim that depression is not a "disorder" at all, but an expression of "problems of living" (e.g., Adler and his following). Still another group claims
that depression is a justifiable emotion, warranted by a situation that
causes a person pain (e.g., Greenspan, 1988; De Sousa, 1987).

This last approach to depression has yet to be fully developed. To
date, relevant studies fall mainly under the heading of the psychology of
career burnout, where conditions in a person's work environment—when
considered in relation to that individual's temperament, values, and
outlook—can be linked causally with ensuing depression. We require a
different framework in which to understand the challenges which creative individuals experience in their efforts to deal with the surrounding
world.[3]

THE PSYCHOPATHOLOGY OF NORMALITY

[T]o write a work of genius is almost always a feat of prodigious difficulty. Everything is against the likelihood that it will come from the
writer's mind whole and entire. Generally material circumstances are
against it. Dogs will bark; people will interrupt; money must be made;
health will break down. Further, accentuating all these difficulties and
making them harder to bear is the world's notorious indifference. It does
not ask people to write poems and novels and histories; it does not need
them. It does not care whether Flaubert finds the right word or whether
Carlyle scrupulously verifies this or that fact. Naturally, it will not pay
for what it does not want. And so the writer, Keats, Flaubert, Carlyle,
suffers, especially in the creative years of youth, every form of distraction
and discouragement. A curse, a cry of agony, rises from those books of
analysis and confession. "Mighty poets in their misery dead"—that is
the burden of their song. If anything comes through in spite of all this,
it is a miracle, and probably no book is born entire and uncrippled as it
was conceived. (Woolf, 1929, pp. 89–90)

Most closely allied to the situational awareness of the artist's experience that is advocated here is an approach to situational depression considerably different from psychological studies of career burnout. Such a situational understanding of the artist widens the acknowledged causal basis of depression beyond an individual's immediate work environment to encompass the society at large. For some people, whose sense of personal identity, life commitments, cultural values, and creative sensibilities place them at odds with their predominantly anti-intellectual and noncultural society, a more specialized variety of depression can result, and it may well have been the mood that Virginia Woolf, who committed suicide, felt when writing the above passage.

We'll explore certain of the ramifications of such depression in Chapters 4–6 in Part II of this book. In these chapters I reconsider the ancient Scholastic idea of *acedia* and place it in a twenty-first-century context as the name for a diagnostic category that includes a group of mental impairments that together result, for many people, in a mental incapacity for culture in its original meaning of *cultus*. Our later discussion of acedia is directly relevant to the focus here on the psychology of creative individuals, so a few words about it are in order.

As we shall see, the Scholastic meaning of 'culture', now largely lost, subordinates mundane and mediocre concerns to a source (not necessarily religious) of higher value. The Scholastics regarded some values as "higher" because they bestow upon everyday life a significance that transcends the workaday world. In the same sense, higher education was called higher because its aim was to encourage cultivation, specifically the cultivation of nonuseful things, having nothing to do with utilitarian pursuits, nothing to do with skills needed to get a well-paying job.

To cultivate such concerns requires leisure—not leisure in the sense of idleness or taking a vacation, but leisure in the sense of an individual's capacity to become aware of a source of meaning that goes beyond the mundane world of everyday preoccupation. Leisure in this meaning was an attitude of mind, of silent affirmation, of active contemplation. To have the capacity for leisure requires that a man or woman affirm his or her own sense of identity, apart from a role as father, mother, worker, or consumer.

To be incapable of this is acedia. In a few words, acedia is an inability to see reality in other than mundane and mediocre ways; it is an inability to perceive reality as it can be transformed through an awareness of "higher values." When this transformative capacity is lost, the minds of people are blunted and they begin to suffer from a disability of values. Acedia is just such a disability, as we shall see in greater detail later on. (For further discussion, cf. Bartlett, 1990, 1993a, 1993b, 1994a, 1994b.)

In the context of the psychology of artistic or creative sensibility, which is the appropriate focus for a psychiatric understanding of creativity, acedia is a widespread disability that afflicts the psychologically normal, with whom the artist must, often reluctantly and out of necessity, deal. In the next chapter, we'll see how the prevalence of acedia in today's college students can lead to a form of burnout among university faculty. The situational basis of the variety of demoralization that affects many artists is similarly to be found in the cultural wasteland that exists, to speak nonmetaphorically, between the ears of the majoritarian psychologically normal and in the society they make up. We often find in the autobiographical writings of creative individuals expressions of loneliness, isolation, and alienation from the normal world. To understand this feeling and the negative mood that results from it is to empathize in a basic way with the "life-worlds" of many "struggling artists," whose struggle is directly attributable to obstacles placed in their way by the psychologically normal, which Virginia Woolf commented on.

Psychological normality has had many unquestioned legitimators—for this is what psychiatrists do when they accept and apply, wholesale, the classification system of the *DSM*. There have been those, however, who have had the courage and the cognitive capacity to "reframe," to step outside the boundaries of familiar categories and to recognize the very real pathologies that are inherent in the psychologically normal constitution. In the history of behavioral science, and in particular in the history of psychology and psychiatry, little effort has been made to study pathologies that afflict not the aberrant neurotic or psychotic individual or social group but the greater population of the psychological normal. Yet, on the odd occasion, an author such as Trigant Burrow (1953/1968, p. 25) will occasionally remark: "a grave error is committed in aligning the usual or average behavior with healthy behavior."

To undertake a study of such "universal pathologies" requires that we focus on the *evil of banality*, a phrase now familiar to readers, and not the considerably more restricted "banality of evil" proposed by Hannah Arendt (1964). I have sought to advance our understanding of a wide range of pathologies that afflict the psychologically normal population in *The Pathology of Man: A Study of Human Evil* (2005). There, I've argued that these *pathologies of normality* have largely been ignored or denied, yet an awareness of the central role that they play in human behavior is essential to our understanding of the psychology of war, genocide, the Holocaust, terrorism, obedience to authority, human ecological pathology, moral stupidity, and cognitive delusion, each of which areas the book explores in detail. A number of the world's leading psychiatrists and psychologists have long urged the need for such a study—clinicians mentioned in Chapter 1, among them Freud, Jung, Menninger, Fromm, and Peck; also quantitative historians Quincy Wright, Pitirim Sorokin, Nicholas Rashevsky, and Lewis Fry Richardson; ethologists Konrad Lorenz and Irenäus Eibl-Eibesfeldt; and others.

The "situation" in which many creative individuals find themselves in the real world of uncreative, psychologically normal people needs to be understood more effectively by psychiatry and clinical psychology— understood, that is, in a more empathetic way that recognizes the importance of situating a therapist's viewpoint phenomenologically from within the perspective of creative individuals, to see the world from the individual's standpoint so he or she may be helped in ways that are appropriate. There is a need to question the categories of mental illness that psychiatry applies to the artistic temperament,[4] and also a place for the detachment and perspective that can come from humor. Earlier I quoted from psychiatrist Louis E. Bisch, who has offered such a desirable blend of humor and seriousness in his all-but-forgotten book about neuroticism. Readers will recall that it was Bisch who exclaimed, "to be normal is nothing to brag about! When I study normals and compare them with neurotics I wonder sometimes whether to be normal is not something to be ashamed about" (Bisch, 1936, p. 32). Relevant to the viewpoint of artists who struggle against the psychologically normal world, Bisch quoted then well-known American author Joseph Hergescheimer, who made this comment: "Normal people are almost invariably without minds or imagination. In the main they are extremely stupid. They are, frequently, widely esteemed and often occupy places of power, grow rich, but they have never produced an elevated written line" (Bisch, 1936, p. 31).

THE PSYCHIATRIC PLIGHT OF THE ARTIST

I began this chapter with the observation that psychiatry and clinical psychology face a dilemma when it comes to diagnosing the extremes of mood experienced by many creative people. Often the depths and heights of artistic mood can be destructive: to the artist, to his or her marriage and family, to professional relationships, and in the end even to the artist's own creative resources. As we have seen, the same intense moods and mood swings can, however, also be vital to an artist's capacity to create. But to go beyond these surface observations, it is important to note that clinical studies of creativity have almost always stopped short of anything approaching a phenomenological understanding of the world as experienced by the artist. There has therefore been little psychiatric or clinical psychological effort to comprehend the situational nature of the despondency into which creative people can sink, depression that at least some of the time, and perhaps more often than we might imagine, is due to the inroads upon their artistic sensibility for which coarse-featured, mundane, and mediocritizing human social reality is responsible. From the artist's own perspective, creative life is very often an ordeal *primarily because of a world that is dominated by the presence of the psychologically normal*, dominated by the physical and culturally deficient environment these people produce, by the superficial values they subscribe to, and by the frivolous interests they advocate. (For further analysis see Bartlett, 2009.)

And here again, psychiatry and clinical psychology have so far failed to take seriously the case that needs to be made on behalf of the artist—to recognize what for many highly creative people is the very real, deadening, creatively destructive pathology of the everyday world and of the everyday people who populate it. The obstacles placed in the way of the artist by a human environment consisting often of a psychologically normal family and normal friends, normal acquaintances and business relations, and a psychologically normal encompassing society are seldom appreciated and factored into a psychiatric understanding of the creative.

What typically happens is that a clinically alleged, and sometimes real, pathology of creativity meets the very real and soul-grinding pathology of normality, and in the encounter it is usually the artist who fares the worst. The conflict is usually thrust involuntarily upon the artist. As Bryron wrote: "I recollect, some time [ago], Madame de Staël said to me in Switzerland, 'You should not have warred with the world—it will not do—it is too strong always for any individual.' . . . I perfectly acquiesce in the truth of this remark; but the world has done me the honour to begin the war" (quoted in Jamison, 1993, p. 178). In a similar vein, Santayana (1920, p. 185) observed of artists that "their unhappiness consists in the sense of their unfitness to live in the world into which they are born." Landau (1980, p. 496) concluded that "artists are people who prefer the open condition of perpetual maladaptation." Hermann Hesse (1973), speaking autobiographically, wrote: "my attempts to adapt myself to the standardized world . . . remain . . . fruitless" (p. 159), and then reflected in more detail:

Are you, mad poet . . . , really mad? Are you sick, suffering so from life that often you scarcely want to go on living, simply because you have neglected to adjust yourself to reality "as it once and for all happens to be"?

And once more, although I was prepared to think realistically even at my own expense, I was compelled to reply as I had so often replied before: No, you are a thousand times right in your protest against this miserable "world as it once and for all happens to be," you are right even if you die strangling on this world instead of accepting it. (Hesse, 1973, p. 213)

Unfitness, maladaptation, warring with the world—they all reflect a state of conflict between the creative individual and a world populated by the psychologically normal.

In reviewing studies of what the majority of clinicians judge to be the abnormal psychology of creativity, we see an overlooked path that brings us to a new perspective on the psychology of normality, for we see that, from the artist's point of view, normality itself can be replete with its own pathologies, pathologies of normality that can contribute significantly to what psychiatrists of creativity have construed to be psychopathologies afflicting the artist. In this, if the observations expressed here are right, there is clearly considerable irony and tragedy. There is good reason to approach creative individuals both with a more circumspect, reflective, self-critical yardstick than psychiatry and much clinical psychology have been accustomed to apply, and with an increased intention and ability to empathize with the predicament of the artist who must cope with a psychologically normal world.

AFTERWORD

As we have noted, the psychology of creative temperament has received comparatively little attention within psychiatry and clinical psychology. Much of the reason for this, I suggest, is that clinicians have failed to recognize that many creative people are different in important ways from psychologically normal people and that, therefore, diagnostic classifications that use normality as a baseline become questionable and even inappropriate when applied to the artist. The so-called "artistic temperament" brings with it values, attitudes based on them, and choices in behavior that often do not coincide with those of the psychologically normal population. We recognize that artists frequently do not bow to the same noble truths as the common person: Creative people can be less nationalistic, considering themselves "citizens of all countries and patriots of none." They may be less inclined to participate in herd warfare, genocides, terrorism, obedience to authority, group-endorsed ideological commitment, bullying, environmental destruction motivated by financial greed (see Bartlett, 2002), and similar acts. But because few psychological studies of the artistic temperament have been made, the foregoing are observations and conjectures based on personal and anecdotal experience not yet statistically substantiated. The paucity of psychological studies of artists is certainly also due to the fact that they comprise such a tiny minority and most especially because, as we have seen, they tend in important respects to be sufficiently "different" that "normal" psychiatric diagnostic categories may fail to apply.

The approach to creative individuals proposed here can be expected to meet a certain amount of resistance. Like all socially applicable disciplines, psychiatry and much clinical psychology are influenced by conformist needs and pressures to adopt prevailing politically correct beliefs. Among these, at the present time, is the widespread political belief among many psychiatrists that all patients should be treated equally or "the same." For such psychiatrists, this means that a uniform system of reliable diagnostic classification *ought* to be applied to each and every patient—to do otherwise would be tantamount to recognizing that individual difference at times should override the application of diagnostic categories defined with reference to a standard of psychological normality. This would not be "egalitarian," and it would also place a heavier responsibility upon the psychiatrist when treating highly creative people, requiring the clinician to think in highly individualized terms outside of the customary, symptom-based *DSM* classification framework.

The artist can be exceptional in ways that put him or her at odds with prevailing normal society. A psychiatrist who wishes to treat creative individuals in a manner that is genuinely appropriate to them must be willing to accept an open-minded, "differential," even "discriminating" approach to psychiatric treatment. But to do this in an honest and fitting way, the psychiatrist is compelled to accept a form of *psychiatric elitism* that recognizes that some people require "special" treatment, unconventional diagnosis, and empathic understanding that recognizes them to be exceptions. This is not easily accommodated by an algorithmic, nondiscriminatory, and impartial diagnostic classification system as currently embodied in the *DSM*, blind as it by definition must be to the needs and values of creative individuals who are exceptions to the norm.

NOTES

1. For the role of harm in pathology, a detailed critique of theories of disease, and the elaboration of a unified theory of disease, see Bartlett (2005, Part I).

2. More than a century ago, psychologist George Romanes defended the thesis that there are certain meaningful and factual observations about the world that do not stand in need of experimental confirmation from empirical science (Romanes, 1883, 1888, 1895). He did not disparage experimental evidence, but he recognized that certain kinds of knowledge are possible, especially in psychology, which do not require experimental validation. We in America especially, with our unbounded drive for experimental substantiation of all observations

however obvious, need to be reminded of this wisdom from the past, as I'll seek to do again in a later chapter.

3. Authors who have made contributions in this area include Pines and Aronson (1988) and Bartlett (1990, 1993a, 1993b, 1994a, 1994b).

4. It should already be clear that I see no validity or legitimacy in medical-diagnostic labeling when it comes to psychological problems that cannot be traced to underlying organic dysfunctions. However, in Bartlett (2009) I consider one diagnostic category seldom associated with creative people, which, if we absolutely must have a diagnostic category to apply to them, might, with a little stretching, serve as a close-to-accurate description, and that is "adjustment disorder." For the *DSM* definition of this disorder and further discussion in other contexts, see Chapters 4 and 6 of this book.

PART II

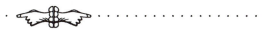

Psychology During a Collapse of Culture

4

Acedia: When Work and Money Are the Exclusive Values

In the last chapter, I urged that a psychologically accurate and clinically appropriate understanding of many creative people requires that we recognize the individualized way in which an artist relates to the world— taking into account the creative individual's sensibilities and sensitivities, how he or she derives a sense of meaning from life and creative work, how the artist reacts to contact with the "normal world" that frequently is unresponsive to the efforts of originality, and related factors. Such a perspective seeks to acquire a *situational understanding* of the creative person and sees psychological problems of the artist as inherently a function of the individual person in relation to a highly individualized context of interests, needs, sources of meaning, and challenges to these.

In Chapter 1 of this book I questioned the psychiatric standard that equates normality with mental health, and in Chapter 2 I sought to make clear how the psychology of definition results in a distorted and unsatisfactory conception of mental disorders. When readers combine the conclusions of both chapters in their own minds, it should make good sense that the *DSM*'s decontextualized and symptom-based diagnostic criteria utterly miss the mark when it comes to the kind of situational understanding of psychological problems advocated here.[1]

In this chapter[2] I want to extend this discussion by examining a certain widespread psychological disability that remains virtually unrecognized and undiscussed. We have seen how a contextually sensitive understanding of the creative individual's "situation" vis-à-vis the psychologically normal world can involve a "mismatch" between self and world, resulting in much of the debilitating *struggle against the world* that typifies the lives of some artists. I now want to turn to a different, more inclusive frame of reference that focuses upon not the small population of the highly creative but rather the general population, which again we'll consider in a situationally relative way. Here, rather than a mismatch, we'll look at the highly adaptive relationship of submission and compliance that has become established between our society's majority—workers who are consumers—and their highly industrialized, commercially driven society. Like the highly creative, today's worker-consumer can experience difficult psychological problems, but they are of an altogether different kind. The particular problem that will concern us here may be called "work-engendered depression."

There has been a general failure among mental health theorists and social psychologists to understand what brings about depression of this kind. Yet the condition is increasingly prevalent in highly industrialized societies, where an exclusionary focus upon work, money, and the things that money can buy has displaced values that traditionally exerted a liberating and humanizing influence. Social critics have called the result an impoverishment of the spirit, a state of cultural bankruptcy, and an incapacity for genuine leisure. From a clinical perspective, the condition has been diagnosed as widespread narcissism and obsessive work. But this misses a great deal.

Acedia, a concept developed by the psychologically astute Scholastics but now virtually forgotten, can throw explanatory light on the origin of this form of depression.

Clinical depression at present is treated in two main, often mutually supportive, ways: by drug therapy and by psychotherapy. Psychotherapeutic treatment may involve any of a large number of alternative approaches, ranging from psychoanalysis to cognitive therapy to behavior change. A few of these therapeutic approaches focus special attention on the central role of a person's attitudes and values in both the genesis and the amelioration of depression.

These psychotherapies include Alfred Adler's individual psychology (1912/1926, 1924, 1929/1964), George Kelly's personal construct theory (1955, 1956/1978), Viktor Frankl's logotherapy (1955, 1959), and Albert Ellis' cognitive therapy (1961, 1973, 1975). A therapist who subscribes to any of these ways of implementing psychotherapy will, to speak in inclusive terms, treat depression by attempting first to make explicit, and then work to strengthen or change, the patient's or client's most basic, relevant attitudes about living. In this perspective, depression is believed to be the result of a fundamental *mismatch* between a patient's beliefs and values, on the one hand, and the realities and goals with which he or she must deal, on the other. Such a state of affairs, it is claimed, brings about chronic frustration, emotional suffering, and potential demoralization. More specifically, these theories of psychotherapy claim that clinical depression is brought about by a group of "basic mistakes" in perceiving the world (Adler), by a self-defeating or self-confounding way of construing the world (Kelly), by an inadequate or unrealized framework of meaning (Frankl), or by an irrational set of expectations (Ellis).

Adler, Kelly, Frankl, and Ellis, among others, situate psychotherapy within the personal framework of meaning or the internal logic and belief system of their individual patients. Their psychotherapies can be likened, in varying degrees, to forms of phenomenological psychology, which began with Brentano (1924, 1925, 1928) and reached perhaps its most direct and explicit development in the phenomenological psychiatry of J. H. van den Berg (1955).

The locus of depression for these essentially phenomenological theories is wholly internal. According to them, depression is born and maintained thanks to an internal dynamic that renders a person vulnerable to demoralization and despair. Here, Adler, Kelly, Frankl, and Ellis refuse to apply the category of disease to psychological disorders: their clients are not "sick," for they believe there is no "disease" there to be treated; the problems they face are problems of living. This was also Thomas Szasz's (1957/1961) view and the basis for his criticism of medical psychiatry: it frequently reifies problems of living into varieties of illness, as we saw in Chapter 2. In doing this, it makes what philosopher Gilbert Ryle called a "category mistake" and falls victim to Whitehead's "fallacy of misplaced concreteness" (which we also saw in Chapter 2). Mistake or fallacy, thinking goes astray when we assert the existence of what has only the rank of phantom pathologies.

In this chapter, we look at a variety of depression first studied by the medieval Scholastics. Their frame of reference resembles that of phenomenological approaches to depression, but unlike them it suggests that a person's attitudes and values do not directly give rise to the form of depression with which they were concerned. Instead, the Scholastics observed that this variety of depression is, we might say, *negatively defined* by a person's values and belief system. It arises, they claimed, due to the *exclusionary* nature of the set of values to which a person is committed: it results, that is to say, from what his or her attitudes *neglect* or *omit*. In other words, this type of depression is, as we will see, brought about by a *deficiency of values*.

WORK AND CULTURAL BANKRUPTCY

The societies of the highly industrialized countries are now firmly in the grip of an obsession with work and its product, money. Work has always been a condition of living, but in the last half century work has become so central in our preoccupations that other values have been displaced.

A single-minded and exclusive focus upon work and the monetary value of time form a social environment in which we increasingly see a certain manifestation of depression. It is a variety of depression whose genesis we've failed to understand clearly and which we have been unable to appreciate for what it tells us about ourselves.

Few concepts drawn from medieval moral theology have direct bearing on the diagnostic vocabulary of the *DSM*. Acedia is no exception. It is a simple idea, one that was apparently not hard to grasp at the height of the Middle Ages. Yet today, though it is still an uncomplicated notion, the meaning of acedia is so remote from our modern daily cares and professional concerns that it is hard to understand. But effort here is worthwhile, if only to help us gain a broader and perhaps a more humane and contextual understanding of depression.

In highly industrialized societies like those of western Europe, America, and now China, the values that have come to supersede all others are money, material comfort, and financial security (the assurance that the first two values will be safely satisfied in the future). The lives of the majority of people in these societies are defined and controlled by a pronounced and single-minded, obsessional concern to acquire and then to remain in a well-paying job. What frequently results is a condition that medieval moral theologians called acedia.

The medieval Schoolmen understood acedia as the cause of an exclusionary focus on the world of work and material gain. In this, they have been followed by Josef Pieper, one of few contemporary thinkers who has given attention to acedia.[3] My interest in this chapter, however, is in the reverse, psychologically important relationship, that is, how an ethic of work and consumption for their own sake leads to acedia. What I examine here is one direction of influence that leads from a narrowly limited preoccupation with work and money to acedia; a complete account would take into consideration the interaction that occurs between the two. Each encourages and helps to perpetuate the other.

According to the Scholastics, acedia is the state of mind that comes about when a person has lost his or her capacity for *leisure*. This seems straightforward. But what they understood by 'leisure' (significantly, they used the Latin word '*scola*' from the Greek '*skole*', the origin of the English word 'school') is no longer familiar to us today. In their view, a certain incapacity to experience leisure develops and becomes firmly established in people whose scope of awareness has become impaired. It is an incapacity whose existence contemporary industrial society is able to recognize only with considerable difficulty.

The values of work and money, like the limited cares of any exclusive preoccupation, blind its adherents to alternative values. They narrow the scope of a person's concerns; he or she becomes wholly and short-sightedly absorbed in immediate gratification and in worry over ensuring future gratification. When this happens, medieval theologians recognized an "impoverishment of the soul." Studies of work-related depression in "career burnout" have pointed to a similar erosion and depletion of personal meaning (e.g., Pines & Aronson, 1988; cf. Rohrlich, 1980), but fail to profit from the insight offered by the medieval understanding.

The logic of usage that underlies the meaning of acedia is alien to us today: A logician would say it is "three-valued," whereas our customary logic is bivalent, recognizing only the two "values" of truth and falsity. In a two-valued logic, a term has one opposite, its negation. In a three-valued logic, a term may have two "opposites," each being the contrary of the other.

Today, we recognize two extremes: On one side, we locate work and the desirable traits that we associated with it, such as diligence, industry, competitiveness, ambition, and so forth. On the other side, we situate leisure, having time on one's hands, being idle, even lazy—in short, having time away from work. Time away from work is useful to the extent and, we now increasingly believe, virtually *only* to the extent, that it serves as a *restorative* that, after the usual two weeks for an American, enables a man or a woman to return to money-making work with renewed energy and zeal.

It is impossible to understand acedia in this context. To understand the medieval conception, we need to think in three-valued terms: Work, diligence, and industry make up one extreme. Idleness, laziness, and time free from the demands of work make up another. And leisure, in the special meaning the Scholastics associated with the concept, is separate from both of these.

In this three-valued context, acedia in the medieval view is an inability to experience leisure. Leisure, as it was then conceived, is opposite to work, but it is also, as we'll see, opposite to idleness or laziness, to merely having time on one's hands. Idleness is of course contrary to work, while leisure is the contrary both of idleness and of work.

In our bivalent attitude toward work, not only do we fall victims to acedia, but we cannot realize that this has happened to us. This is not verbal trickery, but a psychological reality we should be able to appreciate if we will bear with the three-valued medieval view a little longer.

Leisure meant something specific to the medieval mind. It was not synonymous, as we've said, with idleness or taking a vacation. Leisure was instead associated with *culture*, with the cultivation of the spirit, with *cultus*. What is at stake in this conception of "culture" has a radically different meaning than we find in such phrases as "corporate culture," "the culture of the New York Giants," or "U.S. culture." These uses of the word 'culture' are diametrically opposed to the Scholastic conception. In the Scholastics' religiously based standpoint, the human capacity for leisure was one with the ability to be spiritual, to be conscious of the self as a divine creation, to cultivate spirituality within, and to accept one's place in a universe that contains both matter and "higher values," those that transform one's daily life and suffering. Leisure, however, as we shall see in a moment, need not be tied to a religious perspective in order to maintain its capacity to elevate.

The values that the Scholastics thought were *higher* bestowed upon everyday life a significance that transcends the workaday world. In the same way, higher education was called higher because its aim was to encourage cultivation, specifically the cultivation of nonuseful things. The ends of "higher education" had nothing to do with utilitarian pursuits, nothing to do with the acquisition of the technical, social, or other skills necessary to get a well-paying, secure job. Genuinely higher education, as we shall see in more detail in the next chapter, was devoted to those things that are of value "in and of themselves," as it was then commonplace to say.

Leisure, then, was an attitude of mind, an attitude of silent affirmation, of feeling at one in a world in which a person is and cannot but be at home, from birth and throughout his or her life. This form of "letting go" is not inactivity. Leisure is active contemplation, enjoyment, and appreciation of being and of being oneself. To be capable of leisure requires that a man or woman affirm his or her own sense of identity apart from a role as worker, father, mother, or consumer. To be incapable of this is acedia.

Acedia, in short, is an inability to see reality in other than mundane and mediocre ways. It is an inability to perceive reality under the guise of the transformation that "higher values" make possible. During the Middle Ages, these values were rooted in religion—as it happened, in Christianity. But higher values need not be Christian or even theistic. Reality can be transformed by myth, by poetry, by music, art, philosophy, by abstract theoretical research that has no practical application in view, or by imagination. When these powers of transformation diminish or are lost, the minds of the people are blunted, and they begin to suffer from a disability of values. Acedia is just such a disability.

THE SYMPTOMS OF ACEDIA

In the impoverished state of mind brought about by an exclusionary obsession with work and its financial rewards, acedia leads to despair—to an unwillingness and an inability to be fully and richly human. It is a state of mind without hope, a condition of demoralization that is an impasse to realizing one's full human potential.

The Scholastics realized that despair is a block to growth: in the words of Saint Paschasius Radbert, despair "closes the door" (1857–1866, liber II, caput VI, 2). As with the meaning of leisure, the medieval meaning of despair is more comprehensive than is ours today. It is not sadness or grief but a barrier that stands between the man or woman who is slave to the world of work, and higher values. It handicaps a person's ability to transform the mundane, to see beyond and to apprehend what stunted, mediocritized people cannot see or appreciate.

The overemphasis of our society upon work and purchasable things has exactly this stunting effect. Our perspective becomes foreshortened: "greater" and "less than" are reduced to inconsequentialities. The great no longer stand out, the ordinary encompasses all, and indifference and indiscrimination replace the respect that we once bestowed on the extraordinary. We see this in the insistent, exaggerated tendency to make everyone a "hero," to consider everyone a "winner," to "leave no child behind," and to praise every performance with a standing ovation and frenzied cheering. This histrionic and indiscriminate mindset is the product of a psychology that opposes differentiation—the ranking of levels of natural endowment, talent, and attainment—and so loses the capacity to tell and to respect the difference between excellence and the commonplace.

Aquinas identified the other members of acedia's family, the psychological sequelae of this self-imposed narrowing of the human outlook. They are the *filiae acediae*, the partners and companions of despair (Aquinas, 1269–1272/1949, Vol. II, 4; and 1265–1273/1921–1925, Part II of the Second Part, Ques. 35, Article 4, answer to the Second Objection). They spell out, with greater clarity and in more detail than the *DSM*, what work-engendered depression means in human terms.

In addition to despair, acedia leads to what Aquinas called *evagatio mentis*, an uneasy restlessness of mind that expresses itself in

- *inquietudo*—or inner restlessness;
- *verbositas*—a need for the distraction and stimulus of unbridled, mindless talk;
- *instabilitas loci vel propositi*—instability of place or purpose;

- *curiositas*—an unfocused, unanchored, indiscriminate surface interest in any and all things; and
- *importunitas*—the urge to scatter oneself in many pursuits.

In addition to despair and restlessness, the symptoms of acedia include

- *torpor*—repudiation, indifference toward, and neglect of higher values;
- *pusillanimitas*—antagonism toward higher values;
- *rancor*—resentful rebellion against those who represent and seek to cultivate higher ends; and, finally,
- *malitia*—the pure malice that reflects a deliberate choice in favor of evil and a deep-seated commitment to hatred for whatever may be capable of elevating human beings above the trivial, the fatuous, the superficial.

We observe the first three of these—restlessness, the need for distraction, and instability—in frenetic activity, in the exaggerated and fanciful degree that people wish to persuade others, including themselves, that they have successful, meaningful lives in proportion to the degree that their calendars are filled, in the amount of multitasking they pride themselves in being able to handle and with which they are infatuated for the distracting stimulation it provides. When every minute of the day is overbooked in advance, frenzy erects a natural barrier to the possibility of leisure. Inner restlessness and the need for distraction are evident in the public's infatuation for the distractions of emotionally gripping violence and drama and for the adrenalin stimulation gained from extreme sports and thought-dampening loud music. We see instability of place and purpose in the frequency with which Americans move, change jobs and careers, and change marriage partners. Frenzy, restlessness, and the need for emotionally riveting distractions foster superficial interest and the scattering of the self among many pursuits. It's plausible, if a few medieval Schoolmen were alive today, that they would see the accelerating proliferation of attention deficit hyperactivity disorder (ADHD) as yet another, complementary expression of the same condition—and understandably so, since a society dominated by frenzy, distracted attention, and the craving for stimulation can be expected to encourage just such characteristics in its children.

The second set of symptoms of acedia expresses attitudes toward "higher" values—ranging from indifference to such values, to neglect, repudiation, rebellion, hostility and even hatred that is expressed when the victim of acedia is confronted by those who represent values purported to "elevate," values that are claimed to raise a person above the normal level of mundane living. These symptoms of opposition to higher values are expressed in anti-intellectualism, anti-elitism, and an embrace of a thoroughgoing, undifferentiated cultural relativism and multiculturalism, from the standpoint of which there is no "higher" and no "lower."

Together, the psychological dispositions enumerated by the Scholastics form a set of overlapping and mutually reinforcing symptoms. The nine characteristics of acedia promote an agitated, unstable, distracted, and essentially mediocritizing attitude toward living and the purposes of life, the psychology of which we'll examine in detail in Chapter 8.

The list of the symptoms of acedia could easily stand as a psychological profile of industrial society: the medieval terms have their unambiguous correlates in the tense restlessness, angry rebelliousness, embrace of mediocrity, intellectual lethargy, and demoralization that permeate much of our society.

Acedia is, then, a condition that can appropriately be called a disability of values. Higher values are amputated, and yet the amputee is adamant that he or she is sound of mind and body. The dynamic of the person's inner world reinforces this belief. His or her monadic universe becomes self-encapsulated; it is the autistic world of narcissism.[4]

Many who are trapped in this self-imprisoning world of sterile work and trivial pursuits are unhappy—unhappy to the point of clinical depression. Some are unable to sustain their hollow drive to work and consume, and collapse in fatigue, despair, and perplexed disillusionment. Clinical psychology is inclined to say of them that they have acquired a certain disorder of adaptation, and more specifically that they have developed an inhibition to continue working, to which we'll turn our attention in a moment. They are the most evident casualties of a work and consumption ethic gone mad.

ACEDIA: MORAL FAILURE OR PSYCHIATRIC DISORDER?

The psychological result of a society obsessed with work and materialism surrounds us. Acedia is boredom and despair. It takes the form of restlessness and outbursts of impulsive rage and violence. It is an unrecognized form of depression in the face of the monotony and sterility that has permeated the industrialized world, a world in which art, poetry, music, philosophy, and even pure theory and contemplative living have for the majority become no more than distractions and momentary relief from an obsessive compulsion to work, shop, and accumulate things; these distractions offer no more than temporary escape, time out, from a complete absorption of mind and energy in frantic work, the craving for distraction, and the acquisition of things. The disorder we face today might, a century and a half ago, have been called the result of a spreading "moral failure," sustained by a loss of hope before an all-consuming epidemic of work and materialism.

Current psychiatric nosology does not have a place for an expression like 'moral failure', which went out of fashion with the nosology of the influential English psychiatrists D. H. Tuke (1827–1895) and J. C. Bucknill (1817–1897). I'd like to mention their work briefly here, since it can serve as a bridge between the Scholastics of long ago and the present. Bucknill and Tuke (1858/1879) proposed a detailed classification of mental disorders. Their catalog of forms of mental illness included what they called "lesions of the intellect"; such "lesions" included cognitive impairments that they associated with corresponding "moral deficiencies." These, Bucknill and Tuke claimed, were analogous to forms of intellectual deficiency, but instead have to do with deficiencies in the "moral sense" (Bucknill & Tuke, 1858/1879, p. 243). They carefully distinguished varieties of "moral insensitivity," "moral idiocy," and "moral insanity" in an effort to direct clinical attention to deficits or disabilities that can develop in people and cause them to lose sight of a more inclusive value-focused perspective. It was such a perspective that they had in mind when they used the term 'moral'; and it was to develop and strengthen that perspective that they sought to provide appropriate "moral treatment." As they characterized it, this was, on a most fundamental level, therapeutic *education* intended for the individual person; its purpose was humane and liberalizing. We will continue this theme in Chapters 5 and 6, in connection with the psychological objectives of liberal education.

Moral treatment had already been in vogue at the time; Bucknill and Tuke did not originate this approach. It connoted a kinder, more sympathetic treatment of the mentally ill—certainly long overdue and much needed—and it emphasized the importance for physicians to be genuinely compassionate as persons.

The fact that Bucknill and Tuke chose to focus a portion of their psychiatric attention on so-called "moral" matters should not prejudice us today against them, despite the widespread aim of contemporary psychiatry to be value-neutral. Bucknill and Tuke, after all, were not as "soft" as might appear; they were among the first psychiatrists to make the unqualified claim that all mental illness must be organic in origin. Their work has influenced the development of psychiatry through passages like this:

> All disease, therefore, in our opinion, is organic. Not only is this so with diseases which often come under the common observation of the physician . . . but mental and nervous diseases also, of every kind and form.

Not a thrill of sensation can occur, not a flashing thought or a passing feeling can take place without changes in the living organism; much less can diseased sensation, thought or feeling occur, without such changes; changes which very frequently we are not able to detect, and which we may never be able to demonstrate, but of which we are, nevertheless, certain. (Bucknill & Tuke 1858/1979, p. 495)

Today, psychiatry has moved away from the "moral dimension" that concerned both the Scholastics and psychiatrists like Bucknill and Tuke. We have come to believe that this is a sign of progress, to go beyond metaphysics and to make a decisive turn away from religion. Is it therefore possible, in terms of contemporary psychiatric concepts, to make much sense of acedia? Is there a diagnostic classification in terms of which we can situate and understand the depression and related symptomatology we've been discussing?

It is both significant and ironic that contemporary psychiatry has established a category in which, with some stretching, it is possible to accommodate those who, overcome by the barrenness of a world of total work and material acquisition, become conscious of its depressive nature and feel the sapping effect of its superficial, frivolous, and empty gratifications. This is the "disorder" that the *DSM* calls "adjustment disorder, with work inhibition." It is the closest that our current classification of psychological disorders comes to acknowledging, albeit very indirectly, the potential contributing role to human suffering of an exclusionary focus on work that is out of control. The *DSM* diagnostic description is all too short and not especially enlightening:

The essential feature of this disorder is a maladaptive reaction to an identifiable psychological stressor.... The maladaptive nature of the reaction is indicated ... by impairment in occupational (including school) functioning.... [T]he predominant manifestation is an inhibition in work ... occurring in a person whose previous work ... performance has been adequate. Frequently there is also a mixture of anxiety and depression. (American Psychiatric Association, 1987, code 309.23, pp. 329, 331; in APA, 1994 and 2000, absorbed under code 309.9)

"Adjustment disorder, with work inhibition" is a diagnosis that perhaps reveals more about contemporary psychiatry than it does about the correspondingly labeled patient. The label expresses psychiatry's assumption that engagement in the world of work is normal, adaptive, and desirable and that a person who isn't able to be engaged in work, due to "an identifiable psychological stressor," must be afflicted with a "disorder of maladaptation."

Here again we find blinders put firmly in place thanks to the presumption that conformity with what is judged to be normal will lead to positive mental health. With some help from the Scholastics, we can, however, make some constructive progress beyond this limited perspective. It is clear that a life of total work and consumption, along with its resulting cultural impoverishment, can come to be felt as a severe and self-undermining source of stress. When it does, and as seen through the lens of the Scholastics' acedia, work-engendered depression results.

TREATMENT OF WORK-ENGENDERED DEPRESSION

There is indeed, as Thomas Szasz (1957/1961) has protested, a temptation for society to justify its prejudices through its classification of psychological disorders. In a society that believes in the critical value of universal work, leisure in the sense developed here—beyond minimal, regular restorative vacations, which we accept as we do the need for the other type of regularity—inevitably is felt to be a contrary value. In our devotion to utility and technology we can find no room for culture in its root meaning.

Leisure and idleness are therefore equated, and in that equating we have allowed nonutilitarian values, the antidotes to mediocrity, to slip away.[5] Because of our loosened grip on higher ends we live in a time when "culture" is glorified as a kind of trivial pursuit (exemplified with pride in a book such as Hirsch's (1987) *Cultural Literary: What Every American Needs to Know*). In this social context, not only is work-engendered depression promoted, but finding a cure for it is made all the more difficult.

There is a certain naïveté and charm about the views of the medieval theologians; certainly their outlook fit a society very different from ours today. The responsibility fell to men and women in this distant past to try to articulate how people should live in order to live in the best way possible. To do this in a reasonable and convincing fashion, they needed first to have a vision of the meaning of human life. This they did possess, often to a religiously dogmatic fault. Yet perhaps it takes such excess to persuade people who would otherwise have no other criteria with which to distinguish "higher" from "lower" and who would otherwise live in a mundane, one-dimensional world.

Treatment for work-engendered depression requires a meaningful prescription for living. It requires the cultivation of values beyond utility that can balance an unbalanced and now altogether normal obsession with jobs, money, and things. Therapy for work-engendered depression cannot be effective as long as acedia is identified with idleness, as long as we construe depression due to the aridity of work without end as an undesirable maladjustment away from a desirable state of psychological normality, as an "adjustment disorder, with work inhibition." To treat the variety of depression that is acedia, we need to relinquish our fast hold upon the values that constrain us to lives devoted to serving Mammon. As clinicians, we need to lift the blinders from our own eyes in order to help our clients and patients overcome the debilitating blindness that our work- and dollar-obsessed society has produced in them.

NOTES

1. As Robert L. Spitzer recently commented, "*DSM*'s ... criteria specified the symptoms that must be present to justify a given diagnosis but ignored any reference to the context in which they developed" (Horowitz & Wakefield, 2007, p. viii).

2. An earlier discussion of the subject-matter of this chapter was published as an article, "*Acedia*: The Etiology of Work-engendered Depression," in *New Ideas in Psychology 8*(3), 1990, pp. 389–96. The account provided here is revised, updated, supplemented, and the focus changed to fit the context of this book.

3. I am indebted in this analysis to several authors, principal among them Josef Pieper, who, while in his nineties, corresponded with me in connection with research for this chapter. See Pieper (1948/1963, 1977/1986), Jünger (1934), and de Grazia (1962).

4. On the willful self-confinement of clinical narcissism, see Bartlett (1986a).

5. We examine the neglected psychology of mediocrity in Chapter 8.

5

Barbarians at the Door: A Psychological and Historical Profile of Today's College Students

> Modern psychology at its best has a questionable understanding of the soul. It has no place for the natural superiority of the philosophic life, and no understanding of education.
>
> —Allan Bloom (1987, p. 121)

During turning points in history, colleges and universities act as microcosms in which we can sometimes see with particular clarity forces that are less perceptibly at work in the larger society.[1] We face such a turning point today. The values that used to define higher education have been pushed aside to make room for others that emphasize vocational education and the making of money. In the process, not only has the nature of higher education itself changed but so has what we as a society value.

Educators generally see this as a shift away from a traditional conception of higher education in which the liberal arts were central to a more contemporary approach that responds to the dominant role technology has come to occupy. Yet it is more than this; it is not an isolated phenomenon confined to education. The quiet revolution that has occurred in the education offered by our colleges and universities is a symptom of basic and far-reaching change not only in America but in other highly industrialized nations as well. The international emphasis on vocational education is a regressive change that marks, as we shall explore, the reestablishment of a primitive view of humanity and of a fundamentally barbaric attitude concerning the purposes of living. In the process, as we shall see, the standards that once defined the objectives of higher education have been lowered to accord with society's judgment that the average, the ordinary, and the normal should instead be the central concern of university education.

The progressive deterioration in American higher education, which has become particularly acute during the past four decades, has been inevitable. It has come about as a result of commitments that took deep root in the fresh American soil of social and educational policy nearly two centuries ago. On the foundation of these commitments, American higher education has grown: At first its growth was stunted, then became warped, and now it has withered. The historical process described in this chapter has been accompanied by a process of psychological deformity that has culminated in an epidemic of narcissism and its moral counterpart, barbarism.

As we review the history and underlying psychology, we'll find that its past has made the atrophy of American higher education unavoidable, while narcissism and barbarity have spread because they are *appropriate* responses to the psychological forces that animate that history.

WHAT HIGHER EDUCATION MEANT

Higher education is essentially an ideal, an ideal associated with a group of values that for many centuries were thought both to make individual men and women better people and to enrich humanity. Central among them were these two:

First, it was thought that certain intellectual and artistic pursuits have an intrinsic importance to human life. They have no special utilitarian purpose, they do not satisfy particular social needs, they do not tend to bring financial affluence or material comfort, yet they are essential to a fully human life. They are of value in and of themselves, without connection to external gain or vocational advancement.

Secondly, it was accepted that there are comparatively few individuals who are well suited to these pursuits. Only some possess the personal qualities of intelligence, discipline, dedication, and interest to cultivate them. It was nonetheless believed to be important to the well-being of a civilized society that some people devote their lives to intrinsic values of this kind. It was believed that among the students of higher education are some who are destined to become scholars, scientists, poets, artists, and religious leaders: men and women who can offer to others experiences of a distinctive kind that lead to a freer, higher, and richer level of consciousness. The world of pure theory, any genuinely aesthetic encounter, contemplation and meditation—these are experiences that can liberate a human being; they are the experiences that, it was believed, express human nobility and excellence.

They lead to habits of mind and of practice that transcend the workaday world; their importance is wholly intrinsic, for they open doors to an altogether different level and quality of living. Their cultivation elevates humanity as a species, not only those who are members of its elite— provided that one sees humanity as a brotherhood in which those who devote their lives to higher values add to the measure of each. For this reason, when the ideal of higher education was current, even the common worker felt a sense of respect for the liberal arts, however far removed from them his or her own toil might be. This respect expressed a framework of understanding and of values in which life could be situated and lived with dignity and meaning. The average worker had a sense of place in the world, a world in which some learning was clearly "higher" and some "lower."

Culture and leisure for the few: these are essentially the traditional values of higher education. It is a now rapidly disappearing objective, this cultivation of the liberating arts by a small minority who possess the required interests, abilities, freedom from everyday work, and leisure. These are values not of our time, clearly out of place and out of pace with contemporary society.

Our response to an ideal—through allegiance that is given or is withheld—is a psychological event. It is within this psychological, value-laden context that we should look for an understanding of what today's college students, and their faculty, care about, what they value, and what they don't. This psychological substructure is, as we will see, responsible for the decline of higher education, a subject that has been much discussed but as yet not examined in terms of its underlying psychology.

THE DEGRADATION OF THE IDEAL OF HIGHER EDUCATION AS A RESULT OF DEMOCRATIC VALUES

> Materialism, among all nations, is a dangerous disease of the human mind, but it is more especially to be dreaded among a democratic people because it readily amalgamates with that vice which is most familiar to the heart under such circumstances. Democracy encourages a taste for physical gratification; this taste, if it becomes excessive, soon disposes men to believe that all is matter only; and materialism, in its turn, hurries them on with mad impatience to these same delights; such is the fatal circle within which democratic nations are driven round.
>
> —Alexis de Tocqueville, *Democracy in America*

American society today believes that there are three interlinked truths: (1) opportunity should be equal for all, (2) equal opportunity will yield equal results, and (3) equal education for all equalizes opportunity and therefore brings about equal results (van den Haag, 1974). This *myth of egalitarianism* has very little to do with democracy.

Dewey tried to place the myth in its proper place:

> Belief in equality is an element of the democratic credo. It is *not*, however,
> belief in equality of natural endowments.... The very fact of physical and
> psychological inequality is all the more reason for establishment by law of
> equality of opportunity, since otherwise the former becomes a means of
> oppression of the less gifted.... [W]hat we call intelligence [is] distributed
> in unequal amounts.... The democratic faith in equality is the faith that
> each individual shall have the chance and opportunity to contribute
> whatever he is *capable* of contributing and that the value of his contribution
> be decided by its place and function in the organized total of similar
> contributions, not on the basis of prior status of any kind whatever.
> (Dewey, 1949, p. 60, italics added)

Individual variation is a condition of evolution; it is also the spice of life.
Fortunately, we are not all the same. Our intellectual and practical skills as
well as our interests, aptitudes, capacities, and abilities differ. But miscon-
ceived democracy based on the myth of egalitarianism is precisely an attack
on individual variation and hence on individuality. In our zeal for equality
of opportunity, we have mistaken democracy for a commitment to conformity and uniformity, a commitment that elevates normality so that it
becomes a desired standard, in the belief that only when men and women
are homogenized is there real and assured equality: one person is then as
good as any other as an interchangeable part in the social machine, and
democracy and communism find a common point of contact.

The main psychological force that leads to this veneration of equality
by advocates of democracy is their manifest fear of superiority, fear of
the discriminatory entitlements that it is natural to bestow upon men
and women who, in different respects, are our superiors.

In America, the only evidences of superiority that we will comfortably
tolerate are in sports, in the accumulation of monetary wealth, in military
success and rank, and in show business. Celebrities in these areas do not
threaten egalitarianism because the common person is persuaded that he
or she, too, could accomplish such things, if circumstances were right—
that is, if the proper opportunities were assured, and possibly if he or she
possessed the requisite physical capacity. Natural *physical* superiority can
be forgiven in a democracy, perhaps because it has close and familiar ties
with physical labor, which levels differences.

But, if we advance a step further, we tread on thin ice: the performances
of outstanding fine artists, and here I am referring to virtuoso performances of classical music and ballet, though they are physical in nature,
reveal a superiority of accomplishment that is too distant from what the
majority can aspire to. Such displays of attainment are intimidating for

this reason and, as we will see, for another as well, because of the disquieting addition of the ingredient "culture."

The step from athletic proficiency to intellectual superiority puts us in a markedly different universe of uneasy values. To be tolerable in our egalitarian democracy, intellectual superiority must be excused, disguised, and brought down to a commonplace level. The only intellectuals who are really acceptable in America are those with dirt under their fingernails, who speak like any Joe, who possess no unusual qualities of personal distinction, who would, in short, just make good drinking buddies. An article about Bill Bennett, secretary of education for the Reagan administration, is typical: "He holds a B.A. and Ph.D. in philosophy and a J.D. in law, plays a deadly serious game of touch football and is a former rock-band guitarist who is at home with Plato, Shakespeare and Thomas Aquinas. The cozy world of academia never blunted his street smarts; the privileges of his education did not make him an elitist. . . . [H]e not only read classics in Latin, but played on the school's winning football team" (Evans & Novak, 1988, p. 106). Bennett's higher degrees can be once forgiven because he played football, and twice forgiven because he played "on a winning *team.*" In short, Bill is really an all-American guy even if he does have a few degrees.

Similarly, Nobel Laureate in physics Robert Feynman was democratically acceptable because he could play a mean rhythm on the bongos, could handle himself in a fist fight in the men's room of a bar, made quips that entertained the press, and joined a Stockholm students' ceremony for Nobel Prize winners by making frog noises and jumping backward (Grobel, 1986).

The confused equation of democratic equality of opportunity with egalitarianism, particularly during the past 40 years, has led, as we shall see, to a society that prefers the blindness of indiscrimination to the risked sins of discrimination, to a society that favors laxity in its educational expectations and that unquestioningly neglects and repudiates values not closely linked with financial aggrandizement.

The history of higher education and the history of culture and civilization to which it is linked are made up of two kinds of change: we can discern some patterns that, for a time—and perhaps a long time—endure, while many quickly pass. One of the most fascinating challenges for the social psychologist and the historian is to understand the reasons for this difference between the momentary and the comparatively enduring, between the ripples of fads and significant turns in the river.

As we examine the internal dynamic of higher education, we will see that its history has made two interrelated consequences inevitable: the deterioration of the schooling that American higher education can offer and the spread in our society of pathological narcissism and of its result, barbarism. This dynamic is strong and self-reinforcing, so much so that there are convincing reasons to believe that the social and psychological phenomenon of barbarism is here to stay, perhaps for a long time.

THE SELF-UNDERMINING HISTORY OF HIGHER EDUCATION IN AMERICA

> In a single year, America spends more upon higher education than all the people of the world, throughout history, had spent upon the higher learning down to the time of the Second World War.
> What generosity, how indiscriminate, how ineffectual!
> —Russell Kirk, *Decadence and Renewal in the Higher Learning*

From the perspective of the 1830s, the young American republic was enlightened and intelligent compared with Europe. So it seemed to French social critic Michael Chevalier in his study of American society, *Society, Manners, and Politics in the United States*. Speaking of the France of his time, Chevalier says:

> Examine the population of our rural districts, sound the brains of our peasants, and you will find that the spring of all their actions is a confused medley of biblical parables with the legends of gross superstition. Try the same operation on an American farmer and you will find that the great scriptural traditions are harmoniously combined in his mind with the principles of moral and religious independence proclaimed by Luther, and with the still more recent notions of political freedom. (Chevalier 1838/ 1961, Chap. 34)

In retrospect, the schooling offered by American higher education at the time Chevalier wrote supports his judgment. Consider the work still required of freshmen at Oberlin in 1877: The first term, they studied Livy, Xenophon's *Memorabilia*, Greek prose composition, and algebra. The second term, Horace, Lusias, Greek prose composition, and solid and spherical geometry. The third term, Cicero's *De Senectute*, Herodotus, German, and more geometry.

This solid, no-nonsense curriculum that trained both mind and moral sensibilities was quick to give way before pressures that would mock Chevalier's observations. Some of these pressures greeted the Oberlin freshmen virtually upon their graduation: The forces of change were already at work in the 1840s as increasing numbers of Irish peasants and workers came to this country. The influx of the many thousands kindled the fear in America that unless determined steps in educating the immigrants were taken, the settlers would bring with them the seeds of European class conflict and despotic government. As a result of the perceived or imagined threat to the tender new American democracy, reformers like Henry Barbard and Horace Mann argued on behalf of national compulsory education, schooling for everyone.

This was to be the first nail to be driven into the cross-in-the-making for "higher" education. From this time on, education in America, including the so-called higher education offered by its colleges and universities, would succumb to a succession of policies that in time would corrupt academia from within.

Consider. The task of educating the incoming tide of immigrants was above all intended to initiate the settlers into American ways, and so the emphasis of education quickly became nonacademic. By the turn of the century, the schools stressed manual training and vocational education. Their aim was to produce *useful* Americans: efficient workers and politically enlightened citizens. Education in America henceforth would serve the interests of social management.

By 1908, the National Education Association was urged (by a group of businessmen) to include industrial and commercial subjects in elementary schools. Since 70 percent of elementary school students never went on to high school, the best schooling for them ought to be, the NEA pronounced, "utilitarian first, and cultural afterward" (Callahan, 1962, p. 10).

By 1910, public insistence became more widespread that education should not emphasize academic subjects, the ingredients of "a gentleman's education." Manual and industrial training were the needs of the day. Why the protest? Because the American public was incensed at the high rate of failure of its children in schools that still provided academically oriented programs of study. The democratically minded public discerned that higher education must be disassociated from "culture." The interests of the normal population would need to be met.

A second nail was hammered into place. Education would march to the drum of "manpower training." The interests of American industry would increasingly subvert the academic values of higher education. The college curriculum devoted to mathematics, the classics, languages, grammar, history, and rhetoric was transmuted into the baser metals of vocational education, citizenship, health science, homemaking, commercial English, secretarial skills, and accounting—all valued because of their practical utility. "Culture" was to become more and more of an afterthought until, in its original, liberal, and liberating meaning, it occupied no place in the minds of American educators.

It is important to observe that not only did the *content* of education change at this time but, at least of equal and perhaps of greater importance, so did its *tenor*: rapidly disappearing was the sense of *reverence* that characterized the teaching, and the learning, of the older curriculum. This reverence was not transferred to commercial subjects; instead it evaporated. The shift away from a higher learning devoted to culture was in fact, as we can now see clearly in looking back, a shift away from contact with values capable of eliciting reverence. The values of careerism and acquisition of money took their place, but reverence was a thing past.[2] We will return to this subject later on.

In keeping with America's democratically inspired hostility toward social classes, American educators were mulish in their commitment to the integral high school: they rejected the European model that routed some students to universities and others to vocational and technical schools. Democratic equality, the educators felt, was opposed to any form of schooling that discriminated between students who were "college material" and those who were best served through job training. The enthusiastic populace, in their celebration of equality, had discovered anti-elitism, and this mindset drove a third nail in place.

The period from 1910 until the Second World War was one of consolidation. College and university policy makers became more heavily entrenched in dissociating higher education from culture and in enforcing a democratic, anti-elitist integration of manual laborers, tradesmen, professionals, and intellectuals in the schools. Belief in the value of universal compulsory education soon spilled over into the belief that everyone should go to college and, most importantly, that college should be *useful*.

Professor George Boas at Johns Hopkins was a glaring example. During World War II he argued: "If training men in trigonometry and physics and chemistry, to the detriment of the humanities, will win the war, then for God's sake and our own, let us forget our Greek, our Latin, our art, our literature, our history, and get to business learning trigonometry and physics and chemistry" (Kirk, 1978, p. xix).

During the same period, demoniacal Harry Hopkins was especially eager to enlist higher education:

> Every college and university should be turned into an Army and Navy training center. The women, too, should remain in college only while they are being trained for their part in the war effort.
>
> High school hours should be shortened so students will have more time to work, especially on farms. . . . I can see no reason for wasting time on what today are non-essentials such as Chaucer and Latin. A diploma can only be framed and hung on the wall. A shell that a boy or girl helps to make can kill a lot of Japs. (quoted in Kirk, 1978, pp. xix–xx)

Once the war had been won, thanks to these and other more final sacrifices of youth, others had still to be made.

Colleges across the country were flooded with war veterans who, regardless of their academic abilities, were encouraged to enroll under the GI Bill. Enrollments blossomed. New buildings were thrown up.

Unfortunately, in a few years, once the GIs were graduated, the schools were left holding expanded facilities and overstocked faculties, which had to be filled and supported, respectively. The emphasis of higher education therefore turned to "recruiting" replacements for the departing soldiers. To justify their recently expanded "physical plant" and to maintain their now longer payrolls, the schools were forced, or they felt that they were, once again to put academic standards aside and to engage in *attracting* students.

In 1957, the Soviet Union put its first manned satellite into orbit. The Eisenhower administration was alarmed. In 1958, the National Defense Education Act accordingly was passed. Funds were appropriated and distributed to colleges and universities across the country. Teacher training and foreign language programs were given special attention, because the government associated them with national defense.

Here, then, the fourth and last nail was driven into higher education's cross. It was to be a nail of an entirely different sort. It was what general systems theorists call "recursive," since it comprised a self-perpetuating, or self-reinforcing, element in the "system" of higher education. On the one hand, the departing GIs left universities hurting for students; on the other, the government decided to fund the expansion of higher education, adding to the need to find new students. A self-cycling snowball effect was set into motion, one that evades efforts to control it, and one that develops a mind, or more accurately a mindlessness, of its own. As we shall see, this recursive phenomenon was to recur in different forms in the more recent history of higher education in this country. In conjunction with the other three nails that have crucified higher education—the convictions that higher education should be universal, that the education offered should be useful and not "genteel culture," and that higher education should be opposed to intellectual elitism—a system with an extremely stable internal dynamic resulted. It is self-perpetuating, and it is highly resistant to efforts to change it.

Caught with a host of student vacancies to fill, colleges and universities in the early 1960s found the public outcry that everyone has a right to be in college very agreeable. The challenge posed by the student recruitment problem was met by making higher education easier and more entertaining to students. The gates to academe swung so widely open on their hinges that the catchy and candid phrase "open admissions" was added to the advertising vocabulary.

Other events reinforced this trend. There was the civil rights movement of the 1960s, followed by black power. They heightened our democratic sensitivity to minorities and the handicapped. Social consciousness was expanded and equal opportunity education resulted. Colleges and universities embraced a family of nonintellectual functions, ministering to the diminished self-esteem of the poor, the disadvantaged, the handicapped, and the downtrodden minorities. Higher education responded to its new calling by becoming social counseling and therapy for its students.

In 1965, Congress granted $848 million to subsidize higher education. Funds were suddenly available for further physical expansion, for the training of more teachers, and for substantial student financial aid in the form of scholarships and loans. The upshot was that virtually anyone could attend college, without regard to aptitude, preparation, or dedication.

In 1969, the Carnegie Foundation for the Advancement of Teaching asked the Nixon administration for greatly increased funding. Four billion dollars were appropriated in 1970. By 1976, funding would run in excess of $13 billion.

The Vietnam war added another log to the self-fueling blaze. Legions of students enrolled in universities to avoid the draft. In response, faculty whose social consciences were disturbed by the war eased their academic demands on students who, if they received the lower grades they merited, would become cannon fodder. At the same time, the clamoring students insisted that higher education respond to their personal demands for relevance and subjective gratification. The "new courses" that resulted, designed to pacify, lowered standards still more.

The offerings of "higher education" now included such tantalizing attractions as Electronic Existentialism (the "philosophy" of rock groups) and Philosophy of Physical Education, which wormed their way into the pabulum curriculum that offered bachelors' and graduate programs in Food Distribution, Packaging, Agricultural Journalism, Ice Cream and Wine Making, and courses in the then-burgeoning, vague new field of "Communications." From LaMaze Methods for La Leche Mothers to Death and Dying and Hostel Management, the curriculum offered a womb-to-tomb varied diet, not intellectually nutritious.

During the decade of the 1980s, leniency and anti-intellectualism spread more quietly. Declining numbers of students pushed standards lower still, as colleges and universities scrambled to attract even less qualified students to fill their classrooms and wallets. Programs in classics, foreign languages, and even theoretical science dried up and disappeared. As a mass, students and the vast majority of their teachers turned from the more serious and demanding academy, its receding image lingering faintly in the haze, to the radiant, freshly polished idol of financial aggrandizement.

This trend strengthened even more during the 1990s and the first decade of the new century as a menu of university degrees was and continues to be advertised, showcasing the lifetime income each degree can be expected to net. During this period university research in "pure science" has been transformed and harnessed to the financially rewarding interests of such fields as engineering, materials science, nanotechnology, computer science, biotechnology, and telecommunications. Universities now pride themselves on the number of new patents they register each year and the number of spin-off companies their faculty and students establish. _ WAS /

Attending college is now no more and no less than the most direct road to material gratification. Mass education is America's springboard to economic development. The university has relinquished its control to the marketplace. Higher education knows that it now pays only lip service to culture: its real purpose is to cater to students who want, more than anything else, to make money. Students and their parents now commonly apply a two-step decision process in choosing a university: the costs of attending name-brand private institutions are compared with those of less expensive state universities, and the totals are then compared with the projected dollar value of the two varieties of degrees once the student has diploma in hand and enters the workplace. (*Money Magazine* recently ran a feature article that, without a shadow of shame, does exactly this.)

This situation has been a necessary consequence of our history. From the time of the migration to America more than a century and a half ago, education in America, as we have seen, has been forced to respond to public demands that it be useful and responsive to the real world of practical and ultimately financial affairs. Its foundation was universal, leveling, compulsory education. Next came the dissociation of higher education from culture, from the essentially contemplative nature of the traditional higher learning that inspired a feeling of reverence. Elitism, most especially cultural elitism, which would select university students on the basis of their intellectual and creative abilities, was then declared the enemy of the equality-sensitive republic. History has trapped education in a system of self-reinforcing feedback that has turned colleges and universities across America into cafeterias for careerism, with moneymaking heralded as the supreme value.

This is the heritage of American higher education. We turn now to look at its underlying psychology.

THE PATHOLOGY OF NARCISSISM

> No patient I have ever encountered is free of narcissistic problems. At least a third of our patients have this as the leading psychopathology, the central one, the nuclear one around which the tide has to be turned. People argue with me and say it must be two-thirds. Has this always been so, or is this something recent? Is it only that our attention has been sharpened so that we diagnose it more, or is it indeed increasing? I do not know the answer to that but I believe that it may be on the increase, and the question is, "Why?"
> —Heinz Kohut, *The Kohut Seminars on Self Psychology and Psychotherapy*

In the past century there have been three main psychological consequences of the history we have traced, each contributing to bring about the next.

After two world wars against totalitarianism, Americans have been conditioned to feel a reflex arc enmity toward authority. Complete authority embodied in the state is totalitarianism, but authority also extends to the discipline we require of our children and fellow adults, as it does to the values to which we adhere and to the standards of conduct and competence that we respect.

In their rejection of authority, Americans overgeneralized, and they rejected much: values, standards, and discipline were weakened, loosened, rendered vague, or shelved.

When the experience of children, or of adults, is freed from the regulating effects of authority, life takes on a quality of arbitrariness. We come to think of laws and standards as mere conventions; our outlook becomes culturally relativist, tentative, multiculturalist, and ever subject to doubt, reappraisal, and relegislation.

At the same time that American society and most of the free world acquired this antipathy toward authority born of a fully justified fear of its political consequences, the traditional sources of balance in human values began to find themselves in trouble: religion, the classical heritage, and philosophy lost their capacity to elicit genuine reverence. Respect for higher education and for its professors, the transmitters of this cultural tradition, began to deteriorate.

Rejection of authority and loss of respect for the standards affirmed by tradition led to a second psychological consequence: a spreading attitude of leniency that was camouflaged as tolerance—leniency in the home, in the courts, in corporate and governmental affairs, and, of course, in the schools, which concern us here.

At the height of the 1960s, a pamphlet published by Stanford's first-year students, called *Freshmen Voices: Student Manners and Morals*, gave eloquent testimony:

> Our morals, or lack of morals, show our increasing conviction that there is nothing absolute or dependable in this world, that nothing is real and no purpose is valid unless we make it so and believe in it. There is no God, or if there is, the code that people attribute to him is only an invention of man. There is no country in itself worthy of patriotism, unless its ideals coincide with what we personally feel is just. And since Nuremberg, we even feel that a person must decide whether the laws are good and should be followed, or bypassed because they contradict what he believes are right.

The period of the 1960s is of special interest to social psychologists because it shows us how children who have been brought up in an atmosphere of indulgence and leniency will turn in anger on their society to express their pent-up resentment that the guideposts for meaningful living had been stripped away. The children of the 1960s were looking for the authority that had been withheld from them, even if it were only an authority they could challenge:

> No one ever firmly said "No!" As tiny children are said to court punishment, that they may learn definitely what is permitted and what is not, so the college generation of these years probed again and again for solidity, but encountered only flabbiness. Without vice there is no virtue; without folly there is no wisdom. The rising generation could not discover virtue or vice, wisdom or folly: only the phrase of empty consolation: "Do your own thing." Without authority, the world was meaningless. (Kirk, 1978, p. 71)

The loss of firm and respected sources of human values together with the epidemic of leniency led to a third psychological consequence. Clinical narcissism, believed by many clinicians to be a disorder of the self they increasingly find in their clients, goes considerably beyond self-absorption. We will refrain from taking a leap to reification, discussed in Chapter 2, and stop short of making narcissism a form of "mental illness." It is, however, as we shall see, an *appropriate* response to certain of the conditions that have come to make our society what it is.

Freud mentioned narcissism only in passing, and in a sympathetic context: "[A] person who is tormented by organic pain and discomfort gives up his interest in the things of the external world, in so far as they do not concern his own suffering. Closer observation teaches us that he also withdraws *libidinal* interest from his love-objects: so long as he suffers, he ceases to love" (Freud, 1914–1916/1957). Narcissism in Freud's sense is induced not only by physical pain but by chronic illness and disability and by the loneliness and incapacity of old age. Natural narcissism of this kind is tunnel vision brought on by suffering from which there is no escape.

Clinical psychology's description of narcissism has broadened from this early basis in an effort to understand a specific variety of pathology of personality called "narcissistic personality disorder." Central to its study has been the work of Heinz Kohut and Otto Kernberg (especially Kohut, 1971, 1977; Elson, 1987; Kernberg, 1975, 1980, 1984). The pathology of narcissism is most effectively understood if we appreciate both how a person develops the condition and why it has been considered to be a disorder or illness.

Clinical narcissism, which I'll refer to simply as "narcissism" from here on, is often thought to arise as a result of a childhood trauma that drives the child to build rigid fortifications to protect against further pain. In time, these defenses wall the person off from others.

Alternatively, it has been suggested that narcissism comes about in reaction, or as a result of subjugation, to the twisted unreality of a "schizophrenogenic parent." The child attempts to insulate himself from the parents', most often the mother's, confused and conflicting demands, expectations, and distorted style of communication, and isolates himself in a world of his own.

A third hypothesis has gained wide acceptance. It claims that narcissism develops when a child is raised without "confirming" or "mirroring" experience. Again, it is usually the mother who plays the dominant family role: When she is herself self-absorbed, she sees her child as an extension of herself, and so does not really respond to the child at all, but only to her own projected needs. Typically, the child experiences an alternately suffocating and cold or indifferent mother. The father often is absent, physically or emotionally; he either is just not there but, for instance, is always at work, or else he distances himself from the family and remains emotionally uninvolved. The result is a child whose early needs for acceptance and affirmation as a separate and unique person fail to be satisfied. The child then develops a set of symptoms associated with a deficient sense of self.

Writing in the 1960s, before the diagnostic vocabulary of narcissism had been honed, psychologist Salvador Maddi observed:

> All you need to develop a premorbid identity is to grow up around people in significant relationship to you who value only some aspects of you, who believe in social roles and biological needs as the only defining pressures

of life, and who are either afraid of active symbolization, imagination, and judgment, or see no particular relevance of these processes to living. Have these significant people act on their views in interactions with the child, and he will develop a premorbid identity. (Maddi, 1967, p. 324)

Before we look at the symptoms that characterize narcissism, it is worth noticing that the three explanations of the condition agree on one thing: that the early experience of the child leads him or her to erect barriers to further pain. This self-isolation is at the heart of the disorder.

If one were to make a composite portrait of the narcissistic personality from the work of its main contributors, it would look like this:

We are first struck by his or her intense preoccupation with the self. Behind this surface aspect of self-absorption, his (or her, understood throughout) feelings are blunted; his perception of the world is flat and monotonous. He is driven to seek stimulation, "to make life feel real," and so tends to wear masks, to lie, to deny, to blame, and wish for power and infallibility. Megawatt rock music fills his need for a bombardment of noise that can drown out or mask the dullness he feels, what Russell Kirk has called "the tyranny of the auditory nerves": "[T]he scholar's lamp ... glows uncertainly in the blast of cacophony. ... Within nearly all the dormitories and fraternities of the typical American campus, cacophony triumphs insanely" (Kirk, 1978, p. 213).

The narcissist tries, in short, to compensate through excited hyperactivity and self-stimulation for a feeling of inner depression, apathy, and deadness. Because of a feeling of purposelessness, he seeks comfort in conformity. His "chameleon personality" yearns to be "just like others"; only then does he feel affirmed, stable, real. He receives emotional support, social company, and stimulation from being "wired in" at all times through social networking, e-mail, his cell phone, and other devices.

And of course he is attracted to the famous. He seems to gain a strengthened sense of self and personal value through the admiration he directs toward celebrities, whom he sees as extensions of himself. Our society's celebration of the celebrity originates here. But the mirage cannot be sustained: Celebrities "have more" than he does. Their lives are therefore fuller, more real. Like Envy in *Doctor Faustus*, he asks, "Why shouldst thou sit, and I stand?" He yearns for the trappings of affluence, for affluence encourages the unexamined life.

External demands are an unwelcome drain on his energy, and so he evades personal accountability and the judgment of others. As a student and later on in life, he seeks the path of least resistance and, best, the path that can distract and entertain. He wants less work, but even more he wants to evade judgment of its quality.

His psychological world is painfully confined to immediate experience. He cannot appreciate what came before the self—that is, history—or what will come after him—the world he will leave to his descendents. For him, history and the future do not exist as realities; he needs to have the "story" of history portrayed to him in the present tense to make it feel real. He cannot reconcile the demands of the fleeting moment with the sometimes vaguely imagined permanent things that require an attention and care that transcend his cramped world.

Enduring personal relationships—friendships, love affairs, and marriage—demand more than he can give. His substitute is a mania for electronic gadgets and in particular an infatuation for the latest electronic means to fill his time with shallow socializing and the exchange of trivia. His sense of self never solidifies and integrates; the earth moves beneath his feet and he is constantly unsettled by the demands of new experience. More than anything else, he is driven by the desire to be accepted and admired by his peers. He therefore invests his emotional energy in external appearances, extensions of himself. He focuses on money and on career, the two yardsticks that our society esteems as measurements of personal worth. Career advancement and monetary success are expressly *public* ratifications of a person's value. The narcissist hopes to find personal affirmation in the public spectacle of material success.

These, then, are some of the main characteristics of narcissism. They describe a condition that most psychologists today judge to be dysfunctional, a "disorder of the personality." In Chapter 2, I raised a group of objections against the inflationary trend in psychiatry that reifies mental disorders. Reflective readers may therefore want to know how the concept of pathology may be applied within the framework of clinical psychology and at the same time steer clear of an extravagant ontology that populates reality with mental illnesses thought to be disease entities. While many psychologists today consider extreme, clinical narcissism to constitute a "mental illness" à la *DSM*, my intent here is rather to refer to a psychological condition that constitutes a harmful functional impairment—an impairment that does not postulate or assert any type of organic dysfunction, disorder, or breakdown of an inner "psychic mechanism." From this standpoint, to call narcissism pathological is to apply a heuristic conception of problem solving and not a concept of psychiatric nosology: When I refer to narcissism as a "pathology," "disorder," or "dysfunction," this language is intended to draw our attention to a specific set of undesirable, harmful functional shortcomings of narcissistic individuals. To be psychologically impaired is not necessarily in any sense to suffer from a disease or illness.

But in analogy to physical illness (and this is expressly an analogy—that is, only a metaphor), to be functionally narcissistic is both incapacitating and socially and culturally contagious. Narcissism constricts a person's world, undermines his or her personal relationships, and forces him or her into a partial and embittering existence that can never satisfy a hunger for individual acceptance and confirmation. The narcissism that affects America is a disability that constrains a person to perpetual dissimulation, to living a life pretending that a shallow existence of social mimicry and material acquisition is full. And like certain other emotional impairments, narcissism is contagious—that is to say, a narcissistic mother or father will tend to recreate in the upbringing of a child the very conditions that emotionally isolated the parent.

We have traced the outlines of nearly two centuries of the history of higher education in America and sketched a portrait of clinical narcissism. The connections between the two are unmistakable: Our society's history has favored egalitarian homogeneity. It has removed culture from the public's consciousness and appreciation as a result of its single-minded devotion to utility. It has vigorously opposed cultural elitism, which is, despite its unfortunate association with unnecessary snobbery, a public expression of a scale of values with a clearly defined sense of "higher" and "lower."

Not very long ago, Americans and Europeans, like any civilized people, realized that the spectrum from philosopher to menial laborer revealed something important about human life and about the values that make living worthwhile. The distance separating the contemplative from the manual life was conceived not in terms of a leveled range of human abilities, as it is now, but it expressed a hierarchy in which reverence for certain values was natural and meaningful. Culture has ceased to be an *axis mundi*. We have yet to find another that gives men and women direction in living. In place of culture, we have placed well-paying jobs, and even here we are loath to recognize that some ways of amassing money are inherently more meaningful than others. And yet, "working as a brain surgeon is almost certainly more meaningful than working as a salesman of used cars" (Pines & Aronson, 1988, p. 138, who argue that our society's failure to legitimize such discriminations is at the basis of much career burnout).

When the sense of reverence and respect to which I refer is lost, higher education, on the one hand, is brought low; on the other, narcissism is made to spread. Higher education in which the word 'higher' is drained of meaning reinforces on the social level the same phenomenon that

American family life brings about on an individual level. Our sham education takes neglected children who know only leniency and produces sham people—narcissistic, incomplete people who are handicapped for life by their schooling and by a society committed to mediocrity, as we shall see in Chapter 8, none of which can satisfy the narcissist's emptiness.

If we shift our perspective from psychology to human judgment, we realize that narcissism is ultimately barbarism.

BARBARITY AS A STATE OF MIND

> In the space of two or three generations, enormous stretches of the "Judaeo-Christian tradition"... have passed into oblivion. The effective loss of cultural traditions on such a scale makes talk of a new Dark Ages far from frivolous.
> —Christopher Lasch, *The Culture of Narcissism* (1979, pp. 260–61)

To call a man or woman a barbarian is to indict him or her for lack of civilization, for lack of cultivation, for lack of culture. Barbarity is more than the poverty of a loincloth—clothes, at least, have evolved—it is a state of mind. The ancient Greeks and Romans used the term to deprecate men and women outside their civilization who lived in primitive conditions but, in particular and more importantly, to name those with no sympathy for and comprehension of culture.

As we saw in the last chapter, culture is linked to *cultus*, to a public sense of respect and admiration, if only from a distance, toward a source of value that lies beyond the satisfaction of immediate human wants and needs. Culture is free from practical considerations: To be cultivated is to possess a refinement that puts mundane reality in its place, in perspective. It is, in a sense, to have one's head in the clouds while walking on the earth. It is an attitude; it does not derogate the importance of practical things—it is important to emphasize this—but neither is it their servant.

Culture is humanity's link between a world of mortality, finitude, work, and everyday cares, and a world of freedom from these burdens. *Cultus* refers to the capacity to step beyond the immediate and the mundane. Divine worship makes it possible for people to take this step, as do the liberating arts—philosophy, literature, fine art, music, and pure theoretical research.

Those for whom this world of freedom from utility does not exist are trapped in barbarity. Their shrunken sphere of concerns is limited to the satisfaction of immediate biological needs and desires. The only growth of perspective that can be expected of them is that they may develop an anxiety concerning the future satisfaction of those same immediate needs and wants. The result—"the barbarian with a pension plan"—is no more of a contradiction in terms than is "a squirrel that stores nuts." Neither the store of nuts nor the pension elevates.

Barbarity is an impoverishment of mind. It is an exclusive preoccupation with material gratification. It is a blindness to the feelings and autonomy of others. It is a lack of sensibility. And it is all that follows from these: savagery of manners and a desire for stimulation—the excitement of violence and sex, alcohol and drugs, and a sufficiently loud throb in music to permeate and exhilarate a dulled consciousness.

It isn't necessary for us to translate this meaning of barbarism to a higher level to see that today's college students, as a group, exhibit all of its defining characteristics. But then, outside of the ivy-covered walls, so does most of the society at large.

THE MEDIOCRE POPULATION, THE NEW BARBARIANS

Mediocrity, as we shall see later on, often takes the form of an intellectual impairment. The medieval Scholastics would have called it a state of impoverishment of the soul, an ignorant or willful confinement of vision that glorifies the trivial, the fatuous, the superficial.

In the last chapter, we saw how the medieval moral theologians identified an impoverishment and illness of the soul, which they called acedia. The mediocrity and social mediocracy in view here are manifestations of just such a psychological impoverishment. Modern psychology does not yet include mediocrity among its clinical categories, yet there can be no doubt that it is a stultifying and infectious disorder that permanently disables. Mediocrity is a blindness not of the eyes but of the mind, and in particular of that part of the mind in which our special cares and sympathies take up residence. Mediocrity is a disability of values, as we shall see in greater depth in Chapter 8.

The blindness of mediocrity is reflexive, that is to say, when men and women have this blindness, they cannot, for their very blindness, see that they are blind.[3] The world of their cares is hermetic, exclusionary of all that does not gratify consumption, provide an adrenaline fix, or act as a soporific. In short, for the mediocre, culture does not and *cannot* exist.

If we extend the diagnostic vocabulary of clinical practice to include mediocritized consciousness, today's disjointed pieces of the puzzle of higher education become easier to fit together. Assembled, they might look like this:

American education is controlled by an egalitarian distortion of democracy that flattens individual differences and glosses over distinctions. American family life is driven by the themes of money and career. They feed parental narcissism, which widens the emotional distance to children who are raised in an atmosphere of neglect and permissiveness. Family discipline and its social equivalent in the justice of the courts are fumbling affairs of leniency rationalized as tolerance. Caught in this web of laxity, indiscrimination, and materialism, the young, by the time they are ready to enter college, have established within themselves a mental fixity born of fear and disorientation that is strikingly narcissistic in its monadic self-encapsulation, in its fear and resentment of authority, and in its conformist rigidity and intellectual lassitude.

The result is the high-tech barbarian: rude, without appreciation for culture, crude in his tastes, raucous in his behavior, enthralled by the loud pulse of his music, and devoted to the accumulation of megabucks and the amassment of the shining baubles of tawdry affluence. The world of the new barbarian has no place for the ideal of higher education.

As with today's minorities, the handicapped, the disadvantaged, and the deficient, we are tempted to situate the barbarity of college students within a framework of egalitarian charity. We contentedly locate the failure of individual responsibility in these three areas: environment, heredity, and disease. The first serves to dilute individual incapacity and deficiency by spreading them thinly over a culpable environment: in this way, we environmentalize undesirable traits. The second, heredity, allows us to geneticize those traits when they will not abide reduction to environmental causality. The third, attacked by antimedical psychiatrist Thomas Szasz, allows us without misgiving to label as a "disease" what doesn't fit society's proprietary interests.

And so where once we had criminals, bad students, and censurable behavior, we now identify groups of the socially handicapped, culturally disadvantaged, and functionally impaired. We talk of "high-risk students" when we mean those who will probably flunk out or drop out. "Attention deficit disorders" reach epidemic proportions. Every sort of individual shortcoming—in aptitude, sensibility, critical judgment, alertness, manners, intellectual, aesthetic, or moral intelligence (Bartlett, 2005)—is euphemistically labeled and "democratically" excused. Depending on the nature of the diagnosed affliction, special therapists are needed to cope with the newly identified impairments and disorders.

No one is constitutionally *unable* to do anything any more.

We live in an age that, in these dissimulating and camouflaged ways, denies the existence of individual variation, repudiates unequal endowments, and so balks at acceptance of individual limitations. Like mediocrity itself, this denial and dishonesty are reflexive, for they perpetuate a cycle in which laxity is the rule and no one is responsible. This of course fuels the new barbarism.

THE NEW DARK AGE, ALREADY IN PROGRESS, AND THE DISAPPEARANCE OF HIGHER EDUCATION

Mediocrity and the rejection of individual accountability are vicious circles that theoretically can be cut, but it is too late for this. The only institutional solution that could stanch the tide is to place responsibility on college students and on their universities: that is, to brick up most of the breached doorway and to restrict passage to the comparatively few who are qualified and motivated, directing the rest to vocational schools. It would mean a reinstatement of curricular requirements and the detrivialization of higher degrees.

What is missing in our institutions of higher learning and in our homes reflects our opposition, born of a hyperexcited enthusiasm for social equality, to any semblance of elitism. This is an irony, for it is just what we lack that causes our pain. What is missing, ultimately, is that particular species of elitism, of hierarchical valuation, that goes with a recognition of values whose origin is suprapersonal. When right and wrong, better and worse, beautiful and ugly are meaningful in their own right, when we realize that not all is attributable to the subjective, relativist, multicultural eye of the beholder, higher education can get on with its proper task of cultivating and communicating culture, leaving the marketplace to take care of itself.

The elitism that we lack out of fear of social differentiation is identical to reverence for culture, reverence, that is, for certain values that give meaning to the phrase 'higher learning' by putting the world of daily cares in perspective. Without the vision of these higher and fragile things, meaningful living degenerates into crass and disoriented barbarism. When these higher values elicit our respect, a derivative respect is born automatically toward those who transmit culture to us. Only when this basis of respect is established can we appreciate and consciously *choose* the genuinely "higher" learning they represent.

This is elitism, in the original meaning of the Latin *eligere*, to choose. It is not antithetical to democracy, but it *is* incompatible with a society whose indiscrimination has set it adrift in a cultureless sea of narcissistic self-aggrandizement.

The myth of egalitarianism stands in the way of a reawakening of culture. Openness, homogeneity, and indiscrimination have impassioned, narrowed, and impoverished our society; not only will the equality-obsessed majority not question its commitments to devaluation, its members possess the blindly willful pride of narcissists. "Quarry the granite rock with razors, or moor the vessel with a thread of silk; then you may hope with such keen and delicate instruments as human knowledge and human reason to contend with those giants, the passion and pride of man" (Newman, 1852/1960, p. 91).

And besides, it would be too expensive. Our universities, which have grown fat on open admissions, grade inflation,[4] and usurious mass-printed degrees, will resist any effort to restrict the hoards flowing through their doors.

The economic momentum is too great to countenance change away from "universal higher education," the oxymoron that names the great travesty of academia. Individual merit exacts too many costs, and the material benefits are simply not there. To oppose mediocrity, one would need to fly in the face of misguided democracy's fear of cultural discrimination. To resist the ever-increasing momentum is simply too much to expect.

The deck is stacked against the ideal of higher education. We have discarded the natural elitism of unequal ability. And we have discarded the nonutilitarian values of the *artes liberales*; they have been squeezed out in a fervent embrace of money, utility, and homogeneity.

Fads are momentary preoccupations; an age, however, endures for a long time. What is it that accounts for the difference between the transitoriness of a fad and the lingering character of an age?

On the most fundamental level, what appears to be responsible is the presence or absence of reflexivity, the recursive, self-maintaining character of a system that enables it to endure.[5] Both a fad and an age have an internal dynamic. The dynamic of the one lacks equilibrium; it quickly burns out. The dynamic of the other is self-reinforcing and so is self-perpetuating. A fad is transitory because the values and behaviors it excites do not feed back into and diffuse throughout those of an entire society. An age endures precisely because the opposite is true: A society's values and the activity of its members achieve a self-regulating homeostasis that maintains itself more or less efficiently. Lacking this, its reflexive inefficiency, like friction in a perpetual motion machine, ultimately brings it to a stop, and when that happens a new age begins.

The barbarians at the doors of our colleges and universities are not an aberrant and passing phenomenon. They are the symptom, not the cause, of a self-reinforcing period of history in which a psychology of narcissism, mediocrity, and indiscrimination; a mythology of egalitarianism; the raising of normality to serve as a gold standard of desirability; a denial of individual accountability; and a base focus on work and money have combined. They have combined in a remarkably self-supporting, self-reinforcing way.

The dynamic of this interplay of forces suggests the birth of an age, not a passing fad. Only other, stronger forces can perturb its equilibrium, as wars, plagues, and overpopulation do.

The barbarians at the door have now overrun the colleges and universities of America. The same has happened in other industrialized countries. Higher education is history. The ideal remains, but the human response has died with only a murmur.

SOBERING REFLECTIONS

At this point, I want to return to the basic claim made in the Introduction to this book, that people prefer to believe what gives them gratification and equally prefer to reject what does not. We should add to this that the strength of rejection goes up very considerably when confronted by ungratifying *and downright unpleasant* beliefs! We've come face to face in this chapter with a group of observations that many people—according to those very observations—simply do not like because they conflict with the current, conventionally preferred values of industrialized society. For many people, the strength of the perceived conflict is decidedly unpleasant. The psychology of human belief being what it is, we should expect many people therefore not to want to believe such unpleasant observations and to hurry to reject them.

There are different ways to reject propositions that we don't like. One way is to ignore them and go on with our usual lives, retaining our beliefs and practices unchanged. Another is to get mad, feel that we've been offended, and reject the offending propositions not because they're not true but because they've given rise to offense. A third and very common way to reject what we don't like is to summon up in our minds reasons for dismissing the unacceptable propositions, reasons that we very single-mindedly believe to be good, compelling ones—that we don't intend to give up, come what may.

Ignoring what we don't like condemns it to silence. Taking offense gives us an excuse to reject what we dislike, with no other needed justification than the offense taken. Holding beliefs intractably despite challenges to them is the ultimate defensive dodge, one that is typically exempted from rational confrontation when the believer claims they are based on "faith" or "gut feeling."

Underlying all three of these intellectually dishonest responses is, very frequently, a deeply rooted opposition to propositions that, if we should accept them to be true, would take away from us a more cheerful, optimistic view of things. To put the matter directly: we are, most of us, equipped with a mental "circuit-breaker" that kicks in if our need for optimism is short-circuited. It is, to speak diplomatically, "as though" most people cannot bear to live with the real truths about their human condition and so seek refuge in optimism, in the "positive illusion" discussed in Chapter 1. Optimism sugarcoats unpleasant reality so as to make it more palatable. As Nietzsche expressed this in his *Birth of Tragedy* (1992, p. 18), such avoidance borne of a need to maintain illusion is "morally speaking, a sort of cowardice."

Unfortunately, such a self-protective circuit breaker is not adaptive; rather than fostering an accurate perception of reality, it results in denial and illusion. It is, however, an effective means to defend and preserve our existing beliefs. It blocks unbiased processing of new information that conflicts with what we prefer to belief and helps us to continue to believe what we *like*, unimpeded. Unhappily, when we face a challenge that requires a change in our beliefs in order to emerge from a dead-end situation, constructive mental functioning that is subject to such circuit-breaking is fated to fail. One cannot escape from a blind alley if the mind shuts down whenever confronted by a dead end. We have, for some time, been facing just such a dead end and critical challenge in connection with higher education.

If the observations I've made in this chapter are accurate, we face an impasse concerning the future of higher education. Because of the critical importance of higher education to humanity's future, this impasse poses perhaps the most important challenge in the world (foreseen in precisely these terms by Robert Hutchins, 1952, p. 17). But the situation is not a pretty one, and the facts and observations I've brought together in this chapter are a thorn to optimism. Further, they are expressed here in much-needed, direct, no-nonsense language—in just the sort of optimism-deflating propositions that, for many people, are likely to cause their mental circuit breakers to kick in, bringing to a halt their ability to think dispassionately.

There is no easy solution to this. The best that I, and I think any author, can do is to encourage the reader to be reflectively aware of his or her *reflexive* way of reacting to the propositions this chapter has affirmed. There is no shorter route to intellectual honesty than self-knowledge.

If the situation facing higher education indeed does not inspire hope, then at least we have accomplished something in understanding that situation more clearly. To paraphrase Hutchins' point of view in this context, by understanding the psychology and history of higher education as we've sought to do, we may not feel at home in the world of practical affairs in the sense of liking the way of life we find about us, but we will feel more at home in the world in the sense that we understand it more clearly (Hutchins, 1952, p. 4).

NOTES

1. An earlier discussion of the subject matter of this chapter was published as an article with the same title concomitantly in the Netherlands in *Methodology and Science 26*(1) (1993), pp. 18–40 and in the United States in *Modern Age 35*(4) (Summer 1993), pp. 296–310. (Readers consulting the latter publication should see the journal's "Note to Our Readers" printed in Vol. *36*(3), p. 303.) The account provided here is revised, updated, supplemented, and the focus changed to fit the context of this book.

2. An annual survey conducted by the University of California at Los Angeles and the American Council on Education very unambiguously supports this fact. Over the past 40 years, UCLA researchers have studied some quarter of a million entering college students. During the 1960s and early 1970s, when asked why they wanted to go to college, the majority of students said they felt a need to become "an educated person" and develop "a philosophy of life." But starting in the 1990s, there was a significant shift: the majority of students then began to claim that their main reason for attending college was to make "a lot of money" (see Sax et al., 1998). Not coincidentally, as a reminder of the harm resulting from acedia, examined in the previous chapter, this degrading of values has occurred in conjunction with a major increase among college students of psychological difficulties, including depression and suicide.

3. This was Newman's description of the self-inflicted blindness of religious dogma, referring to Catholics' views of education in England during the first half of the last century (Newman, 1852/1960).

4. To cite one example: UCLA receives more freshman applications than any other university in the United States, some 50,744 applicants in November, 2006. The average GPA—note that this is the *average* GPA—of the incoming class for the year 2007, was 4.30 (*UCLA Magazine*, October 2007, p. 12), a veritable *reductio ad absurdum* of inflationary grading policies, still flourishing without check.

The following belief has now achieved near-universal acceptance: the belief that the great majority of children deserve "high" recognition for their alleged superior abilities. One should be reminded of the dictum, rejected by Freud, *credo, quia absurdum*—I believe *because* it is absurd (Freud 1930/1952, p. 786).

5. Reflexivity is a separate and fascinating subject unto itself. See Bartlett (1987 and 1992).

6

Psychology, Culture, and the Demoralization of University Faculty

Work was for him, in the nature of things, the most estimable attribute of life; when you came down to it, there was nothing else that was estimable. It was the principle by which one stood or fell, the Absolute of the time; it was, so to speak, its own justification. His regard for it was thus religious in its character, and, so far as he knew, unquestioning.
—Thomas Mann, *The Magic Mountain*

Without work all life goes rotten. But when work is soulless, life stifles and dies.
—Albert Camus (quoted in Rohrlich, 1980, p. 231)

In Chapter 4, I described a form of depression engendered by acedia, a pervasive psychological deficit in the industrialized countries of the world that has resulted in society-wide cultural impoverishment.[1] In Chapter 5, I turned to examine the psychological and historical background that, in the United States and other Western industrialized countries, has led to the cultural impoverishment of higher education and to a resulting narrowing of outlook and mediocritization of its students. Although we've looked at society-wide cultural impoverishment and the decline of higher education separately in these chapters, we need to be reminded that they clearly are not phenomena independent of one another, for they affect each other mutually.

In our effort to understand the psychology of a society and its higher education, both of which emphasize work and money to the exclusion of consciousness of and respect for culture in its classical meaning, there is a third important part of the picture that remains to be considered: the psychology of university faculty, for it has been upon the shoulders of university professors, in particular liberal arts professors, that the responsibility has rested to communicate the values of culture to their students. The wider society has been severely disabled by the accelerating dissolution of cultural awareness and esteem for culture, and college students have, in a parallel way, been rendered culturally disabled by a system of higher education and by a society in which the meaning of 'higher' has been lost. These two phenomena have had an unexamined effect upon those who serve as the living memory and transmitters of culture: university faculty, to whose psychology we now turn.

Social psychologists hope to take notice of potentially significant changes in cultural values and their effects in personal life while these changes are still subtle. During the last four decades, a gradual trend in higher education and, in particular, in higher liberal arts education, has been a source of concern among people who recognize the influence of the present upon the future of the university. Some of this attention has been directed toward expressions of discontent and high levels of stress among liberal arts faculty. The informal descriptive name for this phenomenon has been 'faculty burnout', which designates a part of more general research relating to career burnout.

    A good deal has now been written about career burnout, less about disillusionment among university faculty, and still less about the specific problems experienced by liberal arts faculty. Most of the more general research dealing with stress in the academic world has held that faculty burnout is due to the gradual erosion of a usually young professor's idealism in an environment lacking in gratification. The reasons given for this lack of gratification are multiple. In general they tend to fall into two categories: the frustrating blocks that young faculty often encounter when they wish to bring about changes in the way higher education is managed and offered to students, and the general absence of direct recognition and approval received by younger faculty from their administrations and older colleagues. Burnout among specifically liberal arts faculty has been viewed from this perspective, emphasizing the frustration felt by young, idealistic faculty who don't receive the acceptance and appreciation they need to sustain them. Without attempting to discriminate problems experienced by faculty in different areas of study, this point of view has been applied in a generic way to burnout experienced by faculty in a wide range of disciplines. There has been no attempt to study the specific psychology of faculty demoralization in the liberal arts, which, as I suggest here, is substantively different from burnout in other professions.

This chapter seeks to widen our understanding of the psychology of faculty demoralization by focusing on its occurrence in the liberal arts. The demoralization of liberal arts faculty in higher education today is a phenomenon that is not on a par with career burnout in other professions. The frustration of youthful idealism and the absence of sufficient, direct, and personal appreciation from one's senior colleagues and from superiors in the college bureaucracy do certainly wear down young liberal arts faculty. But the demoralization that they, as well as many of their older colleagues, feel is more than this.

THE NATURE OF CAREER BURNOUT

Career burnout, inside or outside of the academy, is fundamentally connected with the human need for meaning. When a person's work supports and strengthens the perception of meaningfulness, those who are highly motivated will excel; but when their work detracts from and even undermines their ability to find meaning in what they do, burnout is only a matter of time. Burnout is not the same thing as work stress, depression from overwork, or alienation, though it usually involves these. One of the clearest general descriptions of career burnout has been given by Ayala Pines and Elliot Aronson:

> Burnout is formally defined and subjectively experienced as a state of physical, emotional, and mental exhaustion caused by long-term involvement in situations that are emotionally demanding. The emotional demands are most often caused by a combination of very high expectations and chronic situational stresses. Burnout is accompanied by an array of symptoms including physical depletion, feelings of helplessness and hopelessness, disillusionment, and the development of a negative self-concept and negative attitudes toward work, people involved in work, and life itself. In its extreme form burnout represents a breaking point beyond which the ability to cope with the environment is severely hampered. (Pines & Aronson, 1988, pp. 9–10)

The study by Pines and Aronson suggests that there is a psychological profile which is often typical of people who experience career burnout. More than does the average person,

- they tend to be idealistic, in that they expect their work to give their lives a sense of meaning—"burnout most often happens to people who initially cared the least about their paychecks" (Pines & Aronson, 1988, p. 53);

- they tend to be especially caring about their work and its value, sometimes so much so that they regard their work as a "calling"; and
- they are often highly motivated to achieve, in a way that goes beyond routine high achievement, due to a strong and unquestioned belief that success in one's discipline is closely associated with one's worth as a human being.

People with these qualities tend to burn out when their work environment has these characteristics:

- It frustrates, and may completely block, their aspirations. The frustration they experience, given their high expectations and need for meaningful work, soon erodes their spirit.
- Their work offers minimal personal rewards in the context of inescapable stresses that cannot be lessened or changed.
- Their work load is excessive, or else work itself does not provide sufficient challenge because they are overtrained and do not feel well utilized.

When their work comes to have little or no meaning and the stresses of work day after day outweigh its rewards, burnout becomes inevitable. As mentioned in the above quotation, Pines and Aronson have found that the victims of career burnout experience one or more of the following forms of exhaustion or depletion, which we can distinguish as:

- Mental exhaustion: difficulty concentrating, impaired creativity, and negative attitudes toward one's self, others, one's work, and life generally
- Emotional exhaustion: feelings of helplessness in situations they cannot control, entrapment, and depression
- Physical exhaustion: chronic fatigue, lowered resistance to illnesses, headaches, neck and back pain, eating disorders, and problems in sleeping

Unfortunately, the unreflective tendency among the majority of mental health practitioners is automatically to pursue a course of treatment that encourages the person to adjust to the existing work environment. Pines and Aronson's study opposes this tendency by emphasizing that the major causes of burnout reside in the work environment itself. Their outlook is hopeful, even if unrealistic: "Since we view environments as more amenable to change than persons' personalities, we prefer to direct our efforts to work environments" (Pines & Aronson, 1988, p. 79). They believe that it is the work environment that must be changed, rather than the individual:

> How individuals perceive the cause of their burnout and attribute the "blame" has enormous consequences for action. If they attribute the cause to a characterological weakness or inadequacy in themselves, they will take a certain set of actions: quit the profession, seek psychotherapy, and so forth. However, if they see the cause as largely a function of the situation, they will strive to change the situation to make it more tolerable, a totally different set of remedial actions.... [O]ur work has made it clear that, in the vast majority of cases of burnout, the major cause lies in the situation. (Pines & Aronson, 1988, p. 5)

It is not my purpose to pull the pendulum to one side in this individual versus environment debate. However, it is important to underscore the fact that traditional psychological treatment for career burnout, in its one-sided focus upon individual adjustment, tends to avoid placing responsibility upon the environment.

When career burnout is most severe, the individual becomes clinically depressed and may then benefit from some variety of treatment. However, if, indeed, career burnout is to a great extent situationally caused then treating clinically depressed individuals who have become burned out in their careers exclusively by means of individual adjustment therapies is likely to be both inappropriate and, as we will see, potentially injurious to them.

This is especially true of the burnout of faculty in the liberal arts, as the remainder of this chapter attempts to show.

THE CONCEPT OF SITUATIONAL DEPRESSION

Of the theories advanced to explain depression, among those *least* in vogue among clinicians is the theory of situational depression. To claim that depression is situational is equivalent to blaming the environment for an individual's suffering. This directly conflicts with the individual adjustment bias of psychiatry and most current theories of psychotherapy. Because the majority of psychologists, psychiatrists, and social workers today believe that clinical depression, often associated with serious career burnout, is an *illness* that has its causal basis in the individual, the treatment that is favored by them seeks to change the person—specifically attitudes or other mental and emotional dispositions, or neurochemistry, or all of these. The alleviation of depression, in this view, is a matter of treating the individual—by helping the person better to adjust to his or her environment. The help that is offered seeks to adjust individual attitudes and biochemistry until a more compatible, comfortable fit between individual and environment is accomplished. Seen from this point of view, clinicians serve the purposes of social adjustment, normalization, and conditioning: They help people to continue to carry on with their conventionally endorsed social roles and responsibilities.

So-called "life events research" has been more sensitive to the situational relationship between an individual's depression and his or her life goals, values, perception of obstacles, hopes for success or expectation of failure, and so on. From this point of view, Klinger (1975, 1977) and Nesse (2000) have observed that depression can serve to motivate a person to find a way out of blind alleys, to give up unreachable goals, and to become free from a sense of entrapment in a destructive situation. In this sense, Klinger and Nesse proposed that depression can be *adaptive* because it may serve as a healthy defense against *circumstances* that are harmful and demoralizing. However, such a situational understanding of depression, which claims that an individual's depression is attributable to or largely due to outward circumstances, is relatively infrequent among clinicians; others who have given a nod in that direction include Brown and Harris (1978) and Bowlby (1969–1982, Vol. 3, pp. 254–56).

We should expect that a situational view of depression would be more the province of the social psychologist, who is less directly involved in the treatment of individuals. But even here, situational depression is a concept with comparatively few adherents, perhaps because environmental causes of depression are, Pines' and Aronson's optimism notwithstanding, much less easily changed than may be the attitudes and biochemistry of a particular person. In addition, it can be complex and potentially problematic to evaluate the therapeutic effectiveness of environmental changes in alleviating an individual's depression, due to the absence of comparative experimental controls.

In terms of the question of whether its origin is situational or individual, studies of the phenomenon of career burnout have been both moderate and ambivalent. The majority of researchers who have studied it describe burnout and its treatment in individual psychological terms, although they occasionally and vaguely allude to environmental sources. As yet there has been virtually no clarification of the fundamental questions: to what extent burnout among faculty is a problem due to differing individual sensitivities and to what extent it is contextual. Certainly a more balanced and comprehensive knowledge of burnout requires a better understanding of its situational basis.

THE SITUATION IN THE LIBERAL ARTS

> I consider reality to be the thing one need concern oneself about least of all, for it is, tediously enough, always at hand while more beautiful and necessary things demand our attention and care. Reality is that which one must not under any circumstances worship and revere, for it is chance, the refuse of life. And it is in no wise to be changed, this shabby, consistently disappointing reality, except by our denying it and proving in the process that we are stronger than it.
>
> —Hermann Hesse (1925/1954, p. 67)

Readers may recall this quotation from Hesse in Chapter 3, relevant there in connection with the psychology of creative people. I've quoted Hesse again here because his words are also applicable in a discussion of the psychology of classically oriented liberal arts faculty, as we'll see.

The point of view advanced in this section is phenomenological, a point of view that is fundamentally one of descriptive, definitional logic rather than empirical observation derived from consensus taking. I take for granted as obvious that the nature and goals of the liberal arts can be interpreted in many ways; but my purpose here is to show how, given a traditional, classical conception of the liberal arts, burnout among faculty who hold that conception within the context of today's universities is a phenomenon that is to be expected, is understandable, and, ironically, should be judged as a sign of mental health on the part of the affected individuals. These consequences follow, I submit, strictly from the inner logic of descriptions of the experience of these individuals. But the consequences are essentially human, not merely logical, and they bring pronounced human suffering with them. The purpose in developing the perspective that follows is to provide a clearer context in which the victims of liberal arts demoralization can understand and accept themselves, and in terms of which their sometimes puzzled colleagues and administrators perhaps may acquire a deeper measure of empathy and support for their plight. And, too, it is my hope that you, the reader, will gain a richer and more concrete, person-centered understanding of what "culture" means to a small and specialized population for whom liberal arts values are central.

For this purpose, it would perhaps be helpful if you will agree to suspend (or bracket) your own conception of the nature and goals of the liberal arts (if your idea of these differs) and, for the purposes of argument, to consider with as much intellectual sympathy as you can summon the human sequelae of the stipulative descriptions that follow. These stipulations make clear to you what I presuppose is experienced by the small group of university professors in question:

There is a population of faculty in the liberal arts who, sometimes without self-conscious analysis, see themselves and their discipline in classical terms—that is, they hold a clearly defined set of beliefs about the fundamental purposes of liberal arts study and perhaps a slightly less well-formulated concept of their role in its teaching and scholarship. Among their beliefs are likely to be found convictions similar to the following:

The liberal arts, or *artes liberales*, are, both in kind and in value, essentially distinct from the servile arts, or *artes serviles*, in certain ways.

- The servile arts are mundane and of a chorelike nature, concerned as they are with the impermanent worldly trappings of monetary success and practical effect. The liberal arts, in contrast, intend to liberate the individual from the concerns of the practical, material universe and to open for him or her dimensions of human experience that are qualitatively different.

- These dimensions of experience comprise a separate, distinguishable universe of meaning, one perceived to be a source of the significance of servile life. In this sense, the universe to which the liberating arts provide access is hierarchically superior to the lower-order world of servile pursuits. This is not a matter of marshalling objective and empirical facts but, again, of stipulative, definitional logic. It has the form, "If one understands the liberal arts in their classical meaning, then the above perception is a psychological consequence."

- In the view of the classical liberal arts scholar, human beings are unequally endowed in both their practical capacities and in their personal abilities to gain access to this second-order, higher reality. Their practical capacities differ because of differences in personal taste, inclination, and ability, as well as in their opportunities to develop liberating skills. On the one hand, this can be a simple matter of individual preference, but it can also reflect a poverty of opportunity to attend top-notch institutions of higher learning, to acquire libraries of fine books, of musical recordings, collections of art, and other expressions of culture, as well as the scarcity of time to cultivate liberal pursuits. On the other hand, individual abilities differ as a result of inborn talent; learned interest; discipline and drive; and intellectual, moral, and aesthetic capability.

- Not infrequently, individuals who are particularly well-suited to liberal arts study are ill-suited, or not suited at all, to other professions, just as the opposite is true. Like Thales, who, as legend has it, fell into a well because his eyes were fixed on the stars, traditional liberal arts scholars tend not to be adept do-it-yourselfers in the material world; they tend not to fit the corporate mold; their psychological and personal profiles do not accord with the practical needs of ordinary reality's workforce.

- Partly as a result of their accurate self-assessment, some liberal arts scholars feel drawn ineluctably to their chosen profession with either something akin to a sense of mission or a more self-effacing acceptance that this is all they can do competently. Their sense of mission relates to their perception that meaning in the transitory practical world is ultimately derivative from an enduring universe of more permanent realities.

These are some of the central convictions that define the perspective of the classical liberal arts scholar. From the individual's point of view, it is inherently delimitative and judgmental. The lines of meaning are pre-drawn for such a scholar; he (using the author's gender, but 'she' is also understood throughout) fits into a bipartite reality in a nonambidextrous fashion: Where he can touch his finger to his nose with consummate skill in a higher dimension, he often is completely at a loss in everyday life. On the one hand he is endowed with a gift, and on the other is often the victim of a disability. He can see in the world of the blind, but often blunders blindly in the midst of those whose vision is mundane.

He is furthermore judgmental, since his perspective is essentially elitist and nonegalitarian. For him, however, elitism and the natural rights of humanity are not in themselves necessarily political issues or manifestations of personal arrogance, but facts in a life-world that is constituted as it is. This is the province of phenomenological psychology's descriptive interest in the *logos* of the psyche, a concern to make explicit the regulative principles of a particular, individual life-world. That there exists a higher and a lower reality is as evident to the classical liberal arts scholar as that automobiles emit pollution is to the person on the street. Here, empirical studies with double-blind controls are simply irrelevant. Experienced reality for the classically paradigmatic liberal arts scholar comes with built-in indications of what is higher and what is lower.

Unfortunately for him, the political sensitivity of other men and women is easily ruffled. His in principle innocent perspective, which provides the scholar with a sense of balance and orientation toward what for him is most meaningful, is capable of being used against him by the politically driven. Elitism and a repudiation of egalitarian principles admittedly can lead to overweening pride and abusive social evils, but this fact, with its historical, political, educational, and highly emotional overtones, is out of place in this discussion, where my intent is purely to describe some central characteristics of the experience of the classically disposed liberal arts scholar.

With this descriptive sketch before us, we turn to look at the work environment as it is perceived by the traditional liberal arts professional. As we saw in some detail in the last chapter, higher education in America has changed considerably from the time of Newman, who had less to complain of then. Josef Pieper has come and gone, Allan Bloom briefly stirred a certain amount of dust, but in the end, education today, as we've seen, is no longer "higher" in the meaning that traditionally was attributed to it.

The work environment of university professors has accordingly changed, and it imposes restrictive boundaries on the efforts of the classical liberal arts scholar. A single aspect of his environment affects him most deeply: it is limited by the constricted values, interests, and range of vision of the majority of his students, with whom he is in daily contact. At the same time, the same shrunken perspective is often advocated by his university administrators and many of his colleagues. Like the creative individuals described in Chapter 3, he is impaired, as we shall see, by the impairments of the normal world.

Contact with students comprises the main context for his professional exertions, for it is their talk that fills his ears, their papers that occupy his eyes, and their values and interests that in the end give him pause for reappraisal. To understand the phenomenon of demoralization among university faculty in the liberal arts, we need to consider dispassionately what it is that the majority of students care most about, frequently to the exclusion of all else. In Chapter 4, we examined the phenomenon of "work-engendered depression," a condition due to an exclusionary focus upon work, money, and things. As we saw, many centuries ago such depression was clearly acknowledged and comprehended with a remarkable degree of clarity and was named 'acedia' by the Scholastics. Acedia is no more and no less than a form of psychological malnutrition in which an individual, or an entire people, has lost contact with the very realities that concern the classical liberal arts scholar. These realities may be of an intellectual, moral, or aesthetic kind; they may be highly theoretical and ideal in nature; and as a result, they have the capacity to liberate a man or woman from the confines of an empty dedication to the workplace, social networking, shopping malls, and financial planning. We saw that the culturally depleted universe of people who inhabit a world of total work can lead to a variety of depression little understood today.

Industrialized societies that promote such depression through their exclusionary emphasis on work and money correspondingly promote an approach to college and university education that fosters a culturally depleted mindset among its students, as we saw in the last chapter. During the past 40 years of my professional life, it has been my repeatedly confirmed observation that, more than any other single group, college students exhibit the symptoms of acedia. As the decades have passed, these symptoms have become more extreme, more pronounced, and more prevalent. We recall that acedia serves as a barrier that stands between the man or woman who is a slave to the world of work and money, and higher values. It is an impairment preventing people from transforming the mundane. The result is that their universe of concerns excludes all that is not mediocre. Contact with culture, *cultus*, with the cultivation of liberating arts, is lost, and with this loss has come a certain impairment of mental abilities and an incapacity to cultivate leisure in the sense described in Chapter 4.

Plausibly much of the fault for acedia does not lie with students themselves but with the society and with their families who have encouraged and transmitted to them the incapacitating blinders they wear. And yet it is the students themselves, who are the products of cultural disability, who populate the classes of the classical liberal arts professor. The professor sees before him, day in and day out, legions of students who manifest the symptoms of acedia. Most are young, but acedia has nevertheless already taken firm hold in their minds, hearts, and vocationally compulsive tunnel vision. The consequences upon the classically oriented liberal arts professor are equally pronounced, for he is caught in the neverending ordeal of the classically trained musician forced to perform before audiences who are not receptive, and may be openly hostile, to classical music. The values and skills that he seeks to impart, which define and open access to a reality of a higher order, fall upon ears that have been deafened by loud rock music and upon eyes dulled by the narrowed vision of university education in the service of job acquisition whose purpose is moneymaking.

SITUATIONAL DEPRESSION OF FACULTY IN THE LIBERAL ARTS

I have tried briefly to describe a certain type of individual, whom I've called the classically inspired liberal arts professor and, as seen through his eyes, his audience today. When the liberal arts professor is fully committed to his subject and to the values of its study, and when his audience unquestioningly focuses on vocational and monetary values to the exclusion of all else, the work environment of the professor can lead to situational depression of a particular kind. His environment stands in direct conflict with his sense of self: His students are victims of a disease of the spirit, acedia, an intellectual, moral, or aesthetic disability which blocks them from cultivating the higher learning he would teach. Moreover, the liberal arts professor is trapped by his work environment in the academy, perhaps believing his teaching and research to constitute a personal

calling, on the one hand, while potential alternatives to his academic profession bring him face to face with the shortcomings he experiences in
"lower reality," on the other.

This is the essence of a psychologically double-binding situation: the
liberal arts professor is damned if he does and damned if he doesn't.
A well-acknowledged cause of depression is just this sort of entrapment
in a situation that brings deep pain and from which the only perceived
escape is itself severely painful.

Career burnout in other professions does not involve this complex
dynamic or the distressing and profound conflict both with one's personal
sense of identity and with the conception of one's role in the world.

ADJUSTMENT DISORDERS AND THE LIBERAL ARTS

Earlier in this chapter I referred to the tendency of mental health prov-
iders today to implement individual adjustment therapies in cases of
career burnout, and I mentioned in passing that individual adjustment
therapy for liberal arts professors can be injurious. I'd like to return to this
subject briefly.

The only *DSM* diagnostic classification that seems to apply to the situational depression of liberal arts faculty is "adjustment disorder, with
work inhibition," a classification we also encountered in discussing the
psychology of the artist and the psychology of acedia. Here again is the
relevant *DSM* passage:

> The essential feature of this disorder is a maladaptive reaction to an
> identifiable psychological stressor.... The maladaptive nature of the
> reaction is indicated ... by impairment in occupational (including school)
> functioning.... [T]he predominant manifestation is an inhibition in
> work ... occurring in a person whose previous work ... performance has
> been adequate. Frequently there is a mixture of anxiety and depression.
> (American Psychiatric Association, 1987, code 309.23, pp. 329, 331; in
> APA, 1994 and 2000, absorbed under code 309.9)

Two judgments embedded in this classification need to be made explicit:
first is the judgment that the condition constitutes a "mental disorder," and
second is the claim that the disorder is "maladaptive." These assessments
point to the likely treatment that situationally depressed liberal arts faculty
will receive if they seek psychological or psychiatric help.

If you the reader are willing to move beyond the limits prescribed
by the current classification of mental disorders, perhaps you'll agree
that what certain liberal arts faculty experience today is most akin to

demoralization rather than maladaptive mental illness. This demoralization is a secondary dysfunction, to speak clinically, acquired as a result of the long-term, inescapable exposure of these university professors to acedia, both in their students and embodied in their administrations. Morale is a matter of spirit, certainly of emotional and mental health. When a situation is destructive to morale, it is destructive to an individual's spirit, depleting the energy and desire to realize his or her human potential.

As we've seen, the Scholastics believed that the despair to which acedia leads has precisely this life-blocking effect. In much the same way, the secondary despair of the liberal arts professor is destructive of his potential; he is caught in a work environment in which, in his perception, the members of his student audience—his customers, in this market-oriented society—are functionally impaired in the sense of being mentally handicapped (intellectually, morally, or aesthetically) so as to be incapable of the cultivation he aspires to encourage in them.

The demoralization of liberal arts faculty in question here is not a matter of mental disability; there is no impairment of mental faculties as there is in the condition of acedia. There exist no directly applicable categories in the classification system of psychotherapy with which to label this situational byproduct of acedia. Perhaps the closest is the disorder of demoralization that Viktor Frankl called "noögenic neurosis," his term for existential frustration that occurs when a person's will to meaning is blocked (Frankl, 1955, 1959). The suffering that such frustration brings is the result of a conflict between opposing values—in this chapter, the conflict between the deeply rooted commitments of the liberal arts scholar, understood as essentially absolutist, hierarchical, and elitist—and the vocational, materialist, relativist, multiculturalist, and monetary values that circumscribe the normal interests of the majority of his students and usually also of his university administration.

Other than Frankl's work, George A. Kelly's theory of personal constructs offers a framework in terms of which liberal arts demoralization can profitably be understood. Kelly's therapeutic orientation, like the approach of his contemporary J. H. van den Berg (1955), is phenomenologically sensitive to the world as a person experiences or construes it. Speaking of his clients, Kelly commented: "We have observed only that they do what they do because their choice systems are definitely limited" (Kelly 1956/1978, p. 121; see also Kelly, 1955). The choices open to a person are a reflection, according to Kelly, of the individual's personal constructs, of the "channels of thought" that he or she uses to construe events. Kelly saw these channels as a maze that each person builds and calls his or her own. "The labyrinth is conceived as a network of constructs, each of which is an abstraction and, as such, can be picked up and laid down over many different events in order to bring them into focus and clothe them with personal meaning" (Kelly, 1956/1978, pp. 123–24).

Kelly would probably have portrayed liberal arts demoralization as acute frustration over the narrowed choices that exist from the point of view of the liberal arts professor. When all perceived alternatives are without real hope, demoralization becomes inevitable, appropriate, and understandable. For the classical liberal arts professor, the only alternatives not destructive to the self are to continue to profess a set of values to an otherwise-disposed and deafened audience or to leave the only work environment suited to the kind of person he believes himself to be. It is a dilemma of assured discontent.

'Axiological demoralization', if not such a mouthful, may come closer to an accurate name for impairment due to the experience of incompatibility between an individual's most cherished values and those that define his or her environment. Mircea Eliade refers to the *axis mundi* of certain primitive societies, which both anchors the meaning of the individual lives of members of the society and gives direction to their activities.[2] Axiological demoralization is the experience of the loss of the power of an individual's *axis mundi* to provide life with meaningful direction. Loss of religious faith would be an example, when this loss leads to despair.

For professors whose *axis mundi* is the cultivation of liberating skills and study, such axiological demoralization can assume the character of clinical depression. Yet, because of the uncritical application of individual adjustment therapies to alleviate depression, which I commented on earlier, standard clinical treatment of axiological demoralization is likely to be injurious to such a person.

The reason is straightforward: for anyone whose sense of purpose in living, whose sense of personal identity and capacity for fulfillment, are fundamentally tied to liberating skills and a vision of enduring, ideal, nonmaterial realities, *adjustment to the workplace*, when the academic world of today is involved, is equivalent to destruction of self—literally a form of self-mutilation: Huxley's metaphor applies squarely here—that a person should have his or her eyes put out in order to fit into a society of the blind. This would constitute a destructive form of *prescribed adaptation* that starts with a clinician's perception of misfit between the professor and reality and which then seeks to encourage a normalized, adaptive fit—in the process undermining the individual's source of life meaning.

The application of individual adjustment therapies leads to just such an effect on those whose insight and enlightenment lift them out of the mundanity and mediocrity of the everyday world.

TREATMENT FOR LIBERAL ARTS DEMORALIZATION

Strictly from a phenomenological point of view, two factors play a central role in situational depression among liberal arts faculty: their claim to a higher reality to which the rest of the world is now largely blind and the resistance and even opposition to their values by students and university administrators who are victims of acedia. Outside of the specialized context of the liberal arts to which I'm referring in this chapter, it can be a good deal more conspicuously objectionable when, in some countries, psychiatry is used to label social dissidents—that is, those with politically "maladaptive" attitudes—as "mentally ill." Occasionally, a Thomas Szasz will remark on the similarity closer to home. We live in a society that has become ideologically hysterical about the evils of elitism and the need for a homogenized populace that has been politically purified of standards of cultural excellence. This is the social context within which the situational depression of liberal arts faculty is assessed and treated. It makes sense that our society should be incapable of real sympathy toward the situationally based demoralization of liberal arts faculty. It is understandable that in their response to prevailing social values that prescribe normality as a standard, mental health professionals should classify the demoralization of liberal arts faculty as a maladaptive mental illness. It is the expected reflex of a society blind to liberating values.

If we take the idea seriously that faculty demoralization in the liberal arts is neither maladaptive nor a mental disease, but instead regard it to be a phenomenologically *appropriate* response to a destructive situation, there are, unfortunately, few realistic alternatives for treatment available. Pines and Aronson would prescribe changing the environment. But the environment here is contemporary higher education itself, which, in the perception of the classical liberal arts scholar, has lost the ability to discriminate higher from lower and has succumbed to vocationalism. Today's anti-elitist, relativist, multiculturalist, equality-of-aptitudes ideology offers no socially authorized niche for the liberal arts scholar. His elitism is mistaken as arrogance, his avowal of "higher-order realities" is misconstrued as seditious, and his acceptance in his students of unequal abilities, talents, levels of motivation, discipline, and interest is misinterpreted as a rejection of democratic principles.

From the edge of this precipice, the outlook is grim, for the liberal arts scholar is no more and no less than an anachronism, and for many, an undesirable anachronism. He or she is simply irrelevant to the social order and to the values of the day.

Given that the dynamic of the current social and educational mindset is strongly self-sustaining and resistant to change, as we saw in the last chapter, plausible treatment options for the variety of depression experienced by the liberal arts scholar are few. Two that do not fundamentally compromise the scholar's values and role in living come to mind: The first alternative is to cultivate an essentially private monasticism within the academy, viewing his or her life and work as preserving liberal arts values for a possible future when genuine culture may once again become possible. But walling oneself off is an alienating path to take, and because of its alienating character is a questionably helpful treatment for a depressive condition.

The other alternative—as with any instance of situational depression in which the environment cannot be substantially changed—is to leave the destructive situation that leads to demoralization and to cultivate scholarship outside of the academy. To do so requires an inner capacity to motivate oneself to liberating ends, despite of the mediocritizing and practical obsessions of lower reality. And yet it may be the only true path open that can permit the liberal arts scholar today to maintain his intellectual, moral, and aesthetic health free from despair. Although this choice involves physical distancing from the academic world, for some it may be significantly less alienating than the first alternative, because exposure to the pathology of acedia is reduced.

Liberal arts demoralization is the Huxlean epiphenomenon of the general disintegration of idealism. The values that sustained classical idealism, and the men and women who gave their lives for it, are rapidly disappearing in our consciousness. The increasingly few scholars in whom classical liberal arts ideals remain alive and whose morale has been ground down by a corrosive environment may want to recall Russell's counsel:

> Let us admit that, in the world we know, there are many things that would be better otherwise, and that the ideals to which we do and must adhere are not realized in the realm of matter. Let us preserve our respect for truth, for beauty, for the ideal of perfection which life does not permit us to attain, though none of these things meet with the approval of the unconscious universe. . . . In action, in desire, we must submit perpetually to the tyranny of outside forces; but in thought, in aspiration, we are free, free from our fellow men, free from the petty planet on which our bodies impotently crawl, free even, while we live, from the tyranny of death. Let us learn then, that energy of faith which enables us to live constantly in the vision of the good; and let us descend, in action, into the world of fact, with that vision always before us. (Russell, 1957, pp. 109–110)

NOTES

1. An earlier discussion of the subject matter of this chapter was published as an article, "The Psychology of Faculty Demoralization in the Liberal Arts: Burnout, *Acedia*, and the Disintegration of Idealism," in *New Ideas in Psychology 12*(3) (1994), pp. 277–89. The account provided here is revised, updated, supplemented, and the focus changed to fit the context of this book.

2. Presented by Mircea Eliade in a symposium at the Center for the Study of Democratic Institutions, Santa Barbara, April, 1970. Relevant works include Eliade (1949 and 1963).

PART III

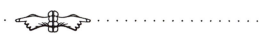

Beyond Long-standing Facts

7

The Psychology of Abuse in Publishing: Peer Review and Editorial Bias

> It has always been true, and it is now more than ever, that the path of wisdom for a young scientist of mediocre talent is to follow the prevailing fashion. Any young scientist who is not exceptionally gifted or exceptionally lucky is concerned first of all with finding and keeping a job. To find and keep a job you have to do competent work in an area of science which the mandarins who control the job-market find interesting. The scientific problems which the mandarins find interesting are almost by definition, the *fashionable problems*. . . . It is no wonder that young scientists who care for their own survival keep close to the beaten paths. . . .
>
> Our Institute here [Princeton's Institute for Advanced Study] is no exception. When I first came here as a visiting member thirty-four years ago, the ruling mandarin was Robert Oppenheimer. Oppenheimer decided which areas of physics were worth pursuing. His tastes always coincided with the most recent *fashions*. Being then young and ambitious, I came to him with a quick piece of work dealing with a *fashionable problem*, and was duly rewarded with a permanent appointment.
>
> —Physicist Freeman Dyson (Roberts, 2006, pp. 268–69, quoting Dyson, 1992, emphasis added)

The emphasized words in this quotation might well serve as a point of entry into the psychology of peer review and editorial bias. But, as we shall see, "tastes" and "fashions" are only surface phenomena that come to light in a psychological inquiry into the ways in which peer reviewers and editors often judge manuscripts submitted to them for publication.

Peer review and to a lesser extent editorial bias have been subjected to considerable discussion in the literature, some positive, some overtly critical. Generally there is consensus on three things: (1) peer review of publications has become the "gold standard" in scientific, academic, and scholarly publishing, in spite of the fact that (2) virtually no serious qualitative or data-based studies have been made to establish, when compared with publications not subject to peer review, that those which are peer reviewed are "better," "more reliable," "more valid," "more accurate," and "more important contributions" to significant advances in any discipline, and (3) for the foreseeable future, peer review is here to stay. (See, e.g., Enserink, 2001; Roy & Ashburn, 2001; Marsh, Bond, & Jayasinghe, 2007.)

The struggle between proponents and opponents of peer review has been anything but quiet. During the past quarter century, hundreds of papers and several books have been published that have, from a multitude of perspectives, endorsed or criticized peer review, in the process often including the behavior of editors. The sheer numerousness of complaints makes evident that these gatekeepers to publication have not been accepted or tolerated with equanimity. If one takes only a fraction of the published complaints at face value, one is compelled to recognize that peer review and editorial bias must be afflicted by serious inadequacies that at times result in unacceptable unfairness and intellectual suppression. These complaints have, among others, included the following allegations (which I mention only as sample *allegations* and as background; the majority will not be the main subject of examination here):[1]

- Peer review has come to dominate journal publishing and grant administration, with a nearly total investment of belief on the part of those concerned, despite the dearth of critical, hard, empirical studies of the extent to which peer review may—or may not—ensure quality and encourage—or suppress—innovation.
- Peer reviewers have frequently been found (by critics) to be incompetent and to lack formal training in the review of manuscripts; much of the time they are chosen from younger and less experienced faculty, scholars, and scientists, who are least qualified to serve as an expert author's "peers."
- In evaluating manuscript submissions there is little agreement in the judgment of reviewers, less than would be expected by chance.
- Many authors find that peer reviewers' criticisms are irrelevant to their manuscripts' intent and content.
- A host of prejudicial factors can play a central role in peer reviewers' judgment, such as the professional paradigm or ideology they embrace; their political and social biases; professional jealousy or vested interest in protecting their own turf (status, reputation, research approach, and results); favoritism toward graduates of their own alma maters, toward colleagues from other institutions they admire, and toward authors who are already well-known; and so on.

- Some peer reviewers seek to gain one-upmanship for their own professional status and research by undercutting an author's work.
- Peer reviewers make frequent mistakes in their evaluations, with little accountability since their identities are generally hidden.
- Peer reviewers tend to reject more clearly written, more simply stated papers in favor of those that are poorly written and clothed in the trappings of technical sophistication; as a result, obscure writing tends to be rated more highly than an author's scholarly or research competence.
- Peer review is costly (time-consuming for authors and reviewers, sometimes also a source of expense) but is between inefficient and meaningless since the majority of papers rejected by one journal's peer reviewers tends to be published anyway by their authors elsewhere, often in their original form.
- There are numerous examples of important, innovative contributions that were rejected outright by peer reviewers, including papers that later received Nobel Prizes and papers that became the most cited articles of all time; for instance, Einstein was so enraged by peer review in the *Physical Review* that in protest he subsequently refused to publish there. (For other examples, see Martin et al., 1986, p. 274; Horrobin, 1990, pp. 1440–41.)
- Reviewers tend to be biased against negative results and to give preferential treatment to submissions that positively bear out what they already believe.
- An extremely small minority of journals has established appeals procedures for authors who complain of the low quality of peer review.
- Approximately half of authors who engage in "dialogue" with reviewers get their papers accepted.
- Peer reviewers are often unable to detect fraud.
- Many peer reviewers as well as editors tend to be "neophobic" when innovative work is concerned (García, 1981, p. 149); papers that lay some claim to being "interesting" tend to be rejected by peer reviewers in favor of papers whose approach is familiar and establishmentarian.
- Peer reviewers tend to focus on the negative in their reports and give little to no attention to the positive features of submissions.
- Peer reviewers often engage in "mean-spirited," "overly caustic," derogatory evaluations of authors' submissions; peer review provides "an avenue for professional nastiness," for "sadistic" abuse (e.g., Holbrook, 1986; Fine, 1996; Levenson, 1996; Rabinovitch, 1996; Hadjistavropoulos & Bieling, 2000).

- Over time, a discouraging pattern of response of this kind can of course undermine the confidence and "submission tolerance" of many authors, disabling their research motivation, and at its worst, ultimately silencing them and causing them to withdraw from intellectual exchange, blocking professional development and potentially original work.
- Editors who oppose an author or his or her paper may intentionally send the paper on to peer reviewers known to hold views antagonistic to the author's; similarly, editors may give preferential treatment by selecting reviewers whose viewpoint ensures acceptance.
- Some authors have complained of peer reviewers who engage in plagiarism: stealing unpublished ideas and/or the research approach of authors whose work has been sent to them for review; there have also been complaints by authors against reviewers who allegedly delayed publication of authors' work when it competes with their own (Rowland, 2002).

This is a fairly long and still incomplete list of complaints that complainants have sought to document and justify. From the sheer length of such a list and the serious nature of the allegations, we should reasonably be persuaded—at the very least—of the need to find a more direct route through the maze, to bypass the impasses created by the many vociferously expressed objections, which tie us up in rhetoric and argument, argument and rhetoric that over the past two decades and more show no sign of abating or of reaching any definite conclusion.

In evaluating the practice of peer and editorial review it would be a step in the right direction if we can get beyond matters of mere belief. One way to get beyond conflicting opinions in this area is to study the underpinning psychology of peer review and editorial bias. Such a study, as we shall see, shows us unequivocally how weak, inadequate, and at times manifestly unacceptable are the prevailing means routinely used to arbitrate the quality of works submitted for publication.

Despite the plethora of publications that examine peer review, it is surprising that none has taken this focus. Martin, Baker, Manwell, and Pugh (1986, p. 4) is unusual even in mentioning this topic and then immediately places an examination of "psychological motivations" to one side, preferring to pay attention to other things. More recently, Frey (2003, p. 208) has noticed that no one has offered "any theory about the behavior of referees ... [n]or is there any well-worked out theory on the behavior of editors." He cites Laband and Piette (from Gans, 2000, p. 119), who state "to our knowledge, no widely accepted theory of editorial behavior has ever been articulated." To be sure, for it to be "widely accepted" it must first be articulated, and apparently no one has (if anyone has, it hasn't successfully passed the gatekeepers to publication). This stands before us as a gap to be filled. Let us therefore look at the emotional and cognitive factors that can play a determining role both in the recommendations of peer reviewers to publish or not to publish manuscripts and in the related decisions and text-modifying interventions of editors.

After devoting four decades to the study of the psychopathology and epistemology of belief, it has become abundantly clear to me that the vast majority of the decisions that people make, in whatever context they make them, are determined largely by belief rather than knowledge. We are a species ruled by our preferred beliefs, and they predispose and control us to an extent that we seldom fully recognize or appreciate.

Adherence to belief is often rigid and recalcitrant to change. Like highly rigid commitments of any sort, inflexible adherence to belief can result in pathology, for strict, blind, or unyielding adherence to belief can, in many situations and contexts, become harmful—that is, destructive and dysfunctional and hence pathological.

In this chapter, my concern is to identify and describe some of these unrecognized *pathologies of belief* that are destructive in today's accepted publishing practice and that are especially dysfunctional in their capacity to block the publication of creative, original research.

Having reached more than the halfway point in this book, readers will likely have developed a sharpened vigilance to some of the ways in which obeisance to the gold standard of psychological normality influences human beliefs, preferences, and judgment. To avoid a needless frequent repetition of the same refrain, I encourage you to share in some of the reframing initiative: to continue implicitly in the background to frame the ensuing discussion in terms of the habitual and uncritical priority given by the normal population to the fashions, paradigms, and disciplinary interests that form the normal status quo—all of which arise and are maintained as a consequence of the high regard invested by the psychologically normal majority in what it judges to reflect its own traits, tastes, and systems of belief.

It is usually thought that "prepublication restraint"—that is, censorship of writing before it can be published—no longer exists to any great degree in the United States or, for that matter, in educated, industrialized countries of the West. But this is indeed far from the case. Peer review and the decisions of editors erect an intimidating, sometimes demoralizing, and often impenetrable wall to authors whose opinions, ideas, research approaches, and research results conflict with the status quo of prevailing, preferred beliefs. Peer and editorial review, by definition, serve as "prepublication restraints": that is their intended and stated purpose, in the presumed service of ensuring greater quality, accuracy, and validity in publications. But that intention, because it has become so diffusively absorbed in our habitual practice, masks a psychology that has long gone undetected and unanalyzed, a psychology that has, once we have made a decision to consider it, obvious shortcomings and realized potentials for abuse.

These potentials for abuse are what this chapter is about. It seeks to show how the abuses that conventional prepublication restraint lead to are manifestly dysfunctional—so much so that it is appropriate to call them symptoms of a specific form of psychopathology that we have allowed to go unexamined for too long, and to exist under the cloak of respectability as the *arbiter elegantiae* of publication.

The abusive use of peer review and editorial judgment are sensitive topics, with a potential to give unintended offense to some readers, peer reviewers, and editors, and so it is important that we step back from the emotionally distracting issues for a moment in order to appreciate the larger historical framework within which peer review and editorial decision-making have evolved. The resulting picture of publishing practice has some intrinsic interest of its own and will help us to gain distance from the subject we wish to consider.

GAG ORDERS THROUGH TIME: SOCRATES, SAVONAROLA, COPERNICUS, BRUNO, GALILEO

[I]t is not permitted to contrive new ideas to defend a conclusion or to use a method of defense that entails new principles. This is a danger to be avoided. I could give many examples to make it clear that, in regard to conclusions, to principles, and to the method of defense, dangers arise from variety, from novelty, and from doctrines that are less than solid.
—Claudius Aquaviva, S.J. (1543-1615), General of the Society of Jesus (from Aquaviva's letter of instruction to all Jesuits, which formed certain of the grounds for Galileo's later condemnation; Blackwell, 2006, p. 210)

We could not wish for more instructive—or sadder—illustrations of prepublication restraint gone bad than in the cases of Socrates, Savonarola, Copernicus, Bruno, and Galileo. All five men were judged by their contemporaries and professional peers, who sought to silence them or change their published views, in three out of the five instances by putting them to death. All five, in different ways, made contributions that we now, with the improved vision of hindsight, recognize to have been major and original. Here are five abbreviated case studies of peer review and editorial tampering from long ago:

1. *Socrates* (c. 470 BCE–399 BCE), who has been called "the greatest hero of freedom of thought" (Laurence Berns, in Cropsey, 1964), is known for having chosen to accept the death penalty rather than cease philosophizing and expressing his ideas publicly. When oral presentation was the main way to communicate to the public, speaking publicly *was* publication. Socrates represents one of the earliest Western martyrs to fall before the power of censorship in the service of orthodoxy.

2. *Girolamo Savonarola* (1452–1498) also challenged the preferred beliefs of his contemporaries. He is known for his passionate social, political, and religious criticism. When the Medicis were overthrown, Savonarola introduced what many historians regard as the best democratic government Florence had every known. His success, his political convictions, and the enmity of corrupt Pope Alexander VI led to a papal gag order, which sought to prohibit Savonarola from preaching. Despite his enlightened and original contributions to Florence, Savonarola was brutally tortured, condemned in a perfunctory ecclesiastical trial, then hanged and burned.

3. *Nicolaus Copernicus* (1473–1543), the Polish astronomer who argued that the planets revolve around the sun and that the Earth itself revolves once a day in its orbit around it, was the victim of what I'll here call "editorial tampering." He formulated his planetary theory in *De revolutionibus orbium coelestium libri vi* ("Six Books Concerning the Revolutions of the Heavenly Orbs"), not published until the year of his death. It was greatly to influence his successors, Galileo, Kepler, and Newton. But its publication was victimized by editorial tampering: The task of overseeing the printing of *De revolutionibus* in Nürnberg was turned over to overzealous Andreas Osiander, a theologian who had tried to persuade Copernicus to represent his theory as no more than hypothetical. With Copernicus living at a safe distance, Osiander made changes in the book without the author's permission. Osiander furthermore had the presumption and arrogance to add an unsigned "Letter to the Reader," inserted in the published work immediately after the title page, informing the reader that the book described only hypotheses that made no claim to truth. As if this were not enough, Osiander proceeded to change the title of the book from the original "On the Revolutions of the Orbs of the World" to "Six Books Concerning the Revolutions of the Heavenly Orbs," a change which he seems to have felt

would weaken the impression that the book described the *real* physical universe. Osiander's editorial tampering did not come to public light until Kepler exposed it in his *Astronomia Nova* of 1609.

4. *Giordano Bruno* (1548–1600) was an astronomer, mathematician, and philosopher, several of whose theories were considerably ahead of his time, among them his theory that the universe is infinite in extent, that there are innumerable planets substantially similar to those in the solar system, and that geocentrism is false and a quasi-Copernican view right (Bruno developed his own version). He was irritated by theological nit-picking, and advocated freedom of speech and thought, for which he was excommunicated in a succession of cities in which he tried to live in both Italy and Germany. He was placed on trial in Venice and then in Rome, where the proceedings dragged on for seven years. His judges demanded his unconditional retraction of his theories. When Bruno claimed that he had nothing to retract and did not understand what he was expected to retract, Pope Clement VIII ordered his execution as an impenitent heretic. Bruno's tongue was bound in a gag—the cruelest and most literal gag order in history—and he was burned alive.

5. *Galileo Galilei* (1564–1642) is well-known for his contributions to astronomy, the physics of motion and strength of materials, and the development of scientific method. He developed and gradually improved his own version of the Dutch telescope, through which he discovered, for example, four of Jupiter's moons and the phases of Venus. His discoveries strengthened his belief in the Copernican view, for which the Church sought to silence him; later he was brought to trial in what lives on in memory as an example of Church narrow-mindedness and infamy, forcing Galileo in humiliation publicly to retract his support of Copernican theory. It was not until 1992 that the Vatican finally expressed regret for its condemnation of Galileo's views.

RELIGIOUS BELIEF, IMPRIMATUR, THE INQUISITION, AND THE *INDEX LIBRORUM PROHIBITORUM*

To be sure, institutionalized religion was responsible for the judgments against Savonarola, Bruno, and Galileo (both the Protestant and Catholic churches in the case of Bruno), and religious dogma was involved in the execution of Socrates and in the editorial tampering that victimized Copernicus. Religious beliefs were at stake (no play on words is intended) so that the "peer review" of the time was dominated by religious commitments and the zeal to defend them.

The Inquisition expressed the resulting mindset of rigid belief and an associated aggressive intolerance toward those not in the fold and is synonymous with many of the atrocities committed in the name of Catholicism. The widespread but false view is that the Inquisition came to a stop centuries ago, but in fact it survived in Spain until 1834, while the term was not formally dropped by the Vatican until 1908, when the congregation charged with maintaining the "purity of faith" was named the "Holy Office." This congregation was then again reorganized in 1965, and called the "Congregation for the Doctrine of the Faith," which persists today. Its task—still—is to promote orthodoxy.

In this context of belief paranoia, the Catholic Church developed its own specialized form of prepublication restraint. *Imprimatur*, which means "let it be printed," was—and still is—required by Catholic canon law. Before permission to publish, authorized by *imprimatur*, can be given, a Church censor must judge that nothing in a work is offensive to Church faith or morals; if the work passes muster, a stamp of approval in the form of a *nihil obstat* is given ("nothing hinders [the work from being printed]").

The first "index" of prohibited books was published in 1559 by the Sacred Congregation of the Roman Inquisition (a forerunner of the Congregation for the Doctrine of the Faith). The *Index Librorum Prohibitorum* ("Index of Forbidden Books"), listing books believed to be dangerous to the faith or morals of Catholics, wasn't discontinued until 1966. Before this, canon law imposed two kinds of restraint on publication: the censorship of books in advance of publication (a practice that continues today) and the condemnation of works considered to be dangerous to Catholic doctrine and faith. The Church focused enforcement efforts on the works listed in the *Index*.

I end this section with quotations from the three peer reviewers commissioned by the Society of Jesus to examine and recommend for or against the publication of a work by Melchior Inchofer, S.J., who was considered an authority at Galileo's trial and strongly influenced its outcome. Inchofer's book was titled *A Summary Treatise Concerning the Motion or Rest of the Earth and the Sun, in which it is briefly shown what is, and what is not, to be held as certain according to the teachings of the Sacred Scriptures and the Holy Fathers* (Rome: Ludovicus Grignanus, 1633). Here is how the appointed peer reviewers judged this work, which we now realize was science at its worst: "My judgment, therefore, is that this treatise is beneficial and should be published, especially since I have found nothing in it that is contrary to sound doctrine" (Fr. Luke Wadding, O.F.M., Commissary General of the Roman Curia). "Therefore we have granted permission for it to be published . . . (Muzio Vitelleschi). "Let it be printed" (Fr. Niccolò Riccardi, O.P., Master of the Sacred Apostolic Palace; quotations from Blackwell, 2006, p. 106).

What I want to suggest here is the hypothesis that only the variety of dogmatically defended orthodoxy has changed since Galileo's trial and not the underlying psychology of many peer reviewers and editors, to which we shall turn in a moment.

SEDITION, TREASON, CENSORS, AND CENSORSHIP

When we look at the extremes to which the adherents of beliefs will go in the defense of their preferred opinions, we see that the many strategies they have used to silence their opponents possess a common psychological dynamic: in the political arena, the condemnation of sedition and treason and the enforcement of censorship manifest a state of mind characterized by *defensiveness arising from insecurity* that closely mimics parallel attempts in organized religion to control beliefs and their expression. Sedition is a crime against a state by encouraging opposition to it, whether through speech or writing. English common law made it a criminal offense to publish seditious writing or to express seditious speech. Treason is closely related: in the United States, treason is considered to be any act of war against the country or any act that supports the beliefs of its enemies. Sedition involves expression; treason, action.

Censorship, in its application to publishing—our focus here—means prepublication control or, to put this more directly, *publication prevention*, often termed "prior restraint" in law. At issue in this context are restrictions imposed by censors that limit what is published and often the way in which authors choose to use language. This is actively imposed censorship. There is also self-censorship through passive acceptance of a prevailing set of values, as when many authors today appear unquestioningly to presuppose the validity of cultural relativism in formulating their results, or accept constraints of political correctness in views they advocate, or comply with gender-neutral uses of language even when doing this can force their use of language to become ungrammatical and terminologically monotonous. This is passively accepted censorship. Together, actively imposed and passively accepted censorship limit what is published. One of the main consequences of publication censorship is to create an atmosphere of anxiety, fear, and resulting conformity in which authors can be blocked from publishing innovative work. It is this phenomenon—the blocking of innovative ideas and approaches—that will particularly concern us later.

Censorship has been present for a long time in the history of book publishing. Freedom of the press has come about in large measure as a result of incremental resistance against censorship. I cannot recount this history here, which includes the role of the Stationers' Company in England; censorship wielded by the Sorbonne in France; Frankfurt's imperial censorship commission; the notorious actions of the British Star Chamber; Milton's eloquent defense of freedom of the press in his *Areopagitica*, in which he argued that there was no possible justification for censorship; England's Licensing Act of 1662; and the eventual abolition of censorship by Sweden in 1766, by Denmark in 1770, and by Germany in 1848. The French National Assembly of 1789 took the strongest position, still often quoted: "The free communication of thought and opinion is one of the most precious rights of man; every citizen may therefore speak, write and print freely."

Let us, however, pause with Milton for a moment. In his *Areopagitica*, he urged acceptance of the principle that censorship blocks "a free and open encounter"; it may sometimes block error, but there is, he believed, *a genuine positive good that comes from exposure to error*, for this is the only way that truth can be tested and strengthened—a principle basic to scientific investigation. It's likely that Milton would have opposed peer review and editorial tampering because of the ways these forms of thought control in publishing can run aground, homogenize and normalize the universe of expressed ideas, and establish obstacles to creative research.

Suppression of publication still continues—worldwide—under the guise of suppression of obscenity, libel, and opinions whose expression might "endanger national security." In this context, censorship has become a way of blocking or forcing changes in writing that is judged to subvert "the common good," writing that can in various ways express what in the history of publishing have been called "forbidden sentiments."

The public's freedom to contest political issues and government decisions can of course lead to unrest and instability, which, while undesirable in themselves, are usually transitory. But, in contrast, the history of censorship has shown us that the abusive nature of publication censorship, in the form of prior restraint or postpublication sanctions, can be much more serious by handicapping the long-term development of knowledge and culture. This, too, as we shall see, applies, *mutatis mutandis*, to the abuses of peer review and editorial control.

ACADEMIC FREEDOM VERSUS PEER REVIEW AND EDITORIAL TAMPERING

In principle, academic freedom provides scholars with the liberty to inquire into opinions, ideas, and theories that are unpopular at the time. Rigid adherence to preferred beliefs by peer reviewers and editors can effectively restrict the freedom of researchers to publish the results of their inquiries and therefore can restrict exchanges among them and communication to the public.

Academic freedom and peer review are seldom recognized to be in potential conflict with one another. Academic freedom is generally understood to provide for the unrestricted liberty of teachers and scholars to study whatever subject or set of ideas or beliefs interests them and to communicate their research to others through publication and teaching without interference from censorial controls; academic freedom equally provides for the unrestricted liberty of students to study the subjects they wish and to think freely and to develop and express their views. Peer reviewers, when their judgments block the access of teachers and scholars to publication, obstruct much that academic freedom stands for.

The values basic to academic freedom are thought to be justified by several interrelated tenets: that education and the growth of knowledge are most strongly encouraged when research, study, and publication are kept free of control by the state, religious institutions, or any special interest group. The judgments of peer reviewers routinely reflect their adherence to the special interests of political, social, or religious bias, and when this happens the control they exert undermines the values of academic freedom.

Ironically, the historical foundations for academic freedom were laid by medieval universities in Europe *despite* the fact that their own professors sought to exercise restraint upon and condemnation of the publications of their colleagues when their manuscripts violated religious beliefs. These censorious faculty colleagues were among history's first peer reviewers. Academic freedom and the freedom to publish have been uncomfortable bedfellows for a long time.

Conflict between peer review and academic freedom can be most pronounced in the humanities, where the lack of an accepted unitary methodology, the absence of a body of accepted results that is built upon incrementally over time, and the proliferation of special interest ideologies characterize much of liberal arts research, teaching, and publication. During the last century, for example, suppression of academic freedom in the humanities has been much more widespread in the communist countries than it has in these same countries in mathematics and the natural sciences, in which researchers have had more freedom of inquiry.

The explosive spread of obsessive sensitivity to "political correctness" has also, as one would expect, affected work in the humanities to a greater extend than in mathematics and science, in which discussions and research results tend to be less immediately applicable to and influenced by inflammatory social and political issues. The adoption by many U.S. universities of so-called "speech codes" during the last two decades of the twentieth century has contributed to higher education's and the general society's

sensitization to political correctness and has provided many special interest groups with deeply felt justification for their increased sensitivity to
offense in connection with ethnicity, race, religion, political persuasion,
gender, sexual orientation, ethnic language and grammar variants, and
general multiculturalism. There is now increasingly a wider and wider
spectrum of issues over which offense can be taken and therefore prepublication restraint imposed.

The complex network of entangled sets of mutually exclusionary
beliefs, whose proponents are frequently hostile toward one another, is a
phenomenon that we see in the worldwide strengthening of ideological
fundamentalism, and this, perhaps ineluctably, has spilled over into the
highly specialized worlds inhabited by research scientists, academics,
scholars, peer reviewers, and journal and book editors. Like the strongly
entrenched believers of other special interest groups, researchers, academics, scholars, peer reviewers, and editors share a sometimes uncomfortable universe of discourse in which those seeking to publish run
afoul of the private censorship that some peer reviewers and editors seek
to enforce by limiting publication to an acceptable range of approaches,
ideas, persuasions, beliefs, writing styles, and choices of terminology.

The effect of such prepublication restraint is of course felt most keenly, as
one would expect, by writers who push the boundaries of acceptability, who
propose ideas and endorse beliefs that at the time are unconventional, and
who have been and remain the main contributors to intellectual progress. It
is perhaps most importantly for their sake that academic freedom to publish
needs to be assured, often in the face of beliefs rigidly held by peer reviewers
and editors. The question is whether this can plausibly be accomplished
given the psychological predispositions of peer reviewers and editors.

RUNNING AFOUL OF THE BELIEF SYSTEMS OF PEER REVIEWERS AND EDITORS: VARIETIES OF ABUSE IN PEER REVIEW AND EDITORIAL TAMPERING

[I]t would be useful to know the fates of daring proposals that failed to
make it through peer review. Were some vindicated with the passage of
time? How prescient were the peer reviewers in judging the promise of
the applicants? Were they better, let's say, than ... a lottery?
—Daniel S. Greenberg (1999, p. 2092)

Let's consider an example of what can happen as a result of rigid adherence
to the preferred beliefs of editors and peer reviewers; it illustrates what did,
in fact, recently occur when an author submitted a manuscript that con-
flicted with peer review and editorial bias.

By way of background, we need to recognize that some 60 million Americans serve as hosts to the brain parasite *Toxoplasma gondii*. In rats, this parasite influences their brain chemistry so they are motivated to seek out cats and so be killed; in this way the parasite can complete its reproductive cycle in the cat. It has been hypothesized that toxoplasmosis infection may also result in changes in human behavior, some subtle, some manifestly schizophrenic. Biologist Kevin D. Lafferty, for example, has correlated high levels of human toxoplasmosis infection with elevated levels of neuroticism in 39 countries.[2]

In the context of this research, parasitologist Jaroslav Flegr of Charles University in Prague has suggested that the consequence of human toxoplasmosis infection may be to unbalance the sex ratio of newborn infants: 104 boys to every 100 girls is normal, but in women who have developed high levels of antibodies to *T. gondii*, the ratio according to Flegr becomes 260 boys to 100 girls. One possible explanation for this effect, again according to Flegr, is that *T. gondii* may suppress the mother's immune system so that the normal tendency of the maternal immune system at times to resist the development of male embryos is neutralized; as a consequence, more boy babies are born.

Flegr's study ran into the prevailing, preferred beliefs of journal editors. He observed: "People don't like the possibility that their behavior and life are manipulated by a parasite." What editors *like to believe* became a block to the publication of Flegr's original research. "Our present study was rejected by eight journals" (Svitil, 2007, p. 14). His earlier study, which showed that toxoplasmosis infection more than doubles a person's risk of having a car accident, ran into the same block to publication.

One could amass many of other anecdotal accounts of similar struggles of authors to publish papers and books that run counter to prevailing preferred beliefs, but it isn't my purpose here to assemble a catalog of the frustrating experiences of authors. What we need instead is to cast light on the underlying psychological reasons for abuses in the publishing process.

Although the following proposition is easy enough to state, and easy enough to recognize when stated, it is often ignored: The "significance" of a paper can't be judged intelligently in terms of its conformity with existing tastes and prejudices. The current "gold standard" of peer review has an unmistakable tendency to equate these, as can editorial tampering.

Let us see in psychological terms how abuses in publishing result. Peer review and editorial bias can become abusive in a number of ways:

1. *Emotional and cognitive gratifications of power and authority.* It goes without saying that peer reviewers and editors are aware that they act as gatekeepers to publication and hence as gatekeepers to

authors' job acquisition, salary increment, promotion in rank, job retention, and professional and research standing, as well as the funding of research grant and fellowship proposals. Furthermore, the judgments of peer reviewers and editors can, in the end, make or break a scientist's or scholar's reputation by limiting his or her access to publication. Within this framework of easily implemented power, which has virtually no oversight to check excesses, a wide range of abuses has been mentioned in the literature, including manifest discourtesy, rudeness, verbal abuse, slighting the significance of a researcher's results, professional snubbing, unsubstantiated destructive criticism, and others (see, e.g., Enserink, 2001; Nicholls, 1999).

2. *Anonymity and malice.* The abovementioned abuses are considerably magnified, as one would expect, by what psychologist Philip Zimbardo (2007) has called "the Lucifer effect." When psychologically normal people are placed in positions of authority and power—and most especially when their anonymity is protected, as the identities of peer reviewers usually are—an opportunity is created in which abusive intent is magnified and the door is opened to its expression. There is nothing like anonymity to give malice free rein.

3. *From belief system defensiveness to psychosis.* Peer review and editorial authority have become authorized, legitimated roles in which it is natural for peer reviewers and editors to seek to protect their own professional positions, research results, and sense of disciplinary propriety. The emotional investment in protecting these sources of personal and professional identity can range from defensiveness to a form of *belief system psychosis* in which believed-in reality is mistaken for the one-and-only "true" reality: turf protection can become delusional identification, reflecting the same psychological dynamic that we see in any rigidly held, exclusionary, self-enclosed system of belief (Bartlett, 2005, Part III).

4. *Emotional gratifications of the familiar.* It is well established that people find emotional security in the familiar and are threatened by the unfamiliar. There is a gratifying sense of safety in which members of the respective disciplines feel "at home" with colleagues who share their disciplinary perspective; who use the same familiar approaches, concepts, and terminology; who are drawn to the same research problems; and who share many of the same beliefs. Peer reviewers and editors are no different in this respect: it is understandable and to be expected that the psychologically normal peer reviewer and editor is emotionally rewarded by his or her decisions that preserve the familiar and that serve professional self- and group interests

which have become comfortable and habitual. The emotional gratification experienced in a research environment made comfortable
through habituation feeds back into the psychologically normal predisposition to mimic and conform to the preferences, values, expectations, and behavior of others. Researchers whose work does not
conform are less likely to be rewarded, as Dyson observed in the
opening quotation.

5. *Resistance, recalcitrance, repugnance, and retaliation.* These are the
"4 Rs" of peer and editorial review. They describe a peer reviewer's
or editor's range of negative response to manuscripts whose content
trespasses beyond the boundaries of acceptable belief. Resistance,
recalcitrance, repugnance, and retaliation have both intellectual and
emotional components. When some peer reviewers and editors are
confronted by opinions, ideas, beliefs, values, approaches, results,
and so forth that they do not like or that they do not believe satisfy
criteria of the conventionally acceptable, their response may be one
of intellectual and emotional *resistance*, in which the submitted
manuscript is passively blocked: a form-letter variety of rejection is
then sent to the author. Should the negative response be more
strongly felt, the peer reviewer's or editor's reaction becomes *recalcitrant:* he or she is repulsed by the views advocated in the offending
manuscript, and then derogating behaviors of the sort mentioned in
item 1 can ensue. The same is true with the last two degrees of
response, *repugnance* and *retaliation*, which are more blatantly hostile
and aggressive, the last expressing a militant judgment against the
offending author, with punitive criticism against the author that
can spill over and be re-expressed in the peer reviewer's or editor's
own publications and communications with colleagues. It is important to recognize that all 4 Rs give a peer reviewer or editor *an opportunity*, which he or she believes is professionally sanctioned, to
gratify defensive needs and at times aggressive behavior as well.

6. *Self-aggrandizement—placing the reviewer's "stamp" on a publication.*
There can be a pronounced and unmistakable experience of self-
aggrandizement when an editor or peer reviewer requires "certain
changes" in an author's submitted manuscript. As H. G. Wells
observed, "No passion on earth, neither love nor hate, is equal to
the passion to alter someone else's draft" (quoted in Asimov, 1987,
p. 57). Some critics of current publishing practice have complained
of the petty, nit-picking mentality to which some editors and peer
reviewers descend (e.g., Greenberg, 1999). Some can only be "satisfied" if, before a manuscript is allowed to pass muster, they require
an author to make a certain minimal number of changes, perhaps

inessential, but still reflecting stipulations that please a micromanaging mindset.

7. *Jealousy and competitiveness.* Critics of peer review have pointed to the paradoxical and self-defeating nature of the current system of publishing, which relies on the opinions of "rival producers" (Albert, 1997, p. 822). It is indeed far-fetched to suppose that one's research competitors are likely to be sources of dispassionate evaluation of research that might equal or surpass theirs. Jealousy is a strong motivating emotion, sometimes sufficient to lead rivals to dismiss without justification competing points of view, approaches, and research results expressed in manuscripts they review. We see the same phenomenon in authors who will intentionally "mis-describe" the work of a rival author and mendaciously seek to subordinate that work to a thesis they have been advocating for a much longer period of time. This is the same dishonest ploy used by Robert Hooke when he attempted to preempt Newton's discoveries by claiming, to paraphrase him, that "whatever is new in Newton's work, I've already done."

8. *Cheapening of authorship.* The value of manuscript submissions has changed over the past several decades as a result of an exploding general population, the consequent explosion of the population of competing scientists and scholars, and the resulting terrific explosion in the number of publications produced annually. Three to four decades ago it was common practice for a journal editor or book editor to *thank* an author for his or her submission, to recognize the *implied compliment* expressed by the author in choosing that particular journal or publishing house as a possible outlet for his or her publication. Today, instead, authors have learned to express their gratitude to publishers, as do interviewees for the *privilege* of having public attention bestowed upon them. The burden to publish or perish placed on the rapidly proliferating population of younger researchers, in a world in which publications are flying off the physical and electronic presses in ever-increasing numbers, has brought with it a cheapening of manuscript submissions and, by implication, a cheapening of respect that was once believed to be owed to the research efforts of authors. Just as life becomes cheapened by overpopulation, so do manuscripts and their authors. This general inversion of values has paved the foundation for many of the specific abuses enumerated here.[3]

9. *Editorial tampering.* This is, I suggest, an editor's, and less often a peer reviewer's, greatest sin. We saw it in connection with unauthorized changes made in the opus of Copernicus; lesser authors also

experience it. Sometimes personal experience should not be con-
signed to silence, while some readers may be interested in an anecdotal story from the author: More than a decade ago, I submitted
an article to a well-known journal, and the paper was accepted.
Before its publication the editor sent me a proof copy. I read, in a
state of shock, a text that had become victimized by extreme editorial
tampering. The editor used his "privilege" to, let us say, "recharac-
terize" my results, apparently making them more palatable to the
beliefs that he *liked*. There was a good deal of this, enough so that
I immediately sent registered letters both to the editor and publisher
saying that, unless my original text was restored, I refused to author-
ize the publication of the paper. There was no answer to either letter.
Some time later, and despite timely objection well in advance of publication, I received author's copies of the printed journal in which my
article was published—with all of the editor's tampering intact. I am
not litigious by nature, but this was simply too much; I retained an
attorney who requested an appropriate resolution. The result? The
journal later published a statement, expressing regret for "numerous
and substantive changes and abridgments . . . to which the author had
not consented," and offered to send readers upon request an offprint
of the text as it had originally been written. My attorney's fee was
paid by the journal, a small satisfaction, since few readers, I feel sure,
ever bothered to request the text as originally written, and the phrase
"editorial tampering" was born in the author's mind.

10. *Expressions of the psychology of stupidity.* The psychology of human stupidity has been little studied in preference to study of its more attrac-
tive big brother, intelligence. The psychology of stupidity is,
however, an area of proper study in itself. Human stupidity is not simply an absence of intelligence; it is characterized by a distinctive set of
psychological predispositions, identified in Bartlett (2005). Many of
these play a role in the psychology of peer and editorial review since,
unfortunately, these characteristics are not rare in the population
nor even within the higher echelons of scientific and scholarly publishing. To make this listing of varieties of peer and editorial abuse
as concise as possible, only three of these predispositions will be mentioned here: There is, first of all, a strong source of human gratification to be found in personal denials both of ignorance and of lack of
specialized knowledge and skills. Many of us resort to denials of this
kind in order to make ourselves feel better when we're confronted
by people who far surpass us in areas in which we are bumbling
incompetents. We may simply deny their superiority, we overlook it,
we do not in fact seem even to notice it. This is a form of denial that

is part of human stupidity. Related to it is intellectual stubbornness and the gratification that comes from pig-headedness. Such a person can pat himself or herself on the back for fidelity to tradition, to "established disciplinary standards," and so on, and in the process be patted on the back by like-minded colleagues. Such pats as these are gratifying to receive, but they have an intellectually stultifying effect. Third, and perhaps most importantly, peer reviewers and editors can, on a fundamental level, lack the intellectual intelligence, skill, and breadth of knowledge that are necessary in order to appreciate a creative author's original work. All of these expressions of the psychology of human stupidity come with built-in gratifications that maintain and preserve a self-limiting outlook. (For a detailed discussion and analysis, see Bartlett, 2005, Chapter 18.)

11. *The presumed equality of opinions.* There is a strong psychological bias today in favor of a presumption of the equality of opinions. It is a bias that engenders hostility toward claims to "intellectual authority" and resentment toward the recognition of elitist expertise. However, the authors of many papers and books know far more about their particular subjects than anyone else does, for many have spent long periods of time—years, perhaps their whole professional lives— dedicated to studying and advancing knowledge in their particular specialized areas of research. Yet, when these authors submit their work for publication, the general disfavor into which elitist expertise and authority have fallen has prepared the state of consciousness of peer reviewers and editors. Like innocents abroad, reviewers and editors can be emboldened to critique and nit-pick in specialized areas in which, to be realistic and to call a spade a spade, they know little more than the crassest amateur. This problem is greatly compounded when an author's research embraces several different disciplines simultaneously, for then it becomes virtually impossible to find, in any single peer reviewer, the qualifications, skills, and breadth of knowledge that are necessary in order competently to evaluate the author's work.

12. *Rejection of novelty.* Advances in knowledge are often made as a result of obsolescence of what was thought to have been known: old beliefs succumb and are superseded. This can be an unpleasant and uncomfortable experience for anyone who has dedicated years of his or her life to theories and results that are now threatened by someone's original, new approach. It is therefore natural to reject novelty and "to do whatever may be necessary" to retain a grip both on the public acceptability of the understanding one has struggled to promote and on one's own resulting professional status.

An even dozen is probably enough in this noncomprehensive description of the psychological basis of abuses to which peer review and editing can fall victim. These abuses obviously do not occur all the time, in connection with every manuscript submission. We still don't know how often they occur, although authors dubious of the value of peer review continue to call for serious, empirical study of the value and effectiveness of this publishing mechanism. Marsh, Bond, and Jayasinghe (2007, p. 33) recently commented: "Given the central importance of the peer review process to science, there is surprisingly little evidence of the use of scientific methods to evaluate the peer review process." Enserink (2001, p. 2187) similarly noted that there is "little evidence that peer review actually improves the quality of research papers," and went on to mention the need for journals to "study their own practices with the scientific rigor they demand of their authors—as should agencies that rely on peer review to dole out billions of dollars in research money." Greenberg (1999, p. 2092) observed:

> It's time for an evidence-based assessment of competitive peer review, the clunky procedure enshrined in science for making choices about who gets money and who sinks into oblivion.... The defenders have fallen back on such tattered lines as "If it ain't broke, don't fix it" and, paraphrasing Churchill on democracy, "It's the worst possible system, except for all others." ... [T]he merits of peer review remain remarkably unexamined, despite complaints about nit-picking assessments, poorly qualified reviewers, clique-ish bias, purloining of ideas, and aversion to risk.... Peer review, however, is one of those subjects about which much is said with certainty but little is known.

But we do—on the contrary—know a good deal about peer review and editorial authority: specifically, we know a good deal about the underlying and chronically ignored psychology of abuse that comes from a system in which reviewers are allowed to hide behind masks of anonymity; are free, if they wish, to engage in destructive and hostile criticism without restraint; and are often chosen precisely because they are research competitors of the author whose work is to be evaluated and hence are *psychologically* the *least* well-suited to pass judgment because their judgment runs a high risk of being prejudiced. Furthermore, we also know a good deal about the dynamics of belief systems and the pathologies to which rigidly held beliefs can give rise. It is plausible to suppose that peer reviewers and editors are usually regular people, and that they are therefore subject to the same shortcomings as the population of psychological normal people.

We do, in short, know enough to be able to *predict* and therefore *expect* the abuses we've identified, even though there have as yet been no data-based studies to tell us their prevalence. But other studies of the prevalence among psychologically normal people of such phenomena as obedience to authority, the "Lucifer effect," participation in state-endorsed wars and group-sponsored genocide, the contagious effect of group prejudice and aggression, the emotional and cognitive gratifications of adherence to the ideology of one's group, and similar pathologies (Bartlett, 2005) would, however, suggest that the abuses we've discussed are far from being rare, and are indeed very common.

There are two remaining issues that I'd like to confront: the hypothesis that the abuses to which peer review and editorial bias are subject constitute, in a certain legitimate sense, "psychopathologies" in their own right, and the suggestion that these abuses present obstacles to the publication of original, creative research.

THE PSYCHOPATHOLOGY OF PEER REVIEW AND EDITORIAL BIAS: BLOCKS TO CREATIVE RESEARCH

The lack of sound judgment among people who have the fate of science and the lives of others in their hands is appalling.... The referee system as currently constituted is a disaster. What is most disastrous is its built-in bias against highly innovative work. The towering achievements of science for the most part have their origins in brilliant individual minds. These minds are exceptionally rare. The concept of peer review is based on two myths. The first is that all scientists are peers, that is, people who are roughly equal in ability. The second myth is that in those rare instances in which someone who is exceptional does appear, the ordinary scientist always instantly recognizes genius and smoothes its path. No one who knows anything at all about the history of science can believe for one second in either myth. Most scientists are not the peers of the very best, and most scientists follow the crowd when it comes to the recognition of brilliance. The concept of peer review is philosophically faulty at its core.

—Horrobin (1982, pp. 33–34)

[W]e must take seriously the possibility that we have traded innovation for quality control.... The numbers of truly important, innovative articles presented to an editor are small. Yet it is this tiny minority of articles that is responsible for [advancing knowledge].... It is my view that innovation is so rare, so valuable, and so central ... innovative articles should be deliberately encouraged and more readily published than conventional ones.

—Horrobin (1990, p. 1439)

[Peer review is an] ... enormous waste of scientists' time, and the absolute, ineluctable bias against innovation.

—Roy & Ashburn (2001, p. 394)

In Bartlett (2005, Part I) I examined the main theories of disease in order to identify, within the existing framework of the science of pathology, the criteria that must be satisfied in order for the term 'pathology' to be applied meaningfully to acknowledged signs of harm. The outcome of that discussion was, in a few words, to recognize that a condition constitutes a pathology if it results in perceived harm in the context of a set of desired purposes, the attainment of which is impeded by the condition. In this sense, for example, a medical patient is judged to be incapacitated by a certain pathology when his physical condition undermines his ability to function as he otherwise would and wants to be able to. In other words, to qualify as a pathology, a condition must be judged to be harmful relative to a set of goals. The concept of pathology has direct application in the context of the psychology of peer review and editorial bias and occasionally has been applied by a few authors, always in passing. Ziman (1982, p. 61), for example, calls the unproved standing of peer review "a gravely pathological situation, calling for serious inquiry and radical remedy," while Horrobin (1990, p. 1441) refers to the suppression of innovation through peer review as a form of "psychopathology" in which the "sophisticated behavior" of "the most distinguished scientists" is "pathological."

The vocabulary of pathology is bandied about with a good deal of freedom, often in applications intended to be only metaphorical. Here, we're not concerned with a metaphor.

Prepublication restraint has, as we've seen, been imposed for a variety of explicit and alleged purposes: to protect religious or political orthodoxy, and in peer review and editorial decision-making to protect scientifically or academically reputable publishing. Peer review and editorial decision-making are *not* established with the explicit and specific end in view of promoting original research. They are inherently conservative mechanisms designed to further the goals of established scientific or scholarly orthodoxy, which is to say, to normalize: to protect against what we might call "secular blasphemy"—dissension from the current prevailing dogma, school of thought, paradigm, and criteria of accuracy, validity, and scholarship. Secular blasphemy, a.k.a. political incorrectness or disciplinary heresy, is the crime of dissenting from whatever is the current dominant system of belief. 'Blasphemy' is the shapeshifting word that is molded to suit the objectives of those who oppose criticism of or departures from the ruling authority's orthodoxy of the moment.

Peer reviewers and editors are not umpires of the truth or falsity of doctrine; their role is to remain neutral. And yet, again and again throughout human history, and continuing today under the guise of relativism, multiculturalism, deconstructionism, postmodernism, feminism, and their cohorts, peer reviewers and editors will often—as it is indeed psychologically normal to do—reflect in their evaluations of prospective publications their favored tastes and prejudices, their ideological and disciplinary preferences, and then will, like religious and governmental censors of times past and present, reject or seek fundamentally to modify manuscripts that diverge from the orthodoxy they advocate. Like religious and government censors, they stand guard before the gate to block the entrance of the "forbidden sentiments" and "false doctrine" that have so threatened the dogmas of the past. All of these are patterns to be expected; they are only human; we can predict these behaviors from our knowledge of the underlying psychology.

And yet we realize that important contributions to the advancement of knowledge in any discipline occur only as a result of the efforts of researchers who are capable of extending, or of breaking free from, the limits of existing understanding. When we see things from this perspective, the 12 predictable abuses to which peer review and editorial bias can give rise will be seen to constitute nonmetaphorical pathologies that can play a destructive, harmful role as obstacles to the goal of publishing original, creative research.[4]

In Bartlett (2005, Parts II & III), a wide range of pathologies is studied, pathologies that result in undebatable harm to countless people, from individuals to entire societies, pathologies that have their basis in normal psychology. Wars, genocides, obedience to authority, human ecological pathology, terrorism, pseudospeciation, psychic numbing, devaluation and dehumanization of others, moral stupidity, and cognitive delusion— to name a few of the principal pathologies—are consequences of the psychologically normal constitution. The theory of disease has usually associated the term 'pathology' only with conditions that are aberrations from normality, and yet there is solid empirical evidence, and solid backing from leading disease theorists, that compels the recognition of pathologies so widespread as to be considered "universal," afflicting the great majority of people.

The abuses that I've described above to which peer review and editorial bias are subject come about as a result of a psychologically normal constitution that seeks, among other things, to defend cherished beliefs, to defend personal and professional identity, and to defend sets of essentially conservative values within territorially protected disciplines. The conclusion we have come to and, I submit, the only rational conclusion to be drawn from this discussion, is that peer review and editorial bias, because they *will* express the psychologically normal constitution, cannot be freed from the abuses to which they are subject. The potential for abuse can only be minimized to some degree through intelligent oversight. A group of much-needed professional guidelines that might accomplish this will be proposed in a moment.

Christine Wenneras and Agnes Wold of Göteborg University, Sweden, have called for "the development of peer-review systems with some in-built resistance to the weaknesses of human nature" (see Morris, 1997, p. 1611). How are we to go about achieving this?

OBLIGATIONS TO WHICH PEER REVIEW AND EDITING MUST ANSWER

As things now stand, most editors proceed in the following way in processing a manuscript submission: They give it a general glancing over and may reject it immediately if the manuscript is perceived to be unredeemable or inappropriate for that particular journal or publishing house. If the manuscript passes this first level of inspection, it is passed on to a small group of peer reviewers, who may or may not have been nominated by the author. The author usually remains in the dark as to the identities of the peer reviewers actually chosen by the editor. Once the peer reviewers have read or at least considered the paper or book, their reports are sent back to the editor, who then reads the reports and makes a decision whether to proceed further. He or she may decide to reject the manuscript, request that "certain changes" be made, or, increasingly rarely, publish the work as it stands. All of this seems straightforward. However it is not, and there are crucial questions that sometimes are, but probably often are not, asked in the process. Here is an imagined exchange between Professor Naïveté, who asks the questions, and Professor Cynicismus, who answers them:

> Prof. Naïveté: Are the peer reviewers truly *qualified* to judge the manuscript? Are they professionally *competent* to judge what is often the work of an advanced specialist, or are they junior faculty whose research experience and expertise are still in the embryonic stages? If the manuscript involves multidisciplinary competence on the part of the author, can the editor find peer reviewers with similarly broad competence?
>
> Prof. Cynicismus: Two things are happening in the growth of knowledge: the increasing specialization of experts and the cross-linking of discoveries in different disciplines. As a result, authors who have the training and professional backgrounds to span several disciplines at once are at a concerted disadvantage when their writing is reviewed by peers who are specialists in single fields. Yet the need for such cross-disciplinary contributions now, more than ever in human intellectual history, is unarguable. Reality no more has disciplinary divisions than does the earth show the territorial borders of nations when it is seen from space. In my experience in publishing numerous papers and books, the vast majority of

peer reviewers are not well-qualified to pass judgment; in fact, many are as ill-equipped as fifth graders saddled with the responsibility to judge the work of a graduate student. Their reports very often reflect ignorance of the subjects and literature treated in a given manuscript, lack of the requisite technical skills, and often, too, ignorance of the author's prior published work to which reference tends, explicitly or implicitly, to be made, and yet their reports express a willful unwillingness to recognize the limits of their own knowledge and competence.

Prof. N.: Are peer reviewers and editors *dispassionate* in their judgment? That is, are their judgments free from bias that favors established practice and theory; are their judgments open to innovative research that extends boundaries, lays the groundwork for new areas of study, or offers new paradigms for research?

Prof. C.: The emotional and cognitive outlook of many peer reviewers and editors was summed up centuries ago in the following passages:

[A teacher or scholar] . . . is not free to devise or present a new doctrine on his own initiative, unless it is supported by responsible and established authors. . . . [I]t is most important, especially in grave matters, that we avoid as much as possible opportunities of devising new opinions. (From a Letter on Implementing the *Ratio studorium* and on Following the Teachings of St. Thomas, from Claudius Aquaviva, S.J., to the Provincials, December 14, 1613; in Blackwell, 2006, pp. 215–16.)

Philosophy professors should not introduce any new questions, or any opinion which is not attributable to some author, to those present who are inexperienced. And they should not defend anything that is contrary to the axioms of the philosophers and the common understanding of scholars. Those who are prone to novelties, or who are too free in spirit, should understand that they will without doubt be removed from the office of teaching. (From "Rules for Philosophers on the Adoption of Opinions," Decree 41 of the Fifth General Congregation of the Society of Jesus, November 3, 1593–January 18, 1594; in Blackwell, 2006, p. 209.)

Prof. N.: Are peer reviewers and editors *free* from egotism, professional pride, envy, and turf-preserving motivation, from the seductions of anonymously wielded power, from the emotional gratifications of imposing or injecting into a publication their own ideological, disciplinary, and stylistic preferences, of pressuring an author to conform in his or her writing style to the politically correct fashion of the time?

At this point, we need to take the last question away from Professor Cynicismus and return to nonimaginary reality: given the psychological likelihood of the publishing abuses identified in this chapter, we clearly are in need of a set of guidelines that could, if followed, help to lessen the psychologically based abuses of peer review and editorial bias. The psychological potential for abuse in publishing is sufficiently great, sufficiently predictable, and sufficiently harmful that, in consultation with journal editors and book publishers, professional organizations should begin serious discussion and pass resolutions on behalf of their members, affirming a code of conduct similar to the following:

A CODE OF CONDUCT FOR PEER REVIEWERS AND EDITORS

1. Journals, book publishers, and granting agencies expect peer reviewers and editors to abide by professional standards of courtesy and respect in reviewing the work of others.
2. Editors are responsible for reading peer reviewers' reports prior to relaying them to authors. Readers' reports that are deliberately dismissive, hostile, offensive, use belittling or sarcastic language, or make unsubstantiated statements will not be sent on to authors but will be returned to the reviewers for revision.
3. Editors will respect the intellectual property of authors by refraining from imposing upon an author's text views or language that are not the author's own, unless authors give explicit permission for such changes in advance of publication.
4. Peer reviewers will similarly respect the text of authors by refraining from acting as copy editors, which is not their assigned job, and for which they rarely have the expertise.
5. The same rigor must be used in the reports of peer reviewers and editors as is demanded of the submitting author—in particular, the use of appropriate literature citations by reviewers and editors to support their statements.
6. Criticism should be constructive and balanced rather than destructive or aggressive.
7. Derogatory statements criticizing an author's alleged misuse of the English language are not acceptable.
8. Gender-neutral language may be encouraged, but in keeping with guidelines formulated by the American Psychological Association, the American Philosophical Association, and the National Council of Teachers of English relating to nonsexist language, these guidelines are intended "to be kept in mind" so that scholars can "take special care to avoid giving needless and unintended offense," but are not intended as "any specific or compulsory set of rules."[5]

(The suggestion for such a code of conduct was made by Nicholls [1999, p. 1853]. I have added to and paraphrased his text.)

REMOVING THE PSYCHOLOGICAL OBSTACLES ERECTED BY PEER REVIEW

[T]he political question par excellence [is] how to reconcile order which is not oppression with freedom which is not license.

—Leo Strauss (1988, p. 37)

Once one has made a decision to take into account the abuse-prone psychology underlying peer review and editorial bias, it is natural to ask what the world would be like if publication decisions were returned to editors without the complex, laborious, time-consuming, and sometimes costly mechanism of peer review. For it would seem that the most efficient way to bypass the majority of the psychologically based abuses in publishing that we have described is simply to give control back to editors so that they can publish what they judge to be worthwhile. It is true that their judgment is sometimes influenced by bias, but this limitation may simply be the minimum "price of doing business" in this less than the best of possible worlds.

Proposals to discontinue peer review have been made, for example by Roy and Ashburn (2001), who note that "most of the best-known scientists such as Nobel laureates, regard peer-review as a great hindrance to good science. . . . An enormous amount of the best science has been and is being run without benefit of this rubric, as is the worldwide patent system." To the objection that no serious alternatives to peer review have been proposed, their response is: "Nonsense. They have not only been proposed but have been in regular use worldwide for a very long time. The users include the world's largest research agency, the U.S. Department of Defense, and industrial research worldwide" (pp. 393–94).

Prepublication restraint—that is, censorship—has always been motivated by the emotional need for security. In human history, its use has shifted from societies gripped by religious paranoia to nations dominated by anxieties over their national security, and now its use has been extended through the growing ascendancy of peer review to safeguard disciplinary and professional security and to defend increased concern for political and disciplinary correctness. The form of censorship embodied in peer review is believed by many to be a necessity. And yet, as Albert (1997, p. 822) observed:

Without peer review, journals will almost certainly reject a small number of papers that should have been accepted, and accept one or two that should have been rejected. But this is what happens anyway. Peer review is inadequate when it comes to spotting downright lies, so what we are really talking about is not so much guarding the gates from evil as directing traffic towards (and away from) various measures of goodness.... Without peer review, [editors] will be forced to take decisions on their own ... on the basis of what they think will inform, stimulate, and entertain their readers. They can still get advice from experts, but it will be on their terms. Some of their subsequent decisions will be wrong, but a lot more of them will be bold, and at least the priorities will be back in the right place.... It could bring some of the passion and excitement back into science.

This is a reasonable point of view. The contrary belief has been rigidly held for centuries, and should by now be recognized as dysfunctional, expressing a true pathology of belief:

[T]he censors must be more conscientious. If we do not contain ourselves within definite and accepted limits, we will face new threats and dangers daily. There is no doubt that we dishonor ourselves when someone wishes to proceed further when he sees that there is permission to hold something about matters that require many distinctions and great acumen, and then others do the same thing, with the result that nothing is ever seen to be stable and uniform afterwards. (From a Letter on the Solidity and Uniformity of Doctrine, from Claudius Aquaviva, S.J., to the Provincials, May 24, 1611; in Blackwell, 2006, p. 211.)

CONCLUSION

Closed-minded peer review and editorial tampering are the main ways that American authors experience censorship, unless they write about sensitive military or political issues, or as Catholic clerics write about Catholic doctrine. Being the victim of straightjacketing peer review or editing provides authors with a firsthand, painful experience of what it is like to be censored. Abuse directed toward what one has written can feel like a personal attack, and in a sense it is precisely that, for one's intellectual property is an extension of the author's self, of work he or she has created on the basis of years of education, later study, research, effort, and perhaps also original thought.

When peer review goes bad and editorial tampering takes place we enter a microcosm of ideological recalcitrance and of the resistance of human belief systems to novelty, a microcosm ruled by a dynamic of conservatism and pettiness that perpetuates prevailing beliefs to the exclusion, as intellectual history often shows, of original, creative work that conflicts with or appreciably extends the boundaries of preferred ideas and fashions. In other words, tastes, dictated by prevailing fashion and coupled with the specific abuses to which normal psychology is prone that we've described here, become blocks to what are unconventional, new, and potentially significant advances in knowledge, when peers and editors take on the serious responsibility—at times in strong conflict with their own self-interests—of judging another researcher's work.

The healthy development of human knowledge and culture requires iconoclasts, rebels, those of independent mind and spirit. Suppressing and blocking creative research and publication is tantamount to choosing, literally, to disable ourselves. The irony is that we do this as a result of normal psychological predispositions which themselves qualify as disabling pathologies.

In our legal system we have preferred to increase the risk of allowing some of the guilty to go free rather than mistakenly punish the innocent. The elimination of peer review could perhaps permit the publication of some outlandish, inaccurate papers and books—which seem, in any event, to appear regularly and unimpeded. We might do well to recall Milton's observation that positive good can come from occasional exposure to error, enabling us to test and strengthen the reliability of what we believe we know: DNA mutation errors are known to be essential to evolutionary advances; the occasional slippage into publication of erroneous results undoubtedly plays a similar role in the evolution of knowledge, helping us to break free of unrealized constraints, to see things in a new light, to question what we have not had the courage or incentive to question in the past. Hysterical peer-review paranoia that "mistakes" may be allowed to slip through the gates is greatly out of proportion to their dreaded danger.

If we are willing to make a conscious, intelligent choice whether to retain peer review or eliminate it, our decision will hinge on whether to open the door a crack through which, perhaps, a few additional unacceptable works may find their way to publication, or whether to continue to use a system predisposed to obstruct the publication of potentially important creative work. If our wish is to advance human knowledge, it should be clear which is the lesser of the two evils.

There is a recognized and legitimate need, prior to publication, for editors to be assured of an author's qualifications—as these are made evident in the quality of his or her research, and not to be confused with either possession of a set of credentials or affiliation with a well-known institution. There is a need for editors to be assured of the satisfaction of a discipline's general standards of proof and evidence—and yet to remain open to persuasion that these standards need to be amended or extended. Solidity of scholarship should be assured—but not at the expense of curbing future work by binding it in slavish adherence to what has been said and done in the past.

Standards of professional certification, criteria of justification for results, and breadth of information do admittedly change with time, and mental space must be reserved to allow for this.

NOTES

1. Nearly every one of the criticisms in this list has its own body of literature; to list references for each would take inordinate space here. My purpose in this chapter is not to review the published literature relating to peer and editorial review, and so I have kept references to a minimum. Readers interested in an overview and discussion of many of the individual criticisms of peer and editorial review that I enumerate, and others as well, may find Campanario's detailed two-part paper (1998) useful and replete with citations; further relevant works include: Albert, 1997; Armstrong, 1996; Bedeian, 1996; Brysbaert, 1996; Enserink, 2001; Fine, 1996; García, 1981; Greenberg, 1999; Hadjistavropoulos & Bieling, 2000; Harnad, 1982; Hojat et al., 2003; Holbrook, 1986; Horrobin, 1982 and 1990; Jefferson et al., 2002a and 2002b; Kassirer & Campion, 1994; Levenson, 1996; Lock, 1985; Mahoney, 1977, 1979, 1990; Mahoney et al., 1978; Martin et al., 1986; Naftulin et al., 1973; Olson, 1990; Peter et al., 1983; Peters & Ceci, 1982; Rabinovich, 1996; Rowland, 2002; Sharp, 1990; Starbuck, 2003; Ware & Williams, 1975; Yalow, 1982; Ziman, 1982.

2. See Kevin D. Lafferty, "Can the common brain parasite, *Toxoplasma gondii*, influence human culture?," http://rspb.royalsocietypublishing.org/content/273/1602/2749.full.pdf+html, accessed May 11, 2011. From the November 7, 2006, issue of the *Proceedings of the Royal Society, Biology*, 273, 2749–2755. News release available from the U.S. Geological Survey at http://online.wr.usgs.gov/ocw/htmlmail/2006/20060802nr.html, accessed May 11, 2011.

3. The number of books and journal papers, and the number of newly established professional journals, are both increasing exponentially, with a current doubling time of about 15 years. There are at present some 30,000 journals publishing 600,000 papers a year (Rescher, 2006, pp. 49–50).

The doubling time of the human population is now about 35 years, so the rate of proliferation of publications far exceeds the growth of the population. The result is a devaluation of publications and authorship, since the value that people place on a product or work of any kind is inversely proportional to its commonness.

Due to this explosive, exponential growth in what is published it is not surprising that the likelihood that any given paper will *not* be cited in future publications is rapidly increasing (Rescher, 2006, p. 52). The pebbles one casts are perceived to be smaller and smaller, the lake larger and larger, while the ripples that are made by cast pebbles disappear faster and faster. The work of authors, the "pebbles" they create and toss, comes naturally and proportionately to be cheapened.

4. On the conflict between the psychology of creative thinkers and the psychology of the normal world, see Chapter 3 in the present volume and Bartlett (2009).

5. Quoting from the "Guidelines for Non-Sexist Use of Language," originally published in the *Proceedings and Addresses of the American Philosophical Association 59* (3) (February 1986), pp. 471–82, and revised and reprinted as a separate report in 2001, and which was based on earlier guidelines of the American Psychological Association and the National Council of Teachers of English.

8

The Psychology of Mediocrity:
Internal Limitations That Block Human
Development

Psychology, as a field, has lots and lots of data, but we don't have very many good ideas.
    —Dennis Proffitt, Chairman, Dept. of Psychology, University of Virginia (Jacobs, 2009, p. 48)

One of the last remaining—and it would seem passionately postponed—frontiers of behavioral and cognitive science is the investigation of *internal limitations* of human psychology, limitations that act to block individual and social development. This area has been a lifelong interest with me. In earlier work, I examined

- Internal limitations of this kind that stand in the way of the meaningful use of many concepts basic to scientific and to everyday thought (which I've called *conceptual pathologies*: Bartlett, 1971; 1975; 1976; 1980; 1982; Bartlett & Suber, 1987; Bartlett, 1992; 2005, Part III);
- Internal limitations that are at the core of the psychology of normality and that result in pathology (called *pathologies of normality*: Bartlett, 2005, 2006, 2009);
- Psychological constraints that block the ability of people to learn from past mistakes and to improve their individual, social, and environmental conditions, condemning people to vicious circles of repetitive, self-destructive thought and behavior (a crucial but entirely neglected area of study, the *psychology of stupidity*: Bartlett, 2005, Chap. 18);

- Handicapping deficits that limit people to a low level and quality of consciousness, conduct, and outlook that are inherently barbaric (Chapter 5 of this book and Bartlett, 1993a, 1993b);
- Limitations that impede individual and group consciousness of culture (familiar to readers of this book in the form of acedia: Chapters 4 and 6 of this book; also Bartlett, 1994a, 1994b);
- Internal psychological limitations that block the continued survival of the world's rich diversity of species as a result of an intransigent human psychology of heedless reproduction and environmental exploitation (Bartlett, 2006 and 2005, Chap. 17); and two more specialized forms of limitation:
- Internal psychological limitations that obstruct the constructive development of the discipline of philosophy (Bartlett, 1986a, 1986b, 1989); and
- Internal psychological limitations that block the human recognition of animal rights (Bartlett, 2002, 2007).

All of these limitations are internal—that is, intrinsic—to normal human psychology, and serve variously to slow, to impede, and at times effectively to halt the advance of human knowledge. These limitations obstruct the development and cultivation of human sensibility, which would otherwise lessen human aggression and cruelty and encourage the broadening and deepening of human compassion. At the same time, many of these limitations are destructive because they block positive, constructive relationships between individuals, between societies, and between human and nonhuman species; and because they are devastating to the environmental conditions necessary not only to sustain life but to make humane, uncrowded, and aesthetic living possible. The majority of these internal psychological limitations function exceedingly well in an obstructive capacity because they remain unrecognized, but more often because their recognition by professional psychologists and psychiatrists and the wider public is strongly resisted and subject to widespread denial thanks to individual and group vested interests and ideological commitments.

In the academic world and in the popular consciousness, the study of "internal limitations" has become familiar only in the field of mathematics, where the discovery of a growing family of theorems of formal limitation is judged by many mathematicians to have been the most important advance in that discipline during the last century. Theorems of formal limitation are proofs of what mathematics cannot, in principle, attain; they are informative results that exhibit the intrinsic limitations of formal systems. Theorems of formal limitation do not describe psychological limitations of mathematicians but rather limitations that are inescapable because they are internal and intrinsic to the subject matter itself of formalized mathematics.[1]

The "internal psychological limitations" that have captured my interest over the years are similar in kind to the formal limitations of mathematics but yet are specifically different. Both varieties of internal limitation, the formal and the psychological, are reflexive in nature. First, such limitations are built into the very fabric of each subject matter, arising as a consequence of the nature of each; and, second, they are discovered and made evident through studies that make reflexive use of the means provided by formal systems themselves, in the case of mathematics, and through investigations that similarly make reflexive use of human psychology, in the case at hand: tools of mathematics are used in order to demonstrate intrinsic limitations in the use of those very tools, and human psychological abilities are relied upon to make evident the limitations of those very abilities. In both these cases, the means of discovery, the tools of analysis, have had to be developed from within the subjects studied, which is to say, self-referentially. An account of the nature and role of self-referential analysis would take us beyond the scope of this book (see Bartlett & Suber, 1987; Bartlett, 1992); suffice it here to say that the psychological limitations I am referring to can be studied by human beings only in a self-referential manner, that is to say—and as cognitive scientists and epistemologists would express this—*reflexively*: we are forced to make use of the means offered to us by our own human psychology in order to study it, and hence when I speak of *internal limitations* this phrase has a literal and concrete meaning which asserts that a very large portion of the human population is internally limited by the psychological limitations mentioned in the bulleted list above.

The varieties of internal psychological limitation that appear on that list are, in different ways, restrictive and handicapping in a sense somewhat parallel to that in which customary psychiatric diagnostic categories are considered to be restrictive and handicapping to those to whom they are thought to apply. But this parallel is a matter of analogy only. Readers will by now be aware of some of my reasons for rejecting psychiatry's concept of "mental disorders." The justification for this rejection, as expressed in previous chapters in this book, rests in large part on the decision to dismiss psychological normality as a valid or enlightened standard of mental health.

The internal psychological limitations that I've listed affect the very great majority of people and are so widespread as to be contrasted rather than compared with conventionally accepted *DSM* diagnostic categories, which, on the contrary, are intended to identify and sort out from the general population special groups of "mentally disordered" individuals. Despite this essential difference, psychiatry and clinical psychology have sought to find therapeutic ways to reduce or eliminate the cognitive, affective, and behavioral obstacles that hinder people psychologically, that cause them distress and disability, that handicap their abilities to reach their personal goals in life. In this general sense, to speak of "internal limitations" within the framework of clinical psychology, as I shall do here, is to make use of an historically appropriate descriptive phrase, while emphasizing that its application is extended beyond a medically narrow conception of psychological disorder.

In this chapter, I continue the study of internal psychological limitations by examining a wholly neglected area of normal human psychology, *the psychology of mediocrity*. Mediocrity, in its multiple forms of expression, is, as we shall see, yet another kind of internal psychological brake that halts both individual and social development. This topic has been so seldom mentioned, much less studied, in the literature that it will not take us long to review what has been written about it, which we'll do a little later.

During the second half of the twentieth century and continuing this trend today, psychiatry and to a lesser extent psychology have been strongly affected by the success of physical science. In taking physics as a model of scientific success, psychiatrists and some psychologists have come to believe that scientific success requires an unemotional neutrality toward values. This interpretation has been reinforced by psychiatry's wish to step beyond any lingering shadows of the value-loaded moral psychology that had been advocated a century and a half ago by Bucknill and Tuke (1858/ 1879) and by their fellow nineteenth-century practitioners—who, it is relevant to remember, inaugurated a much-to-be-appreciated kinder and more sympathetic understanding and treatment of the mentally ill than had previously been the case.

The resulting current fashion, which we now dignify by calling it a "paradigm" and which has been embraced by psychiatry and empirically focused psychology during the past six to eight decades, has sought to emphasize experimentally and behaviorally focused investigation that aims to be purely descriptive, empirically based, and most especially value free. In this framework the preferred paradigm seeks to identify and formulate law-like regularities that govern the psychology of human emotion, cognition, and behavior so as to explain, predict, and gain control over these components of the human psychological constitution.

But this external clothing of psychiatry and empirical psychology, which aims to give the appearance of value neutrality, is only a gossamer-thin outer layer, masking the stubborn persistence of—and indeed the unavoidable need for—value judgments whenever good mental health is differentiated from its lack. As we have seen in earlier chapters, it is an inexorable fact that recognition of disease requires for its very possibility and meaningfulness a context, a framework, in terms of which normative evaluations can be made—in other words, a frame of reference that enables us to distinguish desirable health from undesirable pathology. And so whenever we recognize a condition, a set of symptoms, a disposition, a personality structure, or another construct to be pathogenic, we depend upon a prior acceptance of certain values that determine what we hold to be desirable, in opposition to conditions that we seek to combat, ameliorate, or cure.

In this chapter, we shall examine a set of human traits that, in an unusual and until now unrecognized sense, constitute a widespread pathology—characteristics that are perceived to be manifestly undesirable from the standpoint of a normative frame of reference that is seldom applied and is often neglected. It is, as we shall see, a frame of reference for judgment that is most often resisted with extreme hardihood and rigidity by current psychological theory and practice. This way of looking at and understanding psychological matters arouses uneasy suspicion, opposition, and often obdurate resistance among psychiatrists and many clinical psychologists because (1) it is explicitly and unashamedly based upon a specific set of values that stand apart from those that are conventional and popular, and (2) it is fundamentally opposed to current diagnostic standards that equate psychological health with psychological normality.

Readers who have followed the discussion to this point are by now familiar with the author's Socratic bias. It underlies the following discussion, and so that bias will be repeated: If we cannot abide questioning our most fundamental assumptions, then of course we're fated to be held captive by them, and what we are capable of seeing and thinking will be correspondingly *limited*.

My use of this recurring word 'limited' is central to what follows. My purpose in this chapter is to describe and discuss a set of human traits that are essentially *limitative* in the sense that they comprise, in a variety of ways, traits that stand in the way of the individuals who posses them, traits that block individual and social development by limiting what people can become conscious of and hence appreciate and cultivate. These traits are blinders, constraints, and shackles that straightjacket and confine the individuals who possess them to a partial, impoverished experience of reality. At the same time, they are traits that impede human psychological development and all that this means, including social, political, and, perhaps most significantly, human *moral* development. The traits that

I examine are limitative in both of these senses: They bar the development of both individuals and their societies.

I use the word 'moral' intentionally but with some misgiving since the word is easily associated with the pulpit. But I use the word here not from any pulpit but in the same sense in which it is valid to speak of 'the morality of medicine', when by this phrase we intend to point to the explicit values of combating disease and disability, of seeking to avoid and alleviate suffering, of using the knowledge and means that medical science offers to make human life *better*. 'Better' is at the forefront of morally loaded words, but it is unavoidable as soon as we articulate reflectively the purpose of medical treatment: to resist and combat pathology in an effort to achieve better health.

Psychology is no different from physical medicine in this respect: it, too, aims to improve human life, on both an individual and social level; and it, too, rests upon an implicit morality that seeks to resist and combat pathology. And, as I seek to show in this chapter, the morality that motivates us to oppose pathology leads us to recognize one of the most destructive and handicapping of human pathologies, the stubbornly and almost totally neglected psychology of mediocrity.

The study that follows provides a descriptive psychology of mediocrity, which forms part of the psychology of individual differences. In any science we must begin with description, proceed to taxonomy, and then finally to explanatory or etiological analysis. As H. J. and M. W. Eysenck noted, "No dynamic analysis is possible without a descriptive framework, and the concepts provided within this framework are the stepping stones to a more dynamic analysis and understanding" (Eysenck & Eysenck, 1985, p. 7). Alternatively, William James and many continental psychologists have called this phenomenological psychology. My purpose here is to describe certain of the most fundamental characteristics of the psychology of mediocrity so that they can be readily identified and named. This chapter provides a descriptive framework and offers the basis for a taxonomy. But first our discussion will benefit by a brief historical introduction.

A BRIEF HISTORY OF A MUNDANE TRINITY: MEDIOCRITY, MEDIOCRE, MEDIOCRACY

These three words, proudly self-ascribed by some groups or applied to them in passionate condemnation by their critics, can mean much or little, as we choose. Their dominant meanings have undergone the most extreme changes over time, much like the quaint and today greatly overused word 'egregious', which used to underscore the exemplary standing out or apart from the vulgarity of the common crowd (*e* + *greg* = apart from the flock or herd). But this word—that had once expressed an affirmative judgment that one is distinguished by virtue of *distinctiveness* from one's group—is now, in a politically correct about-face, used to imply an outraged judgment against this very thing, expressing *sotto voce* an affront should anything or anyone have the temerity to stand out from the herd—and those who do are subject to censure. Such temerity is "simply egregious," that is, outrageous, hence an appropriate target for indignation. Here we find one of those insightful, enjoyable (to lovers of language), and telling radical transformations of vocabulary that can disclose much about ourselves and specifically about our psychology.

The three words in our vocabulary that are used to refer to ordinariness, the average, the median, commonness, commonplace, normality, and the social dominance of dullness and triviality—that is, the trinity formed by 'mediocrity', 'mediocre', and 'mediocracy'—have over the centuries also experienced a striking change in the fashion of usage and public intent.[2] The meanings associated with these words have migrated from one end of the spectrum of acceptability to the opposite end, cultural condemnation. As we shall see, they are now in the process of bouncing back again toward their original point of departure.

It was not long ago that 'mediocrity' was used to name a golden mean, an ideal situated contentedly between extremes, to be valued as a goal, to be prized when achieved, to be regretted when out of reach. But with the passing of a few centuries, 'mediocrity' became a label for the second-rate, the undesirably common, middling, and ordinary and, in the distasteful sense, a label for the simply rude, unsophisticated, and vulgar, a word for the uncultivated, the unexceptional, the tawdry, the uninspired, and the nondescript.

And now, the historical course of this trio of words is reversing, as is unashamedly promoted by such books as *The Happy Mediocrity*, or *Embracing Your Inner Mediocrity*, or even *You Take the High Road and I'll Take the Bus: Celebrating Mediocrity in a World That Tries Too Hard.*[3] This "celebration of mediocrity," as we've seen in various forms elsewhere in this book, is real, nonmetaphorical, and actively pursued in an assortment of complementary ways—on the most general level, through adherence to the values behind which the greater society rallies, and in the specific context of higher education, through the content it communicates, the standards it sets, the educational ends it establishes, and the social and political purposes to which it is harnessed.

'Mediocrity' is the English residuum of Old and Middle French, which gave rise, from 1300 to the mid-1500s, to *médiocrité*, which meant an intermediate state, moderation, and moderate fortune. Hobbes, in 1650, assured his readers that it was "[t]he common Opinion, that Virtue consisteth in Mediocrity and Vice in Extreams" (*De Corpore Politico*). In 1681, J. Flavell's *Method of Grace* continued to propose that "A mediocrity is the Christians [sic] best external security." Even in 1878, Thomas Hardy's *Return of the Native* still promoted the view that a well-proportioned mind's "usual blessings are happiness and mediocrity ... enabling its possessors to find their way to wealth, to wind up well."

Despite this proud emphasis on the comforting superfluities of mediocrity, an opposing current began during part of the same period. In 1589, Thomas Nashe would claim: "Which makes me thinke, that either the louers of mediocritie, are verie many, or that the number of good Poets, are very small." By 1669, the word was beginning to point unwaveringly toward a specific meaning—sheer lack of talent and distinction. William Congreve in 1694 would comment, "[m]ethinks he wants a Manner ... some distinguishing Quality ... he is too much a Mediocrity, in my mind" (*Double-Dealer*, II). Here began the second life of the adjective 'mediocre'—to mean an average, unexceptional level of mental ability, skill, endowment, or achievement; and it would soon come to mean even less than this level of attainment.

During the same period, the French became more inclusive in their construction of ideas, turning from the adjective to the noun and using 'les médiocres' in 1658 to denote *people*. Soon 'mediocre', in French and in English, began to imply qualities justifying disparagement, to be contrasted with excellence and superiority. So that by 1987, the October 15 issue of Cambridge's *Weekly News* noticed that "[t]oo little thought and understanding of the audience has produced a new high in mediocrity."

And so to say of something or someone that it, or he or she, is "mediocre" came to express a judgment concerning the quality or merit—from indifferent to downright bad—of the thing or of the person. The adjective was predicated of the perceived low quality of many works of art, music, theatre, and literature; of many levels of ability, education, cultivation, or knowledge; and of many people in terms of their mental competence or other accomplishments. Nehru, in a 1945 letter to Gandhi, would then write, "A few out of the books they send are good, most are mediocre" (*Two Alone*), a twentieth-century refrain of Thomas Jefferson's 1813 comment that "[t]he Latin versions of this passage by Buchanan and by Johnston, are but mediocres" (Oct. 12 letter in his *Writings*).

As for the application of 'mediocre' to people, in 1884 Sir Richard Harrington observed: "The mediocre ... always form numerically the largest portion of every profession" (*Law Times* 77(393), p. 2), and then in 1903 added: "The result would be a kind of nightmare of the mediocre, a universal Brixton" (*The Speaker*, Oct. 17).

By 1991, the fault-finding *m*-adjective flowed unselfconsciously off the tongue: "What emerges is a stream of sad litanies to the mediocre and the ephemeral" (*Time Out*, Nov. 5). The critical, judgmental application of 'mediocre' and 'mediocrity', not just to things and individual persons but to groups of people, meshed well with this usage, and so the third member in our mundane trinity, 'mediocracy', was given room to grow.

The word 'mediocracy' may have come into English existence cloned from the French 'médiocratie', applied in 1869 to refer to political power in the hands of the mediocre. By July 1876, the *Atlantic Monthly* would also use it: "The day which brought the news of the fall of Fort Sumter saw the overthrow of the mediocracy." A century later, psychologist Hans Eysenck would use it in the context of a psychological critique of the human majority:

> The conscious cultivation of a mediocracy, in which the bright, the original, the innovators, the geniuses are held back in order to spare the mediocre the spectacle of outstanding success is to me an abomination. . . . Compassion for the halt and the lame, bodily and mentally, is right and good; it is the hallmark of an advanced civilization. But we must take care that it does not exceed what is right and proper, and lead to the suppression of high intellect and great merit. Even the able have their inalienable right, and a society disregards these at its peril. (Eysenck, 1972, p. 219)

This description of the lexical history of the three *m*-words is an appropriate point of departure; from here on we shall leave lexical definition and seek, instead, a real definition[4] for these terms, that is, an empirically based description of the psychology of most people, putting to one side the historical changes of fashion that stipulate that these words should be defined in certain customary ways.

PAST ATTEMPTS TO UNDERSTAND THE PSYCHOLOGY OF MEDIOCRITY

As I've already mentioned, few researchers in psychology have studied the phenomenon of mediocrity. To my knowledge, only three book-length studies that purport to do this exist; all three works are in Spanish and have not been translated into English. Why Spanish-speaking authors have been attracted to the topic, which has failed to capture the attention of researchers in other countries, is an interesting question to which I have no certain answer. My guess is that the societies with which these authors were familiar were stratified; the social conditions with which they were most familiar were hierarchical, with clear-cut divisions been lower-class manual laborers and the educated and more cultivated upper class.

Societies in which stratification is an explicitly accepted fact of life may perhaps encourage researchers to attend more consciously to the phenomenon of mediocrity since, as we shall see later, the recognition of mediocrity is facilitated when a society perceives individual differences clearly (sometimes with excessive stereotyping), without distortions created by a politically rigid system of belief in universal equality. In a similar way, mediocrity tends to be swept under the carpet or simply ignored in a society, such as that of the United States today, in which the act of acknowledging the fact of individual differences often arouses great hostility. Weighing these two opposing factors—the acceptance of individual differences by some societies and the ideological opposition of others to such acceptance—it may be fair to say that the latter inhibits the study of mediocrity at least as powerfully as the former fosters it.

The first of the three books about the psychology of mediocrity was written by José Ingenieros (1877–1925), who, despite having been born Giuseppe Ingegneri in Palermo, Italy, studied, lived, worked, and published in Argentina under the name for which he has become well-known. He was educated as a physician; he specialized in psychiatry and criminology; the majority of his book-length publications are works in psychology and psychiatry. Ingenieros was the founder of the Argentine Psychological Society and later of the *Revista de Filosofía*, which reflected his interest in philosophical studies, for which he is also recognized.

In 1910, Ingenieros gave a series of lectures on the psychology of character, which were collected together and published in his book *El hombre mediocre* ("Mediocre Man"). The interest that this work aroused was nothing short of astounding, as we look back from a vantage point a hundred years later. It is hard to imagine today that a work about the psychology of mediocrity could excite such interest: His lectures were first published in 1910–1911 by *La Nación* in Buenos Aires, then published by *Archivos de Psiquiatría y Criminología* in 1911, and then were published in book form by the Madrid publisher Renacimiento. For the first edition, in January, 1913, 10,000 copies were printed; only two months later, this was followed by a second edition of 10,000 more copies (Ingenieros, 1913/1957, p. 7). The book has subsequently been published in a number of additional editions and by several publishers. This gives an idea how much attention the topic of the psychology of mediocrity attracted at that time and how neglected, in comparison, it has become today.

El hombre mediocre consists of only about 200 pages. It seeks to describe mediocrity but easily gives contemporary readers the principal impression that the author is engaging in a catharsis and polemic against the psychological characteristics of the common person. The book can tax one's patience; it is unequivocally repetitious and monotonous in its deprecations of mediocrity. But there is a central and significant purpose: to underscore how mediocrity acts as a restrictive block to human development. In this context, "catharsis" and "polemic" are understandable when readers realize that they are expressions of Ingenieros' impatience over humanity's deeply entrenched, stubborn disregard and denial concerning a major psychologically disabling condition which, as we shall see later on, there is good reason to judge to be a form of pathology.

Ingenieros recognized that mediocrity possesses an underlying psychology that is distinctive and in need of explication because, he claimed, it constitutes a critical block to human evolution. Although his description of that underlying psychology is fragmentary and incomplete, what he does say offers a beginning that is worthwhile to consider.

For Ingenieros, mediocrity is fundamentally a psychological incapacity for *ideals* (in much the same way as we saw that acedia is an incapacity for culture in Chapter 4). This incapacity, according to Ingenieros, is tied to the mediocre person's impoverished personality or character. An individual's personality or character is the basis for distinguishing one person meaningfully from another; personality and character are basic constituents of a person's individual identity. Ingenieros calls both the psychological incapacity for ideals and an undeveloped sense of self "mediocrity."

Ingenieros refers to the mediocre as "the obtuse" (*los obtusos*) because "the narrow horizon [*el estrecho trecho horizonte*] of their experience constitutes the forceful limit of their minds" (Ingenieros, 1913/1957, p. 34). He therefore refers to the "obtuse imagination" of the mediocre, which confines them to a limited, partial, and impoverished reality, the result of their limited capacity to have ideals.

Although there is not space here to summarize Ingenieros' conception of mediocrity in great detail, I'd like to draw attention to a set of claims that he makes about mediocrity and its study which are central and which I'll amplify and supplement later on. First, Ingenieros accepts the factual inequality of individuals: individual differences, whatever their ultimate causes, are real and must be taken into account. He agrees with Plutarch's observation that "animals of the same species differ among themselves less than some men from others," and with Montaigne's that "[t]here is more difference between this and that man than between that man and that beast, which is to say, that the animal of highest excellence is closer to the less intelligent man, than this man is to another man who possesses stature and greatness" (Ingenieros, 1913/1957, p. 34).

Second, as a consequence of the reality of individual differences, people vary a great deal, and in their variation, some—and they are rather few—possess a meaningful degree of individuality, a uniqueness of character that is their own, which differentiates them from the mass of other people.

In contrast, mediocre people seek to blend with others, to be like them, and so they are: members of an indistinct, undifferentiated mass. In contrast, genuine individuals, often those who are creative, possess singular personalities that serve to differentiate them and give them distinctness and identities of their own. The mediocre do, of course, believe that they have their own individual personalities, but when observed closely, their personalities are seen to be insubstantial, insignificant, and, as Ingenieros expresses this, they simply dissolve away.

Third, because of the imitative psychology of the mediocre, they suffer from a form of "mental myopia" (p. 62) and are incapable of creating their own ideals, which is precisely what people who develop their own sense of personal identity are able to do; Ingenieros judges such people "superior" in contrast to the mediocre.

Fourth, because mediocrity is threatened by superiority, mediocre people will often go out of their way to resist and block the efforts of those who are superior in ability or attainment.

Fifth, the psychology of mediocrity is "contagious." Despite his training as a physician, Ingenieros did not develop this idea drawn from his background in medical pathology, but perhaps he had in mind the fact that mediocrity brings with it undeniable emotional gratifications, as we shall see later, which attract many people and lead them to embrace it.

Sixth, mediocrity is most at home in a life filled with routine, a fully scheduled existence. The mental life that fits such an existence is similarly routinized; decisions and judgments are facilitated and made a matter of habit through prejudice, stereotyping, and adherence to conventional beliefs, all of which save people the need to think. The mediocre hold their prejudices stubbornly: "their prejudices are like nails: the more they are hit, the deeper they are embedded" (p. 60).

Much of Ingenieros' understanding of the psychology of mediocrity is captured in these six observations. Although his book can be diffuse and repetitive, sympathetic modern readers can perhaps see how each of these six observations relates to Ingenieros' general claim, that mediocrity is an obstacle to human development. He recognized as an inescapable fact that people vary as individuals, that the many copy one another and that some few develop unique, significantly differentiating personal identities. He observed that these few form the world's great, the eminent, the creative— individuals who are able to develop their own values and standards and live according to their own principles. Mediocrity stands as an obstacle to such development and therefore stands in the way of human evolution.

The significance of Ingenieros' study of the psychology of mediocrity perhaps lies mainly here, that he recognized mediocrity to be what I've called an "internal psychological limitation," one that drags down the best that humanity can be, that prevents each mediocre person from developing a genuine sense of self, and, in a society dominated by the mediocre and their mental myopia, that limits and obstructs the future development of the species.

The second book, also in Spanish, purportedly also about mediocrity, was written by Francisco Álvarez González (1986), *El reto de la mediocridad* ("The Challenge of Mediocrity"). Álvarez González (1912–), like Ingenieros, was born in Europe (in Madrid) but spent most of his life in South America, teaching in Bolivia and Ecuador, with a short period in Costa Rica. He was trained in jurisprudence and then in philosophy, studying with Manuel García Morente and José Ortega y Gasset. He made philosophy his career.

El reto de la mediocridad tells us extremely little about the nature of mediocrity; in fact, despite the book's title and its 423-page length, mediocrity as such is seldom discussed. The book is primarily a series of complaints about society and is a rambling, philosophically unfocused description of social and political conditions that the author dislikes. Álvarez González mentions collective human stupidity (*estupidez generalizada*) in Chapter 2, but does not throw light on the phenomenon. The closest we get to anything informative about mediocrity is that it consists of "absence of imagination" (pp. 93 and 423), a claim similar to Ingenieros' but adding nothing to the discussion. I've chosen to mention the book at all for the simple reason that it will come up in any multilanguage search for works about mediocrity.

The third book dealing with mediocrity is Luis Camacho Naranjo's (1992) *Ensayo sobre la mediocridad* ("Essay on Mediocrity"). Camacho Naranjo is a professor in the School of Philosophy at the University of Costa Rica. His *Ensayo* is a short work, a monograph, which, despite its brevity, reflects a serious interest in understanding mediocrity principally from the standpoint of its social psychology. He identifies certain of the social conditions that foster mediocrity, for example, fundamentalism, dogmatism, and lack of openness to ideas. Unusual in the scant literature about mediocrity, Camacho Naranjo raises but does not answer the question whether there may be a biological basis of mediocrity, distinguishable both from the social conditions that foster it and from the personal deficiency that manifests it (p. 52). He bravely writes of the *calidad* of the person—his or her worth or value as a person—which echoes the language of Konrad Lorenz and Abraham Maslow, as we shall see later.

Mediocrity, for Camacho Naranjo, needs to be understood primarily as a phenomenon that affects individuals and not purely as a negative judgment of contemporary society (p. 29). He makes clear that the recognition of mediocrity is relative to an overall context of valuation, of grades of value, in terms of which we make judgments (pp. 34–35). From this point of view, the Peter Principle helps to explain how people can be expected to rise in the ranks of their job or profession until they reach a level at which their performance is incompetent, and then, because they can advance no further, they remain there. As a result, the world falls to the hands of the mediocre, a world in which nothing works correctly (p. 62). Excuses for mediocrity multiply: the mediocre evade personal responsibility, attributing shortcomings and failures to the system or institution in which they live and work, but they are quick to claim credit for any successes and attribute these to their own personal abilities (pp. 56–66). Mediocrity brings about a decline in creativity, behavior becomes routinized, and the way is paved for political repression and totalitarianism (Chapter IV).

Together, these three Spanish works share in the observation that mediocrity is a psychologically limiting phenomenon: for Ingenieros, and even for Álvarez González, mediocrity is a deficiency—an incapacity for ideals and an impoverished personality or a deficiency of imagination. Camacho Naranjo situates mediocrity in a social-political context, recognizing that mediocrity occurs on the individual level, infusing a society with incompetence, absence of personal responsibility, and a readiness to dissimulate through excuses for failure. The result is a society in which creativity declines, facilitating increased repression and loss of individual freedom.

These three books also share a pattern of observation that is inherently multifactorial, identifying multiple, differentiable human traits, all of which express internally limiting characteristics of human psychology. We shall attempt fill out this picture in a more inclusive and unified way in what follows.

MEDIOCRITY AS A SET OF TRAITS

The study of individual differences in the organism, and their interaction with stimuli and responses, is an integral part of scientific psychology, and central to it. Identical stimuli are perceived and reacted to differentially by a bright person or a dull, an extravert or an introvert, an emotionally unstable or stable person. To find the laws according to which this may happen, and to isolate the major dimensions along which we can classify people, seems to me a fundamental and critically important part of psychology.

—Eysenck (1990, p. 195)

Readers will recall the distinction between lexical and real definition in the discussion of the psychology of definition in Chapter 2 of this book. It would be easy to resign oneself to an arbitrary multiplicity of different lexical definitions of the terms 'mediocrity', 'mediocre', and 'mediocracy', and dismiss the range of choice as purely semantical. It is more challenging and constructive to establish real definitions for these words, definitions subject to empirical verification or falsification. My interest here is to describe real and specific psychological deficiencies that can severely limit a wide variety of human abilities, sensitivities, predispositions, tastes, values, motivations, choices, preferences, goals and the means selected to achieve them, and even styles of execution in thinking, feeling, perceiving, and in reflecting about these. There are identifiable forms of mediocrity in connection with any of the foregoing, and, in general, whenever we make evaluations in terms of a scale of value, it is possible to distinguish a lower mediocre range of the scale from a higher range.

In the history of modern psychology, two principal concepts of mediocrity have been suggested. One is the identification of normality with mediocrity, as was done a long time ago by Wile (1940, p. 225): "A central tendency principle establishes normality as mediocrity." The other, more evaluative, was recommended by Francis Galton:

> The meaning of the word 'mediocrity' admits of little doubt. It defines the standard of intellectual power found in most provincial gatherings, because the attractions of a more stirring life in the metropolis and elsewhere, are apt to draw away the abler classes of man, and the silly and imbecile do not take part in the gatherings. Hence, the residuum that forms the bulk of the general society of small provincial places, is commonly very pure in its mediocrity.... Hence we arrive at the undeniable, but unexpected conclusion, that eminently gifted men are raised as much above mediocrity as idiots are depressed below it; a fact that is calculated to considerably enlarge our ideas of the enormous differences of intellectual gifts between man and man. (Galton, 1869/1978, pp. 31–32)

Galton used a ranking system that has become standard in contemporary discussions, the Gaussian or bell curve. As Galton put it,

> the numbers of men in the several classes in my table depend on no uncertain hypothesis. They are determined by the assured law of deviations from an average.... It will be seen that more than half... is contained in the two mediocre classes...; the four mediocre classes... contain more than four-fifths, and the six mediocre classes more than nineteen-twentieths of the entire population. Thus, the rarity of commanding ability, and the vast abundance of mediocrity, is no accident, but follows of necessity, from the very nature of these things.... (Galton, 1869/1978, p. 31)

What Galton meant by the terms 'mediocre' and 'mediocrity' evidently encompasses the largest portion of the human population, and in this I shall follow him, in contrast to Wile's equation of mediocrity with the human average. It is not the average *per se* that we have in view here, but the great majority, who, taken together, as we shall see, make up the population of the mediocre.

More than any other country, the United States has held, often hysterically, to an irrational, empirically false prejudice against the recognition of individual differences. The country's political commitment to social equality has unreasonably spilled over into an unwillingness to recognize individual differences, except perhaps physically—in sports. Diversity of cognitive, emotional, and moral intelligence, variety in literary, artistic, and general aesthetic sensibility, and the presence in individuals of a wide range of traits of personality—all have been resisted topics in American normalized psychology, and often their study has been passionately condemned, demonstrated against, and brought to a halt by the American public.[5] This ideological commitment to social and political equality has obstructed research concerning individual differences, and, as a logical consequence, it has stood in the way of constructive progress in designing an educational system responsive to real differences between one person and another.

From the time of Roman physician Galen's proposal that there are four basic types of personality, the sanguine, melancholic, choleric, and phlegmatic, the psychology concerned with defining traits of personality has, despite American resistance, nevertheless become more discriminating and sophisticated (e.g., Eysenck, 1967; Eysenck & Eysenck, 1985). But in spite of this progress, our recognition of individual characteristics that are responsible for significant differences between individuals and between groups is still fragmentary and partial because what we are prepared to see and study continues to be limited by ideological bias.

Numerous alternative personality inventories have now been developed, but none seeks to measure the identifying marks of mediocrity that concern us here. Given the major role that these gravely limiting traits have had and will continue to have in human development, this state of affairs should strike reflective readers as not only surprising but undesirable.

Most of the empirically based study of the psychology of individual differences has used factor analysis to identify fundamental traits and dimensions (see Thomson, 1939, and Burt, 1940, works that have played a historically influential role). Factor analysis begins with measurements of different variables whose degrees of intercorrelation are quantified; it ends with the extraction of a small number of preferably independent factors that are intended significantly to reduce the number of sources of variance that must be taken into account. Factor analysis ideally condenses the number of variables to a minimal number of common factors and then determines each factor's relative contribution. This can be a great advantage, for example, to psychometrists by providing a minimal conceptual vocabulary shared by researchers. In formalized mathematics, much the same motivation leads mathematicians to expend considerable effort to obtain minimal sets of axioms for which it is possible to prove that each axiom is independent of the others and necessary to its formal system.

J. P. Guilford was a pioneer in the factor analysis of temperament; he sought to identify the major factors in terms of which personality variations can be understood. Guilford's factors comprise such traits as level of general activity, restraint, ascendance (leadership or submission), sociability, emotional stability, objectivity, friendliness, thoughtfulness, personal relations, and masculinity (Guilford, 1936, 1975; Guilford & Hoepfner, 1971). More recently, Eysenck has sought to show that with but three major superfactors—extraversion/introversion, neuroticism, and psychoticism (each encompassing multiple subordinate factors)—an identifying personality profile for any given person can be developed (cf. Eysenck & Eysenck, 1985).

However, a disadvantage accrues to a minimal conceptual vocabulary. We know in color theory, for example, that only the proportions of the three primary colors need to be specified in order to identify any color combination, which can be represented by an ordered set of numbers that quantify the contribution of each of the primary colors. This is in fact how computer graphics software specifies individual colors and how paint stores are able to mix custom-tinted paint to match a color sample. But if one is a fine artist, it can be much more useful—that is, more informative and practical—to be able to refer to viridian, raw umber, Naples yellow, ultramarine blue, Vandyke brown, and other pigment colors by name. For the purposes of human communication, and for the purposes of richness of description, it is often of value to have more than a minimal conceptual vocabulary. In such a context, we care less about the independence of specific factors and more about the adequacy of a description in communicating convincingly and fully what is in view. Such is the case here.[6]

It will not therefore especially concern us when describing traits that are basic to the psychology of mediocrity whether they are independent or may overlap, or whether these traits comprise a unique minimal or complete set. To be realistic and as we've already noted, the psychology of mediocrity has not evolved to a point where psychometric tests for mediocrity have even been proposed, much less designed and implemented. We do not have statistical data concerning intercorrelated traits of mediocrity to subject to factor analysis. Until we do, the best and indeed the only way to proceed is by way of description, using a conceptual vocabulary that is adequate but certainly not minimal.

THE MAJOR DEFINING TRAITS OF MEDIOCRITY

The renowned factorists of human abilities, Spearman, Thomson, Thurstone, Burt, and others, all were interested in identifying factors that represent primary *abilities* of the mind. Here, in contrast, my interest is in identifying certain of the primary *disabilities* of the human mind, to which very little attention has been given.

The description of major traits of mediocrity that follows is a general inventory of traits that typify mediocre people. Not all of these traits need be found in a given person for him or her to be considered mediocre; my intention is to direct attention to different and sometimes overlapping ways in which people manifest mediocrity.

We begin with a manifestation of mediocrity which it is natural to associate with cognitive skills as measured by IQ: *intellectual mediocrity*. Intellectual mediocrity, however, unlike the abilities that comprise cognitive intelligence, consists of a set of *psychological limitations* that constrain an individual's willingness, motivation, and ability to utilize his or her available cognitive intelligence. Although we associate intellectual mediocrity with absence of cognitive ability, there is certainly no direct one-to-one correlation between high cognitive functioning and freedom from intellectual mediocrity, for some of the most intellectually mediocre are to be found among individuals with high IQ. Intellectual mediocrity is decidedly not confined to those of average or low IQ, as shown in Figure 8.1.

Intellectual mediocrity can take many forms, ranging from outright anti-intellectualism to an individual's low reading level and choice of reading; the low value placed by the person on learning generally and on higher education in particular; the individual's choice of occupation and occupational goals; habitual daily concerns, interests, and activities; and lack of both critical thinking abilities and the willingness to apply those he or she may have.

As will become clear, mediocrity in its many forms produces corresponding varieties of *poverty of mind*, and here intellectual mediocrity is particularly obtrusive. The poverty of mind to which intellectual mediocrity contributes is at once experiential and functional: the intellectually mediocre person experiences the world in a flat, one-dimensional, conceptually impoverished way, and is functionally deficient in those intellectual skills he or she uses. Each deficiency of course worsens and

Figure 8.1
Venn diagram showing plausible interrelationships and combinations among psychological normality, abnormality, high intelligence, creativity, and mediocrity. In order to suggest the continuity of transition from psychological normality to abnormality, these two areas are shown as partially overlapping. The diagram does not seek to represent the relative sizes of the populations involved.

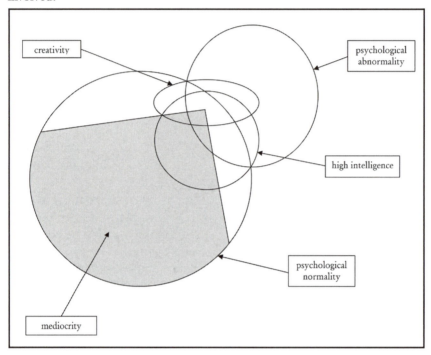

interferes with the others. Ingenieros and Álvarez González saw aspects of this when they wrote of an incapacity for ideals and a deficiency of imagination, but intellectual mediocrity encompasses a good deal more than this. When one compares the experience and intellectual abilities of a peasant with those of a mature, well-educated person, someone who has devoted much of his or her life to intellectual development through depth and breadth of reading and thinking, we may begin to conceive of the two opposite ends of this standard of personal development.

As we continue to describe the psychology of mediocrity, it is central to recognize that we need to maintain sufficient distance from our subject matter to make unbiased description possible. I will not be concerned here to consider how or why individuals and their groups come to be limited by the psychology of mediocrity, or to protest that life is often not fair. It is tempting, particularly at a time when a bias toward environmentalist egalitarianism is dominant, to rationalize or offer excuses (as discussed by Camacho Naranjo) for the limitations of mediocrity. We are reminded that the study of the psychology of mediocrity has not reached a point where it is possible in an intelligent and empirical fashion to explain it in terms of biological, familial, social, or other causes. Before we can begin to determine the sources of the defining characteristics of mediocrity, we first must know what it is we are referring to, and this is the task of systematic description.

The poverty of mind due to intellectual mediocrity is often accompanied by destructive kinds of resistance or opposition to those who excel intellectually. This phenomenon is not limited to plain-vanilla anti-intellectualism but instead frequently includes outright resistance to originality, rejection of creativity and novelty, and a wish to lower great men. Mahoney's (1979) study of the psychology of the scientist draws attention, for example, to the concerted efforts Tycho Brahe made as a lifelong opponent of Copernicanism to block its acceptance. Mahoney points out this has happened many times: "Newton, Mendel, Galton, Planck, Harvey, Lister, Pasteur, Darwin, Helmholtz, Einstein—each experienced the intolerance of their peers, and sometimes the frustration of being prevented from publicizing their views" (p. 357). The reasons most frequently given for the opposition of peers to original work are, as we saw in Chapter 7, the conservatism of peers, their vested interests, professional jealousy, pettiness, and *small*-mindedness, the most literally descriptive of these terms. But the opposition of peers to creative thinking may more appropriately and informatively be described in terms of their intellectual mediocrity, the self-confining poverty of intellectual outlook that has so often impeded and sought to squelch the work of original thinkers.

Closely related, and forming another side of intellectual mediocrity, is the universal tendency of the mediocre to imitate one another. On a cognitive level, imitation takes the form of unquestioning compliance with prevailing conceptual paradigms, the use of the fashionable terminology and writing style of one's in-group, and of course intellectually uncritical acceptance of current standards of political and disciplinary correctness. Originality of thought of course conflicts with some and sometimes with all of these forms of compliance and so engenders antagonism from those whose intellectual mediocrity is dominated by imitation.

Intellectual mediocrity frequently is expressed in the subordinate form of *educational mediocrity*, as vocational education is allowed to infiltrate and take over what used to be genuinely higher education. We encountered some of the central aspects of the mediocritization of higher education in Chapters 5 and 6.

The intellectual mediocrity that has come to dominate much of today's higher education goes hand-in-hand with a recalcitrance to support high attainment and the elitism of high ability. One of the most outspoken, and little-heeded, commentators on such human resistance has been Nobel Laureate in Physiology Charles Richet, who, in his (1919/c. 1925) book appropriately titled *L'Homme stupide* (published in translation as *Idiot Man or The Follies of Mankind*) wrote: "The more stupid and mediocre the masses, the more mercilessly do they persecute those who are simple enough to strive to mitigate their mediocrity and their stupidity" (p. 153). This obstructiveness of the mediocre to original contributions will concern us later.

Intellectual mediocrity includes other subordinate traits. Resistance to culture is evident among people whose capacity to appreciate it is limited, for example, to poster and folk art, pop music, primitive dance, and pulp fiction. Such resistance to culture frequently is associated with an incapacity for refinement—in manners, speech, and general conduct, as we shall see.

There is a close connection between intellectual mediocrity and the inability and unwillingness to attain an effective level of critical reflection concerning the dogma shared by one's group. The cognitive and emotional limitations that come from intellectual mediocrity make it easy to be duped by a group's ideological leaders. Unjustifiable wars and the commission of atrocities are perpetrated by people who are deficient in the capacity to reflect and to evaluate critically and competently beliefs to which they are expected to subscribe.

Intellectual mediocrity leads, then, to a shallowness of views and to the perpetuation of attitudes and behavior that have come to be habitual and comfortable and that do not require the individual to expend effort in serious thinking.

Intellectual mediocrity is often accompanied by a fear of ridicule for being different, for having the initiative to depart from group convictions. As Cioran (1973/1998) noted, "A man who fears ridicule will never go far, for good or ill: he remains on this side of his talents, and even if he has genius, he is doomed to mediocrity" (p. 55).

A second major trait of mediocrity is *emotional mediocrity*. Emotional mediocrity has to do with the preferred content of one's affective experience. The emotionally mediocre person has a need for external stimulation because his or her inner world of experience is limited and impoverished. The need for stimulation can take many forms. It is commonly expressed in the person's wish to be always occupied by external sources of stimulation, and it is most often expressed in a desire for entertainment that is violent and exciting on a primal level. Such need for stimulation is linked, for example, to a love of war for the excitement it produces, for the emotionally gratifying sense of camaraderie that war kindles, for the sharpened consciousness that danger arouses, and for the sense of life purpose that the participants in war experience, often for the first time (Bartlett, 2005, Chap. 9 and Chap. 14). In this sense, war is an anodyne of mediocrity. War "first and foremost . . . gives to mediocre personalities an opportunity to increase their volume and weight by uniting till all sense of mediocrity is lost. . . . It must be an entrancing experience" (Lee, 1920, p. 285).

Emotional mediocrity is associated with low-level affiliative interests and needs. The emotionally mediocre person is indifferent to the second-rate quality—the mediocrity—of his or her friends, acquaintances, and family. When expressed in this way, emotional mediocrity is a form of emotional indiscrimination. Such emotional mediocrity is tied to social mediocrity, which we'll come to later.

Pride in mediocrity reinforces the self-constricting nature of emotional mediocrity. The emotionally mediocre person tends to be proud of his or her mediocrity. This is a self-reinforcing pride: the emotionally mediocre individual pats himself on the back for his "down-to-earthness," she prides herself in being "one of the people," he *likes* being mediocre because mediocrity establishes limits that are comfortable, within which undue effort is not required. These are limits that fit like old clothes— habitual, loose, and unobtrusive in consciousness. "We must remember that a man is not necessarily humble or even modest because has consented to mediocrity. On the contrary, there is a sense of passionate pride among the mediocre" (Finkielkraut, 1996/2000, p. 26). Sartre (1946/1948) also observed this pride of the mediocre in their mediocrity, and singled out the pride felt by anti-Semites, who magnify the perceived value of being mediocre by creating for themselves what Finkielkraut has called "an elite of the ordinary" (Finkielkraut, 1996/2000, p. 26). Pride in mediocrity is now widespread, and can be seen in the enthusiastic celebration of ordinariness, the common, and the vulgar in its pejorative, negative sense.

Jung, too, saw this: "Society, by automatically stressing all the collective qualities in its individual representatives, puts a premium on mediocrity, on everything that settles down to vegetate in an easy, irresponsible way. Individuality will inevitably be driven to the wall" (Jung, 1964, pp. 228–29).

Nietzsche called this phenomenon "the personal arrogance of the self-infatuation of the mediocre" (Nietzsche, 1954, pp. 618–19). He associated such self-infatuation with human stupidity, to which we'll turn a little later.

A subordinate trait of emotional mediocrity should be distinguished. Resistance of the mediocre to those who succeed in developing their individuality is part and parcel of emotional mediocrity. The pride of the mediocre in their own mediocrity takes the form of opposition and often hostility toward persons who have cultivated their own individuality, their own identities apart from groups, their distinctness as persons. We recall that Ingenieros referred to the mediocre person's lack of a developed personality. In terms of the degree of development of their personal identities, the mediocre are characterized by a uniformity that precludes genuine individuation. Those who have been motivated to cultivate a sense of personal autonomy constitute an emotional threat to the comforting commonality of mediocrity, as we'll see in greater detail.

The third major trait of mediocrity is the *aesthetic mediocrity of taste and sensibility*. Aesthetic mediocrity is, like emotional mediocrity, a deficiency in the ability to discriminate: on the most superficial level it is typified by the hearty chorus that "everyone is 'a winner,' " any fireman, policeman, or pilot doing his job is "a hero," and all performances merit standing ovations accompanied by falsetto whoops, whistles, and shrieks of the audience. Aesthetic mediocrity is characterized by a fervent and often exclusive attraction for the primitive: in music, art, dance, film, sensationalist news, literature, and other forms of entertainment. The aesthetically mediocre are limited in their capacity to appreciate cultural beauty. They are blind to refinements of taste because they are deficient in the requisite sensibilities.

Aesthetic sensibility is still a much-neglected area of psychological research. One of the few psychologists to devote himself to its study was Hans Eysenck, who early in his career did research relating to "experimental aesthetics," the study of good versus bad taste in painting, music, culinary art, and so forth. He asked, "given that there is such a thing as 'good taste', do some people have better taste than others?" (Eysenck, 1990, p. 69). He found that this is indeed the case (and before Eysenck, his mentor had confirmed the same thing: Burt, 1940, pp. 121–22). Eysenck observed that people "differed in the degree to which they approximated [an] objective measure of 'good taste' " (p. 70). In the area of "good taste" no less than in that of IQ, it is possible to formulate clear-cut standards, devise tests for the requisite skills, and develop an objective rating scale. And what is such "good taste"? Eysenck found that judgments about the aesthetic merit of individual works of art were generally in agreement, and hence can be used to establish a standard of judgment that is "objective" (p. 69). Of course, a knee-jerk objection to the claim of such "objectivity" can be expected from an egalitarian-minded critic, for whom relativism and "*chacun à son goût*" are persuasive, and to which there is not space here to respond.[7] The identification of traits of mediocrity are, all of them, predicated upon a prior recognition of explicit standards of value, and when this recognition is absent, we're in a situation similar to that in which someone asks "how many meters long is *x*?" and who then proceeds to deny the existence of any metric standard of measurement.

Aesthetic mediocrity is, as we've noted, a form of indiscrimination. It is an inability to judge aesthetic merit: the ability to judge such merit is what aesthetic sensibility means. 'Discrimination' is now a word little used in a positive sense; it has all but lost the meaning of a heightened and refined level of individual taste and judgment that are capable of apprehending *distinction* in the sense of the root Latin *discrimen*.

> Discrimination, once a useful word with a praiseworthy meaning, is now almost always used in a pejorative sense. . . . In everyday life, the ideology of equality censors and straitjackets everything from pedagogy to humor. The ideology of equality has stunted the range of moral dialogue to triviality. In daily life—conversations, the lessons taught in public schools, the kinds of screenplays or newspaper feature stories that people choose to write—the moral ascendancy of equality has made it difficult to use concepts such as virtue, excellence, beauty and—above all—truth. (Herrnstein & Murray, 1994, pp. 533–34)

The psychological incapacity to discriminate is fundamental to many of the traits of mediocrity, as we've already seen and will continue to see in connection with its other traits; indeed, discrimination is plausibly one of mediocrity's main superfactors, were we in a position to perform a systematic factor analysis. Certainly, in polar opposition to cultivated aesthetic judgment and taste, aesthetic mediocrity makes all too evident how central is the capacity to discriminate.

Aesthetic sensibility, and at the other end of the scale, aesthetic mediocrity, have of course been recognized for millennia. In the Orient, for example, Confucius contrasted the *junzi ru* (the noble scholar, assumed by him to be a man) from the *xiaoren ru* (the common scholar), their difference lying in the noble man's sensibility that allows him to recognize the beauty of *ren* (of being human), a sensibility that the "small man" (*xiaoren*) lacks. "Here one may observe the radical difference between the two different universes of *junzi* and *xiaoren*. One is awake to the beauty of *ren*, while the other is not. . . . The *junzi* finds beauty in everything human (*ren*) and accordingly takes pleasure in every expression of the human spirit, namely, in human culture (*wenzhang*)" (Kim, 2006, pp. 112–13). In the West, aesthetic sensibility has been a central and once-revered topic threading through the centuries from Sappho to Plato to Proust.

A century and more ago in the West, aesthetic sensibility was highly valued and was accepted as relatively easy to detect in individuals based on their expressed aesthetic preferences and judgments. Today—except in specialized circles of connoisseurs of arts and letters and among the well-educated—good taste, refinement of aesthetic judgment, and cultivation have become divested of their meanings in a society frantic to assert the universal individual equality of all abilities and therefore insistent upon the relativism of individual taste. When it comes to matters of taste and aesthetic judgment, there now exists no generally accepted understanding of artistic, musical, or literary sensibility and no belief by the American public and by that of other Americanized industrial countries that there are any reliable standards of discrimination that can be relied upon. Sensibility, taste, and aesthetic judgment have been heaped together in egalitarian fashion and dismissed as arbitrary, relative, and purely subjective. This, in itself, is a conspicuous expression of the sway of mediocrity. Ingenieros would again say it reflects the spread of an incapacity for ideals, the inability to recognize nonarbitrary standards of excellence.

Given that "cultivation" has now but a tattered and faded meaning, allow me to quote a short sketch drawn by violinist Yehudi Menuhin of his wife, Diana Gould Menuhin:

> Diana's was a beauty—of mind and soul as well as body—which was the result not only of gifts but of great cultivation, of human endowment worked and disciplined within a tradition to the most refined and durable expression. . . . [H]er upbringing was an interaction of disciplines, her most priceless heritage a strength of selfhood which survived them all and benefited from them. She had the discipline of the English family, whose decorum never slackens, no matter what bombs overhead, no matter what domestic upheavals within. She had the discipline of the ballet. . . . Seeing the pure product, I knew it had been fashioned in the refiner's fire. (Menuhin, 1977, pp. 170–71)

At times, we need to be reminded of what is possible and is sometimes realized by increasingly rare individuals.

A subordinate variety of aesthetic mediocrity is, perhaps surprisingly, financial mediocrity. But financial mediocrity is simply another manifestation of taste, which it is fitting to consider under the heading of aesthetic sensibility. People who express financial mediocrity in their thinking and behavior demonstrate an overarching concern for money and what money can buy. Those for whom life-in-the-pursuit-of-money dominates live a one-dimensional existence of acquisition with no higher purpose that is vital to their daily concerns. The financially mediocre are afflicted by a narrowed outlook that offers little room for cultivation. Like other traits that define the psychology of mediocrity, the financial variety is impoverishing, and it limits self-development. Harnessed to the acquisition of wealth, it paradoxically makes the people it afflicts poorer, limiting them to a single mediocritizing dimension.

The fourth major trait of mediocrity is *mediocrity of conduct*. It can be characterized in terms of (1) the general behavior of the mediocre, and (2) their manners and lack of sophistication. In connection with the first of these, the general behavior of mediocre people lacks discipline and is conformist and narcissistic. Discipline here is the capacity to utilize one's time and energy in a manner resistant to external distraction and on behalf of ends that are "higher." Readers who have gotten this far in this volume will already be aware of the intended meaning of this word, but for others that may join the discussion late, expressed in abbreviated form, the term 'higher' refers here to values that are liberating in the sense of the *artes liberales*—to values, that is, that enrich the human perspective and focus attention on nonmundane matters. Mediocrity is characterized by an incapacity to realize liberation of this kind and is therefore closely related to acedia, discussed in Chapters 4 through 6.

The second characteristic that typifies the general behavior of the mediocre, conformity, which we've already met in connection with intellectual mediocrity and which was recognized by Ingenieros as basic to mediocrity, is the urge of people to copy one another's forms of behavior—to copy their common physical behavior, and most especially their overt expression of conventional attitudes, group affiliation, patterns of response to events, and so on. The third characteristic, narcissism, refers to the self-absorption of the mediocre in the world of their narrowed concerns, interests, and pursuits; a detailed description was given in Chapter 5.

The manners and lack of sophistication of the mediocre make up a second group of characteristics that typify mediocrity of conduct. Here, vulgarity of language and of nonverbal behavior permeate the daily conduct of the mediocre. There is an absence of refinement in language use (as we shall see below in connection with linguistic mediocrity), an absence of physical grace, a lack of polish and a crudeness in nonverbal communication, and often an unrestrained willfulness to engage in verbal and nonverbal offense over trivial matters, the source of the various forms of road rage, shopper's rage, traveler's rage, and related outbursts.

Mediocrity of conduct is closely associated with *social mediocrity*, the fifth major trait of the psychology of mediocrity. Social mediocrity is often expressed in the mediocre person's choice of friends and acquaintances and in the mediocre's enthusiasm to maintain social relationships with mediocre family members. As we have noted in connection with emotional mediocrity, the mediocre person is commonly afflicted by various types of indiscrimination. Social mediocrity involves one of these in particular, social indiscrimination, a disposition encouraged by unquestioning egalitarianism and the refusal to acknowledge individual differences. Social mediocrity is evident in the mediocre person's love for fellow mediocrity, for the undemanding, warm, comforting, bland, mentally relaxing, enjoyable, and emotionally nonstressful herd experience. Social mediocrity is typically exhibited in a low level of quality of conversation: idle chat and prattle about trivia that resolutely exclude concern for "higher topics," the intelligent discussion of which requires a rich cultural experience, education, individual cultivation and refinement, critical thinking ability, and general mastery of language.

The socially mediocre frequently substitute celebrity mania for genuinely meaningful values. Their interests are aroused by the socially trivial and fatuous. Their level of humor is immature and crude, emphasizing reference to body functions, sex, violence, and *Schadenfreude*, pleasure in the calamities that befall other people.

A sixth major trait of mediocrity is *physical mediocrity*, which refers to a low level of care and management of one's physical condition and health and the health of others. The Greeks referred to physical *aretē*, the cultivation of excellence of the body and its functioning. Physical mediocrity is its opposite. Physical mediocrity is characterized by obesity when not due to a diagnosed physiological disorder, by the hypocritical pursuit of dietary fads, by drug and excessive alcohol use, by the placement of a lower value on adequate medical care in preference to material purchases, and by avoidance of exercise and neglect of personal hygiene.

At a critical time of human overpopulation, widespread psychologically based indifference to the physical consequences of adding further to the population qualifies as yet another manifestation of physical mediocrity: it is yet another expression of the inability to engage in reflective critical thinking concerning human reproduction that results in the runaway proliferation of the population. The choice to have children entails the foreseeable physical consequences of bringing more people into a world already characterized by crowding and the consequent impoverishment of the quality of the natural environment. In these senses, physical mediocrity is not only typified by physically unhealthy living but is further characterized by an uncritical, unthinking, and effusive infatuation with the cult of pregnancy and the doting upon infants, by a mindless zeal and unquestioned fanaticism in favor of the bearing and raising of children, in oblivious disregard of the everywhere visible, physical effects of a human population that crowds out other life forms, destroys the aesthetic beauty of the natural world, and poisons itself in the process. In these ways, the lives of the mediocre are dominated by physically irresponsible choices. Living responsibly, on a purely physical level, means living with an intelligent awareness of the consequences of one's physical choices, which include reproductive choices.

On a less globally consequential level, physical mediocrity is also typically expressed in the personal display by the mediocre of an exaggerated lack of personal grooming and shoddiness of dress. We see that physical mediocrity clearly overlaps aesthetic mediocrity, for these traits are clearly not independent of one another. We see both intertwined today, for example, in the young mediocre woman's copycat conformity that gives her voice a forced nasal, duck-like sound, jarring to the few who possess aesthetic sensibility. Fashion rules the mediocre, and this is most especially seen in the choices they make in connection with their personal physical characteristics.

Linguistic mediocrity is a seventh major trait of mediocrity. It refers to mediocrity of expression, that is, to mediocrity of language use. Linguistic mediocrity characterizes those who:

- Exhibit a poverty of expression due to an impoverished vocabulary, through ignorance and lack of retention of the resources of language that make articulate communication possible;
- *Prefer* this limited vocabulary because it is conformist and imitative. Their shrunken vocabulary results in extreme limitation in their expressive ability, and promotes a use of language that makes it most suitable for the expression of elementary emotions, much less suitable for the communication of conceptual complexity, and least suitable for expression that is rich in imagery, figurative, original, eloquent, or in any sense imaginative or evocative;
- Are ignorant of or disregard grammatical refinements of language. Pitkin (1932) called this and the foregoing "linguistic stupidity" (p. 174): "Most people are constitutionally unable to use language in its higher refinements. They live at the mental level intermediate between that of the primordial savage and the superior 1% of modern mankind which has created the subtleties of grammar, rhetoric and style. . . . [W]e say the common man thinks, reads, and talks in catch-phrases and slang" (p. 173);
- Are critically deficient in the reflective metaskills, the linguistic self-consciousness, necessary for competent language use: for instance, subject-verb agreement, distinctions between meaning and use of such word pairs as 'lie' and 'lay', 'effect' and 'affect'; today's mindless repetition of words and phrases such as 'like', 'absolutely', 'y'know', 'unprecedented', and so forth; turning verbs into nouns, as in 'a repeat', 'a mix', and similar manifestations of linguistic carelessness

and indifference. The general lack of *reflective skills* at issue here typifies many of the traits of mediocrity. We shall come back to this issue later;

- Communicate primarily through prattle that has no more lasting value than momentarily excited air, using language principally for the expression of trivia and limited to what is immediate and mundane, without concern or interest in communicating about matters of enduring significance or importance. Related to this is a deficiency in temporal imagination, noted earlier in Chapter 5, which takes the form of an inability to make descriptions of the past or future feel real unless expressed in the present tense;

- Are averse to learning languages other than their native language; who will raise a ridiculing eyebrow when a foreign word, name, or phrase is pronounced correctly; who, as Bertrand Russell once said, condemn to neglect whatever fails to be translated into their own language; and who, through such choices and attitudes, express linguistic provincialism.

In describing these characteristics of linguistic mediocrity, some readers may have the impression that they merely reflect adherence to an intellectually fastidious, grammatically pedantic, rigidly exacting *set of standards* (and it is to be expected that some readers will feel this way about the entire study of the psychology of mediocrity). In a sense, this perception is correct—that is, it is tautologically correct from the standpoint such a reader accepts—but it clearly is not ours here. It is not as though rules of grammar and niceties of speech and writing are hallowed and revered for their own sakes, but they are appreciated as signs of an active, educated, reflective, and disciplined mind, for these are among the qualities that distinguish such a mind from mediocrity. As E. B. White expressed this, "Unless someone is willing to entertain notions of superiority, the English language disintegrates, just as a home disintegrates unless someone in the family sets standards of good taste, good conduct and simple justice" (quoted in Roberts, 2009, p. C3). Certainly the recognition of mediocrity, as it is described in this chapter, is only possible and meaningful from the standpoint of a set of values that accepts the factual legitimacy of what White calls "notions of superiority." We shall return later to consider this issue more explicitly.

Still another major trait of mediocrity is what we may appropriately call *mediocrity of way of living*. Here, I refer to the physical living conditions that the mediocre find acceptable, likable, and even preferable. The mediocre often have low to nonexistent standards regarding the aesthetic qualities of their physical environments and are comparatively insensitive to the presence of noise and crowding. They may have low to nonexistent standards regarding their housing, interior decorating, and housekeeping. They frequently have few standards that are deeply important to them that concern the design of their neighborhoods and the architecture of their towns and cities. They are accepting and tolerant of the degree to which their work is routine and repetitive, of the amount of time that must be given up to commuting, and of the quality and final significance of working in and relating to their community. It is not that mediocre people do not care at all about these things but these things are not for them nonnegotiably important. Relatively few people are willing to undertake fundamental change in their ways of living simply because they will not or cannot tolerate conditions such as I've listed. All of the characteristics that typify mediocrity of way of living involve taste and sensibility and therefore involve an obvious overlap with aesthetic mediocrity described earlier.

Moral mediocrity is the ninth major trait of mediocrity to which we turn. Moral mediocrity is characterized by lack of individual autonomy—specifically, an absence of the strength and independence to set one's own standards; an inability to develop, formulate, and commit to one's own principles; deficiency in critical evaluative ability; and insufficiency in the combined capacity to stand alone in terms of one's evaluative principles, way of life, kinds of experience perceived to be meaningful, and life goals.

In the history of Western thought, Nietzsche has been the most vocal in expressing the importance of rising above levels of moral mediocrity. Through his "anti-mediocre morality" (a phrase used by Ingenieros, 1913/1957, p. 112: *moral antimediocre*) Nietzsche sought to fight back against the mediocre's "general war on everything rare, strange, privileged, the higher man, the higher soul, the higher duty, the higher responsibility, creative fullness and mastery" (Nietzsche, 1972, §212; also §62, §202; 1956, p. xii). Nietzsche described and urged a "final stage of morality" in which "the individual acts in accordance with his own standard with regard to men and things: he himself determines for himself and others what is honourable and useful; he has become the lawgiver of opinion" (Nietzsche, 1989, §94). Nietzsche had no politically correct qualms about recognizing the substantial, real, and inherent distinction between the many and the few, between the noble and the common, between the great and the small (Nietzsche, 1982, §323; 1974, §3, §40; 1968, §984). He emphasized the high worth of individual autonomy, of moral self-sufficiency, and proclaimed that "greatness of soul" involves precisely this kind of independence (Nietzsche, 1974, §55; 1989, Vol. II, §337; 1968, §984; 1972, §§29, 201). In these passages Nietzsche notes that the individual who has reached this high level of morality is indifferent to the opinions to which the mediocre comply and to moral standards which they uncritically accept.

Today, of course, recognition of "nobility of soul," of "the higher man," of "the higher duty," and of "creative fullness and mastery" seldom occurs—in fact, these phrases have lost all pretense of having any definite meaning, and now, for most people, they seem quaint, antiquarian, and when taken with any seriousness are, in an ideological reflex arc, dismissed as unacceptably elitist.

In Bartlett (2005, Chapter 18), a detailed description is given of human *moral intelligence*, to which interested readers are referred for a more comprehensive discussion than can be given here. Moral mediocrity involves a deficiency in such moral intelligence, coupled with an in-built resistance to the moral autonomy that preoccupied Nietzsche. The psychology of morally mediocre people predisposes them to be strongly and rigidly opposed to those who develop and cultivate moral autonomy. Here we again encounter the familiar signature of mediocrity: a psychology of internal limitation that hinders human development.

The tenth and the last major trait of mediocrity that will concern us is *absence of individuation*. As we've seen, Ingenieros referred to the "lack of personality" of the mediocre. In several contexts, we have encountered their lack of discrimination. Both are involved here. The mediocre prefer a state in which they do not feel different from others; they wish not to be fundamentally different since this would erect a wall between them and the comforting warmth of being just like the other members of the herd. This intention to merge the mediocre self with the collectivity of the herd is a *deliberate* internalization of mediocrity.

> This is what constitutes the mediocre man and women, the immense human majority: For the mediocre, to live is to give oneself to unanimity, to permit customs, prejudices, practice, and subjects of concern to become internalized. . . . Beneath the apparent indifference and lack of involvement of the mediocre there always lies a secret fear of having to make decisions for themselves. . . . They dissolve among the multitude. (Ortega y Gasset, 1957/1982, p. 214)

Hence, the mediocre are "indifferent' in the two senses of this word: they prefer *not being different* from others, and they prefer the tepid to the hot or the cold, avoiding whatever goes beyond mediocre acceptability. They dread and resist developing personal identities that would distinguish and differentiate them from everyone else and so render the mediocre person recognizably alien to his or her fellows.

✧

At this point we need to gather together this trait-by-trait description of the psychology of mediocrity. From a level of higher theoretical generality, a level from which we can see the various defining traits of mediocrity as they interact and combine to form the specific phenomenon under discussion, the 10 traits I have identified can be seen to be responsible for a general *mediocrity of values*: They are values that determine and circumscribe the level of a person's everyday consciousness. They determine the objects that receive the person's attention; they determine how his or her life is shaped around these; and they determine how the person makes decisions in a way that displaces or excludes attention to higher alternatives. Such values that absorb the attention of the mediocre frequently have to do with valuing money and things more than time, things more than quality of experience, money and things more than higher realities, imitation and herd commonality more than autonomy and the ability to think reflectively and critically. Mediocrity of values is centered around conformity and compliance and in particular around physical and ideological conformity, shared fashions, tastes, standards, reproductive drives, and doctrinal beliefs. These values motivate the mediocre to gravitate to the menial, the elementary, the undistinguished and hence unexceptional, and therefore to the commonplace; the mediocre accordingly find their most comfortable level of personal challenge and attainment on the humdrum level of ordinariness. And so the imitative and unremarkable identity of the mediocre renders them most contented when in subservience to leaders who themselves share major traits of mediocrity with which they can identify. The mediocre engage in a willful blindness that is both mutually and individually comforting, a blindness that excludes from awareness the experience of the unfamiliar that potentially could challenge, conflict with, or jeopardize accustomed, habitual states of consciousness. As a result, the mediocre live within the boundaries of limited horizons; they lack awareness of other dimensions that go beyond the single dimension of their experience.[8] In the next section, we shall look at the way in which a constrained mediocritizing experience that excludes consciousness of other "dimensions" is intrinsically limiting.

"PEOPLE WHO AREN'T REAL"

"I'm sorry, I certainly don't want to offend you, but, in fact, for me you are without reality. As you present yourself to me, you are without those convincing characteristics that make what we perceive and experience, make what happens, real. You exist, sir, that I cannot deny. But you exist on a level that in my eyes lacks time-space reality. You exist, I might say, on the level of paper, of money and credit, of morality, of laws, of intellect, of

respectability, you are a space-and-time companion of virtue, of the categorical imperative, and of reason, and perhaps you are related to the
Thing-in-Itself or to capitalism. But you have not the reality I find convincing in the case of every stone and tree, every toad, every bird. I can give you
my unlimited respect and approval, sir. I can doubt you or consider you
valid, but it is impossible for me to experience you, it is wholly impossible
to love you. You share this fate with your relations and worthy next of kin,
with virtue, with reason, with the categorical imperative, with all humanity's
ideals. You are magnificent. We are proud of you, but real you are not."
                                           —Hermann Hesse (1973, pp. 153–54)

In Ingenieros' *El hombre mediocre* there is a section entitled "Los
Hombres Sin Personalidad" (Men without Personality) where we find this
claim: "Considered on an individual level, mediocrity can be defined as an
absence of personal characteristics that make it possible to distinguish the
individual in his or her society" (p. 36). We saw earlier in this chapter how
"indiscrimination" and "lack of distinction" can contribute to the mediocre
person's absence of a genuinely individuating identity. The mediocre are,
when considered singly as individuals or as members of the class of mediocre people, not "significantly different." What does this mean?
    In Bartlett (1971, Chapters 1.1, 2.3), I showed how the cognitively fun-
damental concept of an object of reference necessitates that such an object
possess an identity: possession of an identity is an inescapable prerequisite
for any entity. This was the unspoken basis, as I understand Hesse and
Ingenieros, of what both men had in mind: Mediocrity prevents people
from developing a degree of individuation that is genuinely meaningful,
that is significant, that distinguishes them from the masses of other similarly undistinguished people. It is not, of course, that the mediocre are
utterly devoid of personal identity, but when compared with a more fully
developed person who can be distinguished from others by his or her individuating qualities, abilities, and attainments, the mediocre deliquesce
into a undifferentiated mass. As authentic individuals, the mediocre are
not fully real.
    As Hesse might put it, the mediocre are nonentities: there is nothing in
particular that distinguishes them from others who are just as indistinguishable. To make such a claim is to understand the reality of a person
as a function of the level of the realities of which he or she is conscious, that
is, in proportion to his or her exercised capacity to attend to realities that
are "higher." Twice before in this book, I quoted a passage that expresses
what I believe was Hesse's personally defining outlook. That quote begins,
"I consider reality to be the thing one need concern oneself about least of
all, for it is, tediously enough, always at hand while more beautiful and necessary things demand our attention and care" (Hesse, 1925/1954, p. 67).

Those "more beautiful and necessary things" are, for Hesse and others like him, "more real" than the mundane, the ordinary and common. As readers have found presupposed in most of the chapters of this book, there is a frame of reference in terms of which such levels of reality can be discriminated. We'll discuss this presupposition more fully in what follows.

"People who aren't real" is a phrase compatible with Hesse's understanding of the world of mediocrity. The people who inhabit that world are trapped on a level of reality that is—from a "higher," "deeper," "more sensitive," and "more cultivated" perspective—*unreal*: Their world lacks dimensions; they are one-dimensional creatures, with a single, narrowed consciousness that has little depth, little height, and little width. It is only linear, on a single track, confined and impoverished.[9]

This observation is anything but new. Such "levels of reality" were described in detail by Plato, and are basic to many stratified, hierarchical descriptions of human experience. I use the term 'description' with a literal meaning in view: what is described is based on an empirical, matter-of-fact account of what many, but not all, people experience. This is empiricism in its most basic application to the contents of awareness; it is descriptive phenomenology.

Plato wrote: "[I]n heaven, methinks, there is laid up a pattern of such a city, which he who desires may behold and, beholding, take up his abode there. But whether such a city exists, or ever will, is no matter; for he will live after the manner of that city" (Plato, *The Republic*, Chap. XXXIV, ix. 591–2). This "higher level of reality," which for the majority is not real (just as these people themselves are unreal for the Hesses of the world), can become the dominant and most real center of one's concern, of what one values, of one's attention and care. It can then form one's dominant "mental space." Seemingly bordering on metaphor, but yet not metaphorical, that space possesses more dimensions than the mental space inhabited by the mediocre. It is a genuinely "extra-ordinary" space, and access to it and the cultivation of it, on an experiential level, is what most distinguishes the mediocre from those who are not similarly limited.

RESISTANCE TO ACKNOWLEDGING INDIVIDUAL DIFFERENCES IN ABILITIES

It is in the most unqualified manner that I object to pretensions of natural equality.

—Galton (1869/1925, p. 12)

Unfortunately, even to give utterance to such observations as I've just made concerning "levels of reality" is for many people today, just as when

Francis Galton wrote more than a century ago, objectionable and subject to condemnation and intellectual suppression. In his justly famous *Heredi-tary Genius*, quoted above, he admitted: "At the time when the book was written, the human mind was popularly thought to act independently of natural laws, and to be capable of almost any achievement, if compelled to exert itself by a will that had a power of initiation" (p. vii). Later in his book, he commented:

> Our race is essentially slavish; it is the nature of all of us to believe blindly in what we love, rather than in that which we think most wise. We are inclined to look upon an honest, unshrinking pursuit of truth as something irreverent. We are indignant when others pry into our idols, and criticize them with impunity, just as a savage flies to arms when a missionary picks his fetish to pieces. (Galton, 1869/1925, p. 189)

We recall that Ingenieros quoted Plutarch's observation that animals of the same species differ among themselves less than some men differ from other men, and Montaigne's opinion that there is more distance between some men than between some men and animals (Ingenieros, 1913/1957, p. 34). Galton's study of genius bore out such judgments. He wrote: "To conclude, the range of mental power between—I will not say the highest Caucasian and the lowest savage—but between the greatest and least of English intellects, is enormous. . . . There is a continuity of natural ability reaching from one knows not what height, and descending to one can hardly say what depth" (Galton, 1869/1925, p. 22).

Much more recently, psychologist Arthur Jensen ran painfully aground on the most bitter resistance to an acknowledgment of individual differences, shouted in protest with a degree of impassioned hysteria almost beyond belief by his professional colleagues as well as by the general public. About the series of personal attacks and professional abuses he endured, he wrote:

> To a psychologist observing all these phenomena [of ill-treatment], the question naturally arises as to why so many otherwise objective and dispassionate intellectuals display such vehement moral indignation and even zealous combativeness toward any explanation of human behavioral differences. . . . We all feel some uneasiness and discomfort at the notion of differences among persons in traits that we especially value, such as mental abilities, which have obviously important educational, occupational, and social correlates. There are probably no other traits in which we are more reluctant to notice differences, and if circumstances force us to notice them, our first tendency is to minimize them or explain them away. (Jensen, 1972, p. 55)

A colleague of Jensen later commented that some people were unable to consider individual differences dispassionately because they are committed to an unquestionable belief that *unless* it is true that human beings are equal in abilities, a democratic society simply cannot succeed, therefore such equality *must* be a fact. He drew an analogy from religion: "If there weren't a Heavenly Father to sustain me in my agonies, I couldn't go on living; therefore God exists" (Jensen, 1972, p. 57).

A diversity of individual abilities is a fundamental fact of our present human reality. At this time, it is an inescapable given. Perhaps in the future this fact can be replaced with another more to the majority's liking, but if our task is to describe the *present human psychological constitution*, we are stuck with the facts; whether these facts turn out to be due largely to genetics, or chiefly to environment, or to a certain contribution of both is irrelevant insofar as the psychological description remains the same.

THE EPIDEMIC OF MEDIOCRITY

As we have seen, each major psychological trait of mediocrity is associated with psychological gratifications that cause mediocrity to be *self-constraining*—that is, literally to limit the *self* of the person who possesses that trait, preventing the individual from developing further, analogous to the way in which a mechanical governor limits the speed of a motor: as the motor rotates faster, the governor exerts more and more braking force. We have recognized that there potentially exists a level of mediocrity corresponding to every imaginable ability, capacity, sensitivity, or sensibility. Those forms of mediocrity that I have selected to describe are among the most insidious and infiltrating, working their ways into the lives and concerns of the majority of people. These traits of mediocrity enter a person's life often in unobtrusive ways, insinuating themselves into habits of thinking, feeling, and behaving that are essentially constraining, restricting the mediocre person's experience to the lowest levels that he or she finds gratifying. In this sense, mediocrity can accurately be described as *contagious*, a fact that Ingenieros also recognized.

A set of traits can become psychologically contagious—in a literal and not a metaphorical sense—when those traits bring people deeply felt gratifications of the kind this chapter describes; these gratifications, in turn, encourage people to make them habitual. This is a contagious process that results in addictive habituation. In Bartlett (2005, Chap. 7), I described the contagion of "psychic epidemics" in which mass infection or mass pathology occurs and to which rationality succumbs. Are we in the midst of an unrecognized "epidemic of mediocrity"?

More than half a century ago, Jung observed that through such contagion mental illness can come to afflict an entire society. It happens especially, according to Jung, in war. Discussing Germany's part in World War II, he wrote of the "mental contagion that threatened every European," a nonfigurative kind of psychological infectiousness, an "all-engulfing force of attraction" in which "each man clings to the next and each drags the other with him" (Jung 1946/1967–1983, p. 230).

As this occurs, the capacity of people for independent and reflective response is blotted out, their moral sense is diminished so that the larger the social collective in which the mediocre person establishes his or her identity, the lower its moral standards. "Any large company composed of wholly admirable persons has the morality and intelligence of an unwieldy, stupid, and violent animal. The bigger the organization, the more unavoidable is its immorality and blind stupidity" (Jung, 1916–1917/1967–1983, p. 153). "Hence every man is, in a certain sense, unconsciously a worse man when he is in society than when acting alone; for he is carried by society and to that extent relieved of his individual responsibility" (Jung, 1946/1967–1983, p. 228).

During this process, capacities for individual thought and independent response are wiped out. As they are lost, the individual's moral sense (to whatever degree it may exist) is dissolved, so that the larger the herd in which the individual is absorbed, the less is moral restraint observed. Actions that an individual would abhor when acting on his own initiative and conscience then become commonplace: "[T]he greatest infamy on the part of his group will not disturb him, so long as the majority of his fellows steadfastly believe in the exalted morality of their social organization" (Jung, 1946/1967–1983, p. 229).

It is important again to stress that in Jung's judgment the pathology he had in view is not a literary fiction but real: The infection takes place in the minds of people, it sweeps away their capacities for individual, independent thought and action, and it attributes ultimate importance to the social herd. When the collective comes to assume ultimate significance, then the contagion "puts a premium on mediocrity," elevating the ordinary, the mundane, the common, so that "everything . . . settles down to vegetate in an easy, irresponsible way. Individuality will inevitably be driven to the wall" (Jung, 1967–1983, Vol. 7, p. 153).

This phenomenon of contagion unfortunately is not confined to war but is an everyday occurrence. The psychology of mediocrity is a magnet for people who wish to be relieved of the burdensome responsibilities of independent thinking, self-governing morality, and autonomous feeling and behavior. The traits that characterize the psychology of mediocrity are among the most seductive, insidious, and subverting, working their way into the lives and concerns of the majority of people.

MEDIOCRITY: ARRHOSTIA OR SPANDREL?

As I use it here, the word 'arrhostia' (derived from the Greek, meaning "ill health") refers to a normal condition or trend in development or evolution that is recognized to be pathological.[10] The other word, 'spandrel', harkens back to the construction of the domes of Gothic cathedrals, where triangular spaces below the dome came about as the unintended, adventitious results of the way the dome was mounted on the surrounding arches. Gould and Lewontin (1979) picked up the word and applied it to accidental characteristics that fall between the cracks of natural selection and confer no evolutionary advantage. Somewhat less descriptively, Jensen (1972, p. 160) chose to call such conditions "polymorphisms." Hence, the question this section raises is whether the psychology of mediocrity is simply a "spandrel" (or "polymorphism") that bestows no advantages upon human survival, or is instead an "arrhostia" that has become a normal condition and acts as a pathology.

Readers will anticipate my answer to this question, since mediocrity has been described in terms of traits that constitute functional impairments that are inherently limitative for individual as well as to general human development. From this standpoint, the psychology of mediocrity focuses on a specific, pathological branch of human psychology, a branch characterized by a group of self-perpetuating disabilities.

We should note that there is no *necessary* association between low levels of ability, sensitivity, sensibility, and refinement, on the one hand, and the mediocre's willful determination to limit those who excel, on the other, for—after all—the compliant and imitative worker ant performs an obvious social function, and yet does not resist or attack either other workers who excel in their jobs (if among ants "workers of eminence" exist), or, hopefully, the preeminent queen. There is no necessity that low levels of ability, sensibility, and the other characteristics described in this chapter should take the form in people of hostility toward the new and the different, or hostility toward supramediocre levels of attainment. And yet among human beings this plainly does happen, and very often. The psychology of mediocrity not only limits the individual development of those who are mediocre but it would place fetters on others who excel, and, when mediocrity becomes dominant in a population, it turns society into mediocracy, obstructing its advancement.

Needless to say the mediocre serve many functions in human society and fill many useful niches. Ingenieros recognized their socially important role: much of social stability and functioning depends upon people who fill the common ranks (Ingenieros, 1913/1957, pp. 45–48). Unfortunately, the psychology that dominates them brings with it inherent limitation. When the psychology of the majority of the human population involves traits that handicap them in critical ways, we are justified in judging that psychology to be to be pathogenic. In a better world, low levels of ability and achievement in some people need not be associated with the deeply rooted resistance that we see in the mediocre to their own self-development and the development of others.

TRAITS OF EXCELLENCE AND SUPERIORITY

As we have seen, many of the traits of the mediocre set them in antagonistic opposition against those who possess superior abilities; have more cultivated tastes; and show a higher level of education or manners, a broader cultural awareness, excellence in linguistic competence, greater originality, greater concern for physical health and for aesthetic physical surroundings, heightened moral sensitivity and development of moral autonomy, richer personal individuation, and freedom from conformity. In all of these ways, we see the psychology of mediocrity sharply divided from traits that define such qualities as excellence and superiority of ability, achievement, and sensibility.

The branch of psychology dealing with such positive traits has not been as neglected as the psychology of mediocrity. It would take us beyond our present subject to describe these characteristics in detail. Many have already implicitly been named in the course of this chapter, often preceded by the adjectives 'higher', 'better', or 'superior'. There are different routes that language provides to refer to these traits: we may choose to speak of "levels of reality," "dimensions" of awareness and concern, "higher" as opposed to "lower," "richness" as opposed to "poverty" of mind, an "elevated life" in contrast to a life of mundanity. Proust (1913–1927/1981, Vol. III, p. 698) spoke of having "another plane" in one's life; alternatively, we can refer to imagination that goes beyond selfishness, beyond ordinary life and its attendant concerns, beyond routine, job, family, and the mundane necessities that surround us on all sides; and then we encounter a willingness, even a need, to go against the tide.

But when such qualities are found in an individual person, and he or she is called "superior" in certain respects, a rumbling of protest begins. The taboo of individual differences reacts quickly in a prereflective reflex, and then ideology comes into full swing. Nietzsche's most deeply felt concern,

I believe, was the creation of conditions necessary for genuinely superior individuals to develop and achieve greatness. He believed that he foresaw a future—which there is evidence to believe has become the present of today—in which there could develop "a general war on everything rare, strange, privileged, the higher man, the higher soul, the higher duty, the higher responsibility, creative fullness and mastery" (Nietzsche, 1972, §212, cf.§62, §202). He wished for a world in which the long-standing dominance of the mediocre would be replaced by the ascendancy of people of genuinely superior abilities. Like Galton, he did not hesitate to take note of distinctions between the many and the few, between the common and the noble, between the small and the great (Nietzsche, 1982, §323; 1974, §§3, 40; 1968, §984).

Nietzsche has admittedly received bad press, thanks in part to editorial tampering with his writing at the hands of his sister and through the Procrustean stretching of his ideas by the Third Reich. It does of course require independent and clear-headed thinking to break free from such associations that can prevent us from considering an individual's thought on its own merit. More recently, Konrad Lorenz and Abraham Maslow have tried to do this. Lorenz (1940, p. 71) wrote of "the man of high value," "the fully superior person," and "the fully valuable person" (*Vollwertige*). He had in mind many of the traits mentioned in this section and was intellectually and emotionally at ease as an ethologist in accepting the variability of human abilities. He saw no reason to suppress a recognition of the superiority of some people and urged appreciation and respect for outstanding abilities and achievements when they are found in individuals. (For more on this subject in Lorenz, see Bartlett, 2005, Chap. 10.)

Like Lorenz, Maslow also used the language of "superiority" in connection with the factual inequality of human abilities. Since for many people Nietzsche has become "tainted," and perhaps even Lorenz as well (because of uncertainty concerning his early association with the National Socialist environment of his time), I'd like to pause for a few minutes to consider Maslow's thoughts on this matter. Fortunately, he seems to have had no potentially compromising political affiliations that we might hold against him. Maslow is known as a humanistic psychologist with a gentle touch and engaging style. It may surprise some readers that he was unreservedly outspoken about the "superiority" of some people. One of his papers, which is almost never cited—for obvious politically correct reasons—bears the title "The Superior Person" (Maslow, 1964). Since this paper is apparently little read, I'd like to quote some sample passages from it:

> None . . . dares to lock horns with the problem which is so unpopular in any democracy: that some people are superior to others, in any specific skill

or—what is more provocative to the democrat—in *general* capacity. There is evidence that some people tend to be generally superior, that they are simply superior biological organisms born into the world. . . . No society can be really efficient unless its superior persons are preferred and elected by the other people. (p. 10)

Maslow calls this a "delicate problem . . . docked by democrats" (p. 10). He goes on to say, obviously without mincing his words: "[T]here must be a good 10 percent of the population, at least, whom we simply tell what to do and whom we care for as if they were pet animals. Our society has never squarely faced the question of the objective superiority of some people and the inferiority of others" (p. 10).

This topic—for constructive research or for public discussion—is swept under the table: "It is permitted me to say in public what my weaknesses are, but it is certainly not permitted to me to say what my superiorities are. This is a real weakness in our society" (p. 10). He expresses the observation: "The unselected differentiated population at large has a fair proportion of very sick people, very incompetent people, very psychopathic people, insane people, vicious people, authoritarian people, immature people" (p. 11). He then goes on to refer to the "constitutional endowments" of individuals, which these facts reflect (p. 13).

Readers would expect that, in a paper bearing the title it does, Maslow would tell us what the "superior person" really is, what main traits one should expect to find in such an individual. In the paper from which I'm quoting, he uses the phrase "psychologically healthy" to refer to the superior person, but we learn little more in this publication. But it would come later. Maslow concluded his "superiority paper" with these words:

> In an ideal society is seems very clear that people must be able to admire, to choose, and to follow the superior leader with a minimum of antagonism toward his superiority. I am stressing this because I am so aware of the fact that real factual superiors tend to be strongly resented as well as admired, and that therefore they are less apt to be chosen on the basis of a democratic vote.
>
> We must work out some better criterion for selecting leaders than popularity. . . . The good society is impossible unless we develop the ability to admire superiority. (Maslow, 1964, p. 13)

We do find a more fully detailed description of human superiority in Maslow's (1971) *The Farther Reaches of Human Nature*. There, he makes a good deal clearer what he has in mind: a "small and selected superior group" (p. 7) who share his now-famous trait: they are "self-actualizing," that is, they have developed what I've called moral autonomy (Maslow:

"They do not get confused just because 95 percent of the population dis-agrees with them" [p. 9]). They are "psychologically healthy" and hence "psychologically 'superior' " (p. 6); the "psychologically healthy" person is the "more highly evolved" person (p. 96); they are "better cognizers and perceivers" (p. 6); they have a "mission in life" that is meaningful because of "principles which seem *intrinsically worthwhile*" and which "are not abstract to the self-actualizing person; they are as much a part of them as their bones and arteries" (p. 192). Such people are "our (fac-tual) superiors," and for this reason often they are abused by people who are envious of them (p. 219). Superior individuals are more resistant to the pressures of conformity and enculturation (p. 270). And the last char-acteristic of self-actualizing people that I'll mention from Maslow's work is that they are "more responsive to beauty" (p. 287).

Unlike Nietzsche and Lorenz, Maslow wished to be very specific about these traits; in fact, he recognized that they can be defined operationally and measured through psychological testing, as the Personal Orientation Inventory (Shostrom, 1963) attempts to do. Maslow was intellectually and emotionally relaxed, was secure in accepting the factual, wide varia-tion in individual differences, and was no more hesitant to call one person another's "superior" with respect to specific qualities than he was to rec-ognize that one person was taller than another. He accepted the unfair-ness of unequal natural endowments: "Neither would it be fair that one [child] is more talented or intelligent or strong or beautiful than another" (Maslow, 1971, p. 224). He chose to study "remarkable human beings," and about them he wrote: "It was as if they were not quite people but something more than people" (p. 42). Of the total population, perhaps they make up "the healthiest 1 per cent or fraction of 1 percent" (p. 92).[11] And he recognized that some people will feel "deep conflicts over the 'elitism' that is inherent in *any* doctrine of self-actualization—they are after all superior people whenever comparisons are made" (p. 289).

What of the rest of the people, the majority? I don't recall that he used the word 'mediocre' to describe them, but he did use the phrase 'less evolved' (p. 313). Despite the fact—which we may not like but to be real-istic must accept—that the great majority of the population is stupid, cruel to each other, and falls between shortsighted and blind (p. 288), Maslow appears to have been hopeful: "[W]e must be very careful to imply only that the higher life is in principle *possible*, and never that it is probably, or likely, or easy to attain" (p. 326).

Others beside Maslow, Lorenz, and Nietzsche have tried to paint accu-rate portraits of the superior person. As we noted in Chapter 1 of this book, Fromm (1941, 1947, 1955) developed the concept of the "autono-mous person," Rogers (1961) the concept of the "fully functioning person," and Jung that of the "individuated person" (e.g., Jung, 1958, p. 81; for a general discussion of such approaches, cf. Jahoda, 1958). What was their motivation in studying the traits of human beings that make up such a tiny minority? It is of course impossible to answer this question about other authors without speculation, and so I'll bring it home to bear on myself: Why study the psychology of mediocrity? Certainly the framework that I have presupposed in describing the major traits of mediocrity is elitist in precisely the sense that it is elitist to identify and promote traits of human superiority.

And so why do this? I gave my own answer to this question at the beginning of this chapter: "to make human life *better*." If we don't recognize and fully comprehend how major psychological traits that characterize the majority *limit* us, we will remain correspondingly limited and unable to shake off our shackles. The traits that together contribute to the psychology of mediocrity are compelling in their conformist attractions and in the gratifications they bestow, and so not only is it difficult to focus attention on them in a climate of denial but difficult to summon the willingness to repudiate them and then hopefully grow beyond them.

REJECTING NORMALITY AS A STANDARD OF MENTAL HEALTH

In 1932, Columbia University professor in psychology and philosophy Walter B. Pitkin, who studied with Edmund Husserl and Georg Simmel at the University of Berlin and who was influenced by William James, published a lengthy work with the intentionally ironic title, *A Short Introduction to the History of Human Stupidity*. In that hefty volume, he wrote:

> To select as a standard the present normal member of a social group strikes me as itself evidence of imbecility. I should incline to reject normality in the social sense altogether; for the entire social life of our age seems to me . . . sickening in its innumerable deviations from good sense, the rules of health, and the broader principles of human happiness. (Pitkin, 1932, pp. 502–3)

As I've noted in the course of this chapter, the psychology of mediocrity has been almost completely neglected. The same has been true of the study of the psychology of stupidity, to which Pitkin sought to contribute. And the same has true of the study of the psychology of what I have called "pathologies of normality" that characterize much of typical human behavior. In Bartlett (2005, Chap. 18), an attempt was made for the first time to identify major factors that combine to form the familiar phenomenon of human stupidity, one that psychology has failed to study as a disabling condition with its own special traits and a dynamic not captured merely by labeling it a deficiency of intelligence. In Bartlett (2005, 2006, 2008, 2009), similar attempts were made to fill what I consider to be a major loophole in clinical psychology, to study characteristic traits of the normal population that predispose people to engage in destructive thinking, emotion, and behavior. And in this chapter, an equally broad net has been cast in an effort to focus attention, again, on traits possessed by the majority of the human population.

In terms of the purpose of this book, these three foci of study that I've mentioned—human stupidity, pathologies of normality, and mediocrity— are intended to serve a single main purpose, to encourage readers to begin to doubt whether the largely unquestioned equation of psychological normality with mental health is desirable; whether this equation, in the light of what we know about human behavior, is justifiable; and whether there is not a more theoretically plausible, rationally valid, and empirically convincing alternative model for good mental health.

In the course of his principal book on this subject, Maslow admitted: "[W]e are confronted with the very saddening realization that so few people make it. Only a small proportion of the human population gets to the point of identity, or of selfhood, full humanness, self-actualization, etc." (Maslow, 1971, pp. 25–26). In addition to the most obvious reasons for this failure, which include poor parental care, impoverished environments, dietary deficiencies and inadequate medical care, and—the bitter pill for egalitarian environmentalists to swallow—intrinsic constitutional limitation, there is another complementary perspective which we can, if we choose, adopt, and that is heightened awareness of the role of the psychology of mediocrity in holding people back. If readers come away with anything from having read this chapter, I hope they will recognize some of the main ways in which the traits of mediocrity serve to restrict the mind, encouraging imitation, unreflective thought, a narrowed range of concerns, and deeply vested resistance against novelty, originality, and the recognition of eminence.

Such a recognition requires, as I've tried to underscore, a prior recognition of "higher standards" and perhaps of "higher orders or levels of reality" (if one acknowledges the legitimacy of these concepts). It has not been my purpose in this chapter logically to *compel* readers' acceptance of such "higher standards," since this task isn't one of logic but rather of sensibility, whose development cannot be compelled and perhaps not even encouraged. And so the prior acceptance of "higher standards" has been something I have no other alternative but to presuppose. Once presupposed, logically and empirically this follows: "From the point of view that

Table 8.1
Three varieties of internal human limitation.

Mediocrity—focusing attention on:	*Pathologies of Normality*—focusing attention on:	*Stupidity*—focusing attention on:
limitative characteristics that function as self-chosen blocks to development	psychologically normal characteristics that are explicitly harmful, therefore pathogenic	characteristics that involve a wide range of deficits and impairments, whether intellectual, emotional, moral, or aesthetic

I have outlined, normalcy would be rather the kind of sickness or crippling or stunting that we share with everybody else and therefore don't notice" (Maslow, 1971, p. 26). The mediocre typically share a great deal of psychological normality among one another, while those who are not mediocre share much less.

Mediocrity, pathologies associated with psychological normality, and human stupidity are not coextensive but overlap in various ways, as shown in the earlier Venn diagram. The following table may make some of their interrelations clearer.

The distinctions suggested by this table are intended in part to allow us to change the perspective of analysis, that is, to concentrate attention on different areas of study and in part to denote specific populations. In this chapter, I've described major traits of *mediocrity* in some detail; here, a few words are in order in connection with the other two headings in the above table. *Pathologies of normality* include a psychologically rewarding set of emotional and cognitive gratifications provided by vicarious or direct participation in aggression and violence, by ideological rigidity and abso-lutism, obedience to authority, prejudice and persecution, sheer self-defeating stupidity and low levels of moral development (with obvious overlaps with mediocrity and stupidity), and their many sequelae in geno-cides; terrorism; wars; school, domestic, social, and political bullying; pub-licly approved imprisonment, torture, and executions; an unappeasable appetite for human reproduction (another evident overlap, and there are others); the unquestioned placement of human interests above those of all other life forms on the planet; the enforced subservience of nonhuman life to human wishes and convenience; and the resulting devastation of global biodiversity. In addition and central to the subject of pathologies of normal-ity is human resistance to an awareness of it. "Denial" would be an under-statement, for the forces that stand in the way of mankind's reflective consciousness of the pathogenicity of the species are incredibly strong, tenacious, and self-preserving. (For a book-length analysis and discussion, see Bartlett, 2005.)

The third category in the table, human *stupidity*, can be understood in terms of the interaction of a group of affective and cognitive functions:

- Forms of behavior and thinking that are frequently known perfectly well to be harmful and wrong
- Unstable and quickly forgotten knowledge of these forms of behavior and thinking
- Frequently, deliberate evasion of facts

and it commonly involves the following:

- Suggestibility, gullibility, and intellectual laziness, especially in connection with critical, independent appraisal and judgment
- Conformity in thought and feeling (overlapping with mediocrity)
- Disinterest in lessening stupidity itself and unwillingness reflectively to recognize one's own stupidity
- Willful opposition to clear thinking and a preference for reality-denying fantasy
- Disinclination to deal with problems until they have reached crisis proportions
- Inability to make the future or the past real, and hence a mental inflexibility in which only what is perceived to be immediate is real (again, shared with mediocrity)
- Projective thinking (for a more complete discussion see Bartlett, 2005, Chap. 18, especially pp. 286–88)

Understood in this way, human stupidity is both a pathology and a set of characteristics pervasive among the psychologically normal population, found to varying degrees in the majority of people.

We should immediately see that stupidity plays an implicit role in pathologies of normality, as do some of the traits of mediocrity identified in this chapter (e.g., ideological myopia, social compliance, and conformity). Recognizing cross-linkages and overlaps among psychologically limitative traits is not inherently undesirable when these interrelations are informative. As I remarked earlier, at this stage of our knowledge of the psychology of mediocrity it is not useful to become bogged down in sharpening our pencils to determine the independence and theoretical completeness of categories of classification. At present, a truly minimal conceptual vocabulary consisting of the smallest number possible of major independent trait-factors stands more of a chance of handicapping communication rather than of increasing its effectiveness. But we should be self-consciously aware that the three categories in the preceding table significantly overlap.

Among the many memorable maxims attributed to Einstein is the remark, "To keep doing the same things unsuccessfully is insanity." Using the vocabulary of this chapter, we might say instead, "To keep doing the same things unsuccessfully is stupidity; refusing to see this, despite adequate cognitive ability, is mediocrity; and remaining in this unnecessary and destructive cycle is most certainly pathology."

THE TRANSMISSION OF MEDIOCRITY

We have already noted implicitly how the psychology of mediocrity promotes its own transmission: since the mediocre gravitate to imitation, they copy traits of mediocrity from others. And since many of these traits provide emotional gratification, their transmission is virtually assured.

In making these claims, it is not necessary for us to become needlessly embroiled in the debate whether such traits are biologically based or environmentally promoted, in order to reach the assured conclusion that the spread of mediocrity, once firmly established in a social group, is difficult to contain. It has been argued that "human beings in our world today have no more, or little more, than the absolute minimal intellectual endowment necessary for achieving the civilization we know today" (Harlow & Harlow, 1962, p. 34), and this "minimalist thesis" is probably also true in the encompassing sense that takes into account not only intellectual abilities but moral and aesthetic sensibilities that are the foundation of the meaning of civilization.

Readers are no doubt familiar with the bell curve distribution of intellectual ability, with a high bulge in the middle where most of the population is concentrated and tapering to the opposing tails of the curve where we find, at one end, those who are sorely impaired, and, at the other end, those who excel. If one were to draw a curve to represent the distribution of mediocrity, however, it would most plausibly look like only the right half of a bell curve—as though the curve had been cut vertically down through its center and the left side thrown away. Only in the progressively slim right tail of the curve would be found those who are comparatively free of the traits described in this chapter. (By way of comparison, see the chart in Appendix III, which depicts the estimated overall distribution of mental health in the population.)

Biologically focused researchers in the area of cognitive intelligence—such as Galton (1869/1925), Jensen (1972), Herrnstein & Murray (1994), Eysenck (1998/1999), and others—have all voiced warnings of the predictable dysgenic tendency of any population in which, for whatever reasons, the population of those with lower-level abilities increases disproportionately in relation to the population of those with high-level abilities. We are not yet in a position to determine the extent to which the traits of mediocrity are genetically transmitted, and for purposes here we need not be. It is enough in laying a purely descriptive basis to recognize (1) the very large *distribution* and *prevalence* of mediocrity in human history, and (2) its very large *distribution* and *prevalence* today. Recognizing both of these is enough to remove any sense of surprise in observing (3) the increase in the *incidence* of mediocrity in the past several decades. (These are central terms in the theory of disease: The *distribution* of a disease typically relates to the extent of its geographical diffusion; its *prevalence* relates to the proportion of a population that has contracted the disease; and *incidence* refers to the rate at which new occurrences of the disease develop during a specified period of time.)

As readers are sure to be aware, we live at a time when the doubling rate of the population is becoming shorter and shorter. To whatever extent mediocrity is heritable or environmentally conditioned, we should expect its contagious and internally limiting psychological traits to be expressed in an increasingly prominent way as the human population continues to double, with resulting crowding and the undermining of many of the environmental and intellectual conditions that eminent individuals rely upon for personal development, to which I will turn in concluding this chapter.

Harry and Margaret Harlow's hypothesis, that people today have no more or little more than the absolute minimal endowments needed to attain our present civilization, becomes an urgent warning when applied to the future. If my own observations during four decades of research in this area are right, then we are already bemired in our own kind of Dark Age—dark because the heavy atmosphere, fixated on "correctness" and "normality," resists critical questioning.

This observation isn't idiosyncratic on my part, though it is not often made.[12] Lee McIntyre, for example, expresses much the same perception in *Dark Ages: The Case for a Science of Human Behavior*: "Political ideology is today doing to social science what religious ideology did to natural science in the ... Dark Ages. ... Afraid of what we might find out about ourselves, today's academics have stood in the way of a science of human behavior in precisely the same way that religious clerics attempted to stunt the scientific revolution of Copernicus and Galileo" (McIntyre, 2006, pp. xviii–xix).

Resistance to self-criticism is intellectually regressive and feeds the internally limiting dynamic of an infectious, invasive, self-perpetuating psychology of mediocrity that brings about a dark age. When a globally distributed population doubles increasingly rapidly and is characterized by a psychologically contagious mindset that limits that population to one-dimensional concerns and thought, we have the ingredients for a potentially long-lasting dark age, literally an Age of Mediocrity. The future shape of such a world's "half-bell-curve" of mediocrity would show a swelling in the height of the bell as it comes to incorporate more and more people, and a diminishingly thin tail to the right, as the comparative size of the population of those who have been spared, or have freed themselves, from mediocrity dwindles.

"A ROOM OF ONE'S OWN": THE VIEW FROM THE THIRD FLOOR

I've described mediocrity as a pathology that essentially limits the mediocre person, obstructing the individual from becoming—in important, higher, ways—more than he or she is, a pathology that condenses the person's experience around narrowed concerns framed within a limited horizon. It is a pathology that motives the person to associate with others who are similarly limited, erecting mental and emotional barriers in the mediocre person to recognizing, accepting, and wishing to affiliate with others who are superior in any of numerous abilities, and erecting similar barriers to ideas that conflict with those that are familiar, habitual, and therefore preferred. My focus here has been on the nature of mediocrity in limiting self-development, accompanied by observations of the effect upon society when a majority of its members are mediocre. To conclude this chapter, I turn to examine the reverse effects of a mediocre society upon those whose preeminence of ability, moral and aesthetic sensibility, and breadth of concerns place them outside the category of the mediocre.

In Chapter 3, I quoted briefly from Virginia Woolf's *A Room of One's Own*. In that passage she commented on the "poison of fear and bitterness" that the external—we would now say "mediocre"—world inflicted upon her. The mediocrity to which she was exposed and which she could not avoid felt soul-destroying to her, "like a rust eating away the bloom of the spring, destroying the tree at its heart" (Woolf, 1929, p. 64). I went on to discuss similarly severe difficulties set in the way of creative artists by a society that we are now justified in characterizing as profoundly mediocre.

In Chapter 6, I described a variety of depression experienced by some university faculty in the liberal arts, the result of their unavoidable contact with students and university personnel who are afflicted with acedia, an impairment that is an incapacity for culture, and which we now can recognize as an essentially mediocritizing disability.

In the present chapter, I've tried to provide a description of major traits of mediocrity, and to do this have made use of what might be called a "two worlds" or "two-storey" classification of human experience. Maslow devoted much of his professional life to studying "remarkable human beings," and he wrote about them, as I've quoted earlier: "It was as if they were not quite people but something more than people" (Maslow, 1971, p. 42). In a nonfanciful and real sense, such remarkable people can be unlike mediocre people in considerable and far-reaching ways: from their own points of view, it can be very much as though they belong to another species. And so I've talked about "higher standards," "elevated lives," and multiple "orders" or "levels" or "dimensions" of experience, in contrast to the one-dimensional scope of concerns that characterizes mediocre consciousness.

If we are prepared to recognize the existence of "people who are something more than people" (admittedly a big 'if' today), and *if* we are willing to recognize the existence of "upper storeys" of human experience and attainment that some human beings are able to reach (also a sizeable 'if'), then perhaps we can see, for such remarkable people whose mental space includes levels above the mundane, how living among the mediocre can be oppressive, discouraging, and depressing. This is a phenomenon similar to the predicaments of the artist and of university faculty in the liberal arts, but it concerns a greater number of people, even though they still make up a very small minority in relation to the total population.

The world of the mediocre is increasing, strengthening, and becoming more dominant before our eyes, and as it does, the freedoms upon which many of the exceptional have relied are vanishing. Mediocrity overrides many of these freedoms: the freedom to develop one's own ideas, principles, standards, and tastes without the tyranny of the restrictive judgments of mediocrity; the freedom to coexist with natural beauty, unspoiled by human crowding and the many forms of human invasiveness; the freedom to think, work, and live without intrusive noise from increasingly loud and inconsiderate neighbors and from the society at large (cf. Bartlett, 1987; Hempton & Grossman, 2009); the liberty to pursue one's aesthetic, cultural, and intellectual interests in an environment not subject to intellectual suppression, and hence the free ability to give expression to creative conceptions, views, judgments, and theories, to publish with freedom from editorial and peer mediocrity, in an intellectual and cultural environment that is uncrowded by mediocrity that competes with and often willfully displaces genuinely original and significant work.

When the mediocre deprive these conditions from those who are superior in ability and sensibility, not only are the latter often blocked in their development and creative work, the world losing in the process, but they suffer on a personal level as a result. We find hints of this recognition in Maslow:

> Hospital staffs have learned the unloved babies die early from colds. Do we need truth in the same way? I find that if I am deprived of truth, I come down with a peculiar kind of sickness—I become paranoid, mistrusting everybody and trying to look behind everything, searching for hidden meanings to every event. This sort of chronic mistrustfulness is certainly a psychological disease. So I would say that being deprived of truth results in a pathology—a metapathology. . . .
>
> The deprivation of beauty can cause illness. People who are aesthetically very sensitive become depressed and uncomfortable in ugly surroundings. . . .
>
> How much the ugliness affects you depends on your sensitivity and the ease with which you can turn your attention away from the obnoxious stimuli. To carry the point further, living in an unpleasant environment with nasty people is a pathological force. If you choose beautiful and decent people to spend your time with, you will find that you feel better and more uplifted.
>
> Justice is another [case in point], and history has given us plenty of examples of what happens to people when they are deprived of it over a long period of time. (Maslow, 1971, p. 193)

My concern here is with a range of emotion, attitudes, and critical judgments of and by the very small minority of the nonmediocre, whose state of mind and state of feeling about the rest of humanity is predominantly negative. Disappointment, discouragement, and depression felt by a small number of people, because of restrictive and destructive traits of the larger society in which they find themselves, is not unusual. History is full of examples of the justifiably discontented. Recently, to mention one professional group, lawyers have expressed dissatisfaction and estrangement due to what they perceive as a general decline in their profession. In the 1990s, a RAND study sponsored by the California Commission on the Future of the Legal Profession and the State Bar showed that a majority of attorneys despaired of the decline in the sense of integrity and honor of their profession; half admitted they would not choose to become attorneys in today's world (McCarthy, 1994). A study by the Maryland Judicial Task Force (2003) revealed the same kind of distress among attorneys in that state, who feel that their profession has degenerated and given way to rudeness, impatience, and an atmosphere of verbal abuse. A further sign of the inroads that mediocrity is making on professional integrity concerns professional ethicists, whose testimony as experts is relied upon during judicial proceedings in such issues as patient rights. Some among this very group of people who are appointed to be experts in ethical decision-making have become discouraged over increasing paradoxical breaches of ethical integrity by their ethicist colleagues, as explained by the title of a recent article, "Moral Expertise: A Problem in the Professional Ethics of Professional Ethicists" (Crosthwaite, 1995).

These are, however, only faint signs of the seriousness and magnitude of the spread of mediocrity and of the powerful effect this has on the needless struggle of the eminent, who cannot avoid contact with the mediocre population that willfully, steadfastly, and with great stamina and commitment will block their way. As Eysenck remarked:

> Faced with such truculent opposition, unreasoning at best, vehement at worst, creative people need personality traits that help them to cope with such opposition. Such traits are not always approved of by the majority. Persistence, bloody-mindedness, nonconformist behaviour, even asocial and antisocial behaviour—these are some of the protective devices needed by the creative person to cope with the obstacles society, and specifically the society of his peers, throws in his way. If you want to be creative, you might be prepared to fight; if you are a genius, the fight may be even more deadly. Sometimes genius shuns the fight. Copernicus did not publish his heliocentric theory till he was dying. Gauss did not publish his work on n-dimensional geometry; he knew how it would be received. (Lobachevsky, who was the first to actually publish his results in this field, was considered insane, and banished to remote parts of Russia!) (Eysenck, 1998/1999, p. 185)

To say of such remarkable people merely that "they suffer" as a result of mediocrity would be an irresponsible understatement, for their work, their lives, and that of their families are often painfully torn apart by the self-assured and self-chosen limiting nature of mediocrity. In this light, we should be able to appreciate and respect the superior person's *frustration and anger* over the prevalence of mediocrity—because it suffocates him, with a capacity to prevent him from doing what he is convinced he is here for. The mediocre person, in contrast, acquiesces in his acceptance that large portions of his life must be spent in petty matters of daily existence, in competition and struggle with others, in time spent to defend the narrowly perceived beliefs and interests of his group against others who are equally small-minded, in laboring to rectify the stupidities and incompetence of others, and so on. The mediocre person *accepts* such realities of everyday living, and is not thrown off course and out of balance because he has nothing higher that can be brought lower by them. But the same mediocritizing life makes a world of difference to the superior person. The anger and frustration he feels *because* of the intrusion of the mediocre in his life are clearly defensive. They express the superior person's awareness that mediocrity is a threat to his life purpose, and that he is forced to waste much of his life in dealing with, coping with, and combating the persistent invasion of mediocrity in his experience.

Above the ground floor of the common, the everyday, and the mundane, on which the mediocre live, think, and feel, there is a second floor or order of reality on which the remarkable, the eminent, the creative set their sights and establish what concerns them most. From a temporarily rented room on the floor above that second storey, from which we may have a view of the two floors below, we should be able to develop a more sympathetic and supportive understanding of the great effort that outstanding people must often summon—unnecessarily—not to develop their abilities or to advance their work, but simply to survive successfully amid mediocre people. The degree to which the mediocre stifle, obstruct, and oppress, and of course fail utterly to support and encourage individuals with unusual and invaluable capacity, talent, ability, and sensibility is seldom recognized, less often appreciated, and virtually never explicitly opposed, as one chooses to do once we realize that a condition constitutes a widespread and handicapping pathology.

NOTES

1. The most thorough and clear discussion of the internal limitations of mathematics is still Jean Ladrière's (1957) *Les Limitations internes des formalismes*, a major 700-page work still unfortunately untranslated into English despite my offer to do this in 1971. It was M. Ladrière's belief that Anglo-American publications relating to the foundations of mathematics and the theory of formal systems were considerably ahead of publications in Latin languages, and he therefore preferred to make the book available in French and in Spanish translation only.

2. My discussion of the history of use of these words relies in part on the resources of the *OED*'s recently instituted detailed online search service.

3. Related to the appearance of this genre of reading is another recent telling title, *Idiot America: How Stupidity Became a Virtue in the Land of the Free*, which relates to the topic of the psychology of stupidity, discussed later in this chapter.

4. On the difference between lexical and real definition, see Chapter 2.

5. One of the most exaggerated examples of this kind of professional and public protest took place in reaction to Arthur Jensen's genetically focused research on intelligence (Jensen, 1972); much the same thing occurred years later in connection with similar research by Herrnstein & Murray (1994). There are, unfortunately, many other examples.

6. Another way of expressing this is to see that while a purely theoretical orientation can profitably emphasize minimal conceptual simplicity, a practical orientation will often benefit from a useful, maximally rich vocabulary. Burt recognized this when he wrote: "[T]he attitude of the practical psychologist shows a curious contrast to that of the theoretical investigator. The theoretical

investigator wants to describe a maximum number of tests in terms of a minimum number of factors. The practical psychologist would rather aim at *deducing a maximum number of factors from a minimum number of tests*" (Burt, 1940, p. 76, his emphasis).

We gain still another reinforcement for this view by realizing that the fewer the number of factors used to describe an individual, the greater the variability that each factor must account for, and hence the less that we will actually know about the individual. If understanding the individual is the therapist's primary goal, then limiting his or her therapeutic evaluation of the client to a minimal number of descriptive traits will provide minimal information specifically about the individual.

7. An adequate response requires a refutation of relativism, for which see Bartlett (2005, Chap. 20).

8. Again, it is essential to underscore that the traits I have described characterize people *to varying degrees*: few people possess all of the traits of mediocrity to a maximal extent; most people possess a fair number of them; and very few people have none at all. We saw how Confucius perceived "a radical difference between the two different universes" inhabited by those who are awake to beauty and those who are not. One of the disadvantages of a descriptive psychology of traits is that it is easy to form the incorrect impression that possession of a certain set of traits by any given individual is an either-or proposition—in this example, that the "two different universes" can be readily distinguished with respect to any given person. But this is not always the case, for people possess the traits we've distinguished to varying degrees, *on a continuum*. However, the situation changes when we have entire classes of people in view. Then it makes sense to distinguish between the large class of the mediocre and the small class of the distinguished, cultivated, or eminent, and then it makes good sense to speak of the "two different universes" that these people experience. It is important, then, to be aware, on the one hand, of the *continuity* of degrees to which individuals may possess traits of mediocrity, and, on the other, of the *disjunct* nature of distinct populations. And so when I refer to "the population of the mediocre" we should have in mind individuals who express traits of mediocrity to a pronounced, typifying, degree.

9. We need to bear in mind that in expressing observations of this kind we're not deficient in compassion toward those of lesser ability or sensibility; but the focus of our interest here is purely descriptive, to recognize psychological limitations of which we are little aware.

10. This seldom-encountered word is sometimes used to refer to a condition that only "resembles" or "simulates" a diseased condition, as in Henderson (1960/1963, p. 43) and Knight (1948, p. 12). Here, I use it without this qualification.

11. Maslow's estimate of the rarity of such remarkable individuals has a proper place within the panoramic perspective offered by Charles Murray's systematic, comprehensive study of human achievement. There, Murray studied the incidence of genuine human eminence, which is truly rare. In his words: "When we assemble the human résumé, only a few thousand people stand apart form the rest. Among them, the people who are indispensable to the story of human

accomplishment number in the hundreds. Among those hundreds, a handful stand conspicuously above everyone else" (Murray, 2003, p. 87).

12. A decline of civilization has been recognized from a variety of perspectives, from Arthur de Gobineau's *Essai sur l'inégalité des races humaines* (1853–1855), to Nietzsche, Burckhardt, Spengler, Sorokin, and Toynbee, and pointed to most recently by Charles Murray, who observed: "If the question is how much art and science has been produced relative to the people who had a chance to produce it, the West has been on a downhill slide since the end of the Renaissance" (Murray, 2003, p. 434). For studies of the decline of civilization, see also Brander (1998) and Herman (1997).

9

Normality, Pathology, and Mental Health

> If the status quo is presented as natural and normal, then deviation or criticism is by definition unnatural and abnormal. The definition of abnormality thus depends on one of normality which is never itself questioned or justified.
>
> —Cannan (1972, p. 253)

In the first chapter of this book, I quoted a few passages from psychiatrist Louis E. Bisch, who, readers with good memories will recall, thought that the psychologically average make a dismal model of psychological health. He defended the important place in the world of nonnormal people "who have the courage to stress their individuality and sensitiveness and make it outstanding and telling" (Bisch, 1936, p. 28). He did not believe that the world needs more "normals"; it rather needs more exceptional people, remarkable people, people who are not, as we've seen in earlier chapters, afflicted with acedia or are mediocre, barbarous, or stupid.

There are two ways we can take the similar recommendations of Bisch, Fromm, Rogers, and Maslow. Either they are pointing toward unrealizable ideal fictions or there is a need to reassess what we mean both by psychological health and mental disorder. To do this, there is no getting around the need to remove the primary obstacle that has, with obdurate stubbornness, blocked the way toward a more enlightened and realistic psychology and psychiatry. The obstacle that I refer to is of course the equation of psychological normality with mental health.

It is important to remind readers what I mean by 'psychological normality'. Toward the beginning of this book, I affirmed an open and accommodating understanding of the meaning of 'psychological normality', using this phrase to refer to "the set of *typical* and *socially approved* characteristics of affective, cognitive, and behavioral functioning, a set of characteristics derived from the reference group consisting of the majority in a society's population, and relative to which clinicians understand 'deviations from normality' and hence 'mental disorder'. I use the term 'normality' in its commonly accepted meaning of 'customary' and 'typical', and 'norm' in its ordinary meaning of 'an authoritative standard'." In this chapter, I continue to understand psychological normality in this sense.

THE ROMANES PRINCIPLE

In Chapter 3, I referred to psychologist George Romanes, who in his own informal way defended the thesis that there are meaningful, factual truths about the world that do not stand in need of experimental confirmation by empirical science (Romanes, 1883, 1888, 1895). For convenience let us call this "the Romanes Principle." It expresses a point of view that today borders on the heretical, given that we've become adamant in distrusting virtually any claim, however obvious and factually based, unless it has been subjected to double-blind, statistically sound, and replicated studies. There is surely a place in science for caution, but not for thickheadedness. Human history is already a readily available laboratory that is able, in keeping with the Romanes Principle, to provide us with reliable information about how human beings feel, think, and behave, and are likely to continue in the same old patterns.

Here are some of the historically established facts that we should have at our fingertips and at the forefront of our consciousness when we equate psychological normality with mental health:

- Human history, as any schoolchild knows, has been dominated by wars, revolutions, genocides, persecutions, and the varied brutalities of martyrdoms, judicial executions, political assassinations and murders, imprisonments, torture, and the many other signs of human aggression and self-destructiveness in which psychologically normal people routinely have been and continue to be involved. In wars, they play the role of active participants, nearly always uncritically willing, indeed enthusiastic, to do the bidding of their leaders. The ranks of the psychologically normal are never in short supply, whether to *serve* as members of a country's armed forces, to *serve* as jurors whose decisions send others to imprisonment or a sentence of death, to *serve* as public prosecutors, judges, wardens, jailors, and public executioners, or in any other capacity to *serve* in the defense of the ideology of their group. The willingness of the psychologically normal to "serve" obediently in all of these ways does not stand in need of further confirmation from empirical science; history is more than enough.[1] (For those who would like a detailed discussion and justification of all of these claims, a separate book is required: see Bartlett, 2005.)

- The psychologically normal make up the great mass of the mediocre, as the previous chapter made evident. The internal psychological limitations to which this greater part of humanity is subject are powerful and increasingly dominate and check the development of the human population. We see this in the history of higher education, the history of the liberal arts, and in evident changes in the public's level of consciousness of culture, literacy, aesthetic sensibility, language competence, manners, and other expressions of taste.

- The closely related traits of acedia, barbarity, mediocrity, and human stupidity taken conjointly, that is, adding the respective groups together, designate the greatest portion of the human population. At the same time, the dominant portion of this population is, by virtue of the customary definition we are applying, characterized by psychological normality. The total size of the population of individuals who fail to be psychologically normal and yet who exhibit the characteristics of acedia, barbarity, mediocrity, or stupidity is, in comparison, extremely small (the size of the set of the psychologically nonnormal is itself small).[2]

- In their thinking, beliefs, and attitudes, the psychologically normal make use of a vocabulary of ideas and cognitive patterns that are permeated by forms of projective thinking that are self-destructive. It does not take a sophisticated level of conceptual analysis to show any historian or ethologist precisely this conclusion from the available record of human prejudice, ideological commitment, pseudo-speciation (the willful propensity of human groups to identify, or manufacture, group distinctions that give them a basis to differentiate and distance themselves from other groups), and ethnocentrism (a group's insistence that it is special and uniquely good). (Again, for a detailed discussion of these observations, see Bartlett, 2005.)

As human history has abundantly shown, the above are some of the typical and socially endorsed ways in which typical, normal people think, feel, and behave. And yet, despite these overwhelmingly indicting expressions of psychological normality, psychiatry and much psychology persist in equating psychological normality with mental health! To do this is similar to a pulmonary specialist who uses tubercular lungs as a model for pulmonary health, or an oncologist who uses samples of cancerous tissue as a standard of healthy tissue, or a cognitive scientist who finds in imbecility or dementia a standard of fully functioning intelligence. And yet we do not and will not see this. Using psychological normality as a measure of psychological health is to use a defective measuring stick. Bisch tried humor to correct this deeply rooted mistake, but his small readership probably only laughed, and the point he sought to make has yet to be made.

It should go without saying that psychological normality is functional in many ways, as we saw in connection with mediocrity, which also serves its functions, many of them useful. But the pathology of normality has almost always been neglected, evaded, or denied.[3] It is true that the tubercular lungs of the still-living patient continue to perform a function, as may cancerous tissue, or the imbecilic individual. But the functional deficits that are involved far outweigh the functional advantages and make evident to us that pathology is present and treatment needed.

It is difficult to learn from history: Each new generation has no memory and so must depend upon education to transmit what can be learned from the past. When education fails adequately to do this, and the psychological constitution of people from generation to generation does not itself undergo fundamental change, people can be expected to continue to exhibit the same patterns. When it comes to the pathogenic traits of normality, psychology and psychiatry have not learned from human history. As disciplines, they are not alone in their failure to pay sufficient attention to evidence drawn from the past; however, they *are* unique in establishing a standard of mental health that *fully ignores that past*.

Clinical psychology and psychiatry that are historically well-informed would need to recognize that there is no *brake* or *restraint* in the psychologically normal person to prevent him or her from engaging in behavior, thought, and affect that are so *typically normal* as found in the above bulleted list. In looking as far back as we can see in the human historical record, we see behavior, thought, and affect that are mediocre, stupid, afflicted by acedia, barbarous, and self-destructively projective—exemplifying precisely such things as we find in the above list. These patterns constitutive of the greater part of human history have become so familiar that they are not only accepted and tolerated but have come to be ignored, while at the same time psychological normality has been raised on a dais of its own and then used to define and act as a standard of good mental health. This is Kafkaesque absurdity; it is to turn reality on its head and to mistake the typical but regrettable for the good and desirable.

Acedia, barbarity, mediocrity, stupidity, and projective thinking that is self-destructive—all of these are ingredients of the normal psychological constitution. It can only reflect shortsightedness and an unwillingness to face the paradox at the core of the mental health disciplines for us to continue to dig ever deeper the ruts in which we're entrenched in our stubbornly persistent equation of psychological normality with psychological health.

TWO PROMISING DIRECTIONS AND TWO KINDS OF PATHOLOGY

As I see the situation we face, there are two main directions in which mental health theory can constructively develop; they were introduced to readers in the first chapter of this book. There are good grounds for us to recognize that both are therapeutically promising. Both avoid the misplaced emphasis traditionally invested in psychological normality as a standard of mental health, and both are more realistic, more accurate, and more insightful in their understanding of human psychological problems.

The first seeks to understand mental health in terms of special, smaller populations that exhibit signs of healthy, benign—nonpathogenic— mental functioning. Such special populations show identifiable marks of good mental health that can be distinguished and pried freed from the context of pressure to conform to the majoritarian larger population. Abraham Maslow offers one of the best examples of this approach through the detailed descriptions he has given of characteristics possessed by exceptional people, people who, as he put it, are "meta-motivated," or who, as I've expressed this, succeed in living a life above the mundane, an elevated life, individuals whose awareness exceeds the boundaries of the common limited horizon, who are morally intelligent, capable of independent critical thought, culturally enlightened, aesthetically sensitive—who, in a word, are truly "civilized."

A second approach, which can easily be employed in conjunction with the first, involves a return to an individualized, human-centered, nonregimented, nontaxonomic understanding of psychological problems— dispensing with technically structured, algorithmic catalogs of constructed diagnostic codes and avoiding the theoretically ungrounded notion of "mental disorders." As noted earlier in this book, such an approach was proposed by psychiatrist J. H. van den Berg; he called it *phenomenological psychiatry* (van den Berg, 1955, 1972, 1980; de Konig, 1982). It opposes standard psychiatric classification and diagnostic pigeonholing and instead seeks to help individuals through nonjudgmental support of the client by the therapist, support that is situated from an empathetic standpoint that recognizes the reality and legitimacy of the person's own experience. Rogers expressed this well:

> It is the counselor's function to assume, in so far as he is able, the internal frame of reference of the client, to perceive the world as the client sees it, to perceive the client himself as he is seen by himself, to lay aside all perceptions from the external frame of reference while doing so, and to communicate something of this empathic understanding to the client. (Rogers, 1965, p. 24)

Therapy offered from such a point of view consists in helping the individual to deal more effectively with his or her own individualized situation in terms that involve the person's values, goals, competences, abilities, sensitivities, and temperament. Successful living through self-adaptation becomes the focus, rather than adaptation to the normal and normalized world.

In this way we could, if we chose, change the reference group in relation to which we understand mentally healthy functioning from the population of the psychologically typical and average to special, smaller populations that demonstrate traits of psychological health. Alternatively, we can choose to understand psychologically healthy functioning in highly individualized terms. Both of the resulting conceptions of good psychological health suggest corresponding and mutually compatible approaches to psychological therapy, the first by enabling us to establish a set of ideal standards of mental health and the second by recognizing that the psychological problems experienced by individual people are best understood and helped on a situationally relative and individualized basis.

Were we to make either choice, or both, how should we then understand pathology in the context of mental health?

There are, as I see this, two distinct psychological senses in which it is meaningful and justifiable to call a condition a variety of pathology. In Chapter 2, I made the case to restrict the meaning of psychiatric pathology to confirmable organic disorder; this meaning of 'pathology', in itself and as far as it goes, tends to be unobjectionable to both the medical-psychiatric and the clinical-psychological communities (both of course are not content with this but want to include varieties of pathology beyond the organic). As readers will recall, I oppose the reification of symptoms and syndromes into distinct "disease entities" that simply reflect our predisposition to engage in projective thinking.

There is a second legitimate meaning of the term 'pathology' that I'd like to introduce at this point, and will give only a brief sketch here of this concept (for a detailed discussion, see Bartlett, 2005). Suppose that we're especially interested in cognitive intelligence as measured by IQ. If a person's IQ can be shown to be very considerably lowered, for instance by dietary deficiency or an abusive home environment while he or she is a child, it makes good sense to characterize this destructive lowering of IQ as a consequence of pathology. There may or may not be evidence of organic damage, of any physical "lesion," but still it conveys useful information to speak of pathology in this context. Our justification for using this language is that we share an objective means for measuring IQ, and more importantly, we base our judgment of pathology of the observed desirability and preference to be given to a state of higher IQ. To attribute individual pathology in the context of IQ, we need to be able to measure or estimate a given individual's IQ; to do this in an objective manner, we must share the use of a common IQ standard and scale; and we need to be convinced that an individual's level of desired cognitive functioning has been harmed.

In more general terms, the judgment that pathology is present in a given individual is relative then to (1) an expert group whose members share an agreed-upon standard and scale of value; (2) one or more ways of establishing by formal measurement or informal appraisal, *where* on such a scale, applying the given standard, an evaluative measurement is to be located; and (3) an evaluative judgment, giving greatest weight to the individual's own judgment, that his or her level of desired functioning has been harmed. When these conditions are met, we have established a reference frame in terms of which we can meaningfully speak of "pathology." And, in this, we note that we do not projectively reify "disease entities" or go beyond empirical evidence.

To give another illustration, in my book *The Pathology of Man* (Bartlett, 2005), I examined a wide variety of human pathologies, including mental, social, and conceptual, none of which are, at least at present, known to be linked to verifiable organic dysfunctions. Such pathologies include psychological gratifications obtained from hating, injuring, and killing others; aggression against others for the sole reason that they are perceived to be different; persecution of those whose beliefs differ from our own; and so on. All of these can appropriately be called pathologies because there is an informed, perhaps I should say "enlightened," group of people who agree that such acts are undesirable, and there are standards of harm which they can apply to identify and rank the kind and degree of pathology involved.[4] Here again we note that calling such psychological predispositions "pathological" does not entail any sort of projective reification of disease.

In the present book, I've used the language of pathology to describe varieties of harm that we can recognize as undesirable thanks to our possession of the relevant standards, but the use of such language does not imply that (1) we are referring to disease entities inferred or assumed to lie behind complexes of symptoms, or (2) equate such pathology with deviations from normality (see Chapters 2 and 3).

As far as I can see, the two concepts of pathology that I've outlined above are the only two fundamentally distinct ways in which judgments claiming that pathology is real (and not merely stipulated by definition) can be solidly defended by psychiatry and clinical psychology. Earlier in this book (Chapter 2), I described one of these ways through an analysis of the traditional psychiatric concept of mental disorder; the result of that discussion was to recognize that it is crucial for legitimate psychiatric pathology to be correlated with a detectable organic basis.

The second variety of nonarbitrary pathology is the subject matter of Bartlett (2005). There, diagnostic judgment rests on the solid basis offered by the shared values of a specific reference group chosen because its members possess traits of exceptional psychological health. As we have seen, our recognition of pathology is essentially a matter of evaluative judgment and hence is a matter of values. Our ability to recognize pathology, in the specific sense intended here, involves the "morality of medicine" or the "morality of psychology." I referred to the morality of medicine in the preceding chapter to emphasize that, in recognizing pathology, we intend "to point to the explicit values of combating disease and disability, of seeking to avoid and alleviate suffering, of using the knowledge and means that medical science offers to make human life *better*." With the meaning of this kind of "morality" in mind, it will make good sense to some readers that the reference group whose evaluative judgment is presupposed when the "morality of psychology" is at issue consists of people who have what elsewhere I've referred to as a high level of *moral intelligence* (see Chapter 1 of this book, and in more detail Bartlett, 2005, Chap. 18). They are "extraordinary" people; "remarkable" in Maslow's sense; "egregious" in the root meaning of that word: they stand apart from the crowd.

CREATING MENTAL DISORDERS BY BALLOT

The counsel men agree with is vain: it is only the echo of their own voices.
—George Bernard Shaw (1934, p. 184)

In contrast to the two concepts of pathology that I've just described, contemporary psychiatry (and clinical psychology to the extent that it has surrendered to *DSM*-defined practice) has set down classificatory criteria that define "mental disorders" through a complex, committee-driven process that *votes into existence* those symptom clusters that are judged by appointed committee members, now numbering more than a thousand, to be undesirable, harmful, disabling, and then further judged to entail psychological dysfunctions that express underlying "mental disorders." (Note that it has never taken a thousand physicians voting together to decide that tuberculosis is a bona fide disease!) We need to dwell for a moment on the inescapable *psychological implication* of this process:

Since large numbers of appointed mental health practitioners are involved, it will follow, as a consequence of the law of large numbers, that their preferences and the judgments to which they arrive will reflect the statistical average as communicated by the vote of the majority.

"Ontology by plebiscite" is the result: psychiatry brings mental disorders into existence through the casting of votes by increasing large committee groups. The result of this process is the creation *ex nihilo* of "mental disorders" that seldom, as we have seen, have any known underlying organic basis. At the core of this process is the unquestioned acceptance that psychological normality is equivalent to mental health. We need to see that this core commitment is the automatic reflexive effect— whether intended or not—of any plebiscite whose voting members subscribe to the legitimacy of a process that stipulatively defines "mental disorders" by the majoritarian preference of an exceedingly large group.

Here is the essential point: The uncritical acceptance of the standard provided by psychological normality is not merely an unexamined assumption of the dominant psychiatric nosology, it is a *symptom* of the very process used by diagnosis-oriented psychiatry. The consequence of seeing this is to realize that it is not enough for us to discard an unwarranted and indeed historically absurd assumption that places normality in the role of a standardized norm, but we must bring a halt to our toleration of a professionally endorsed process that votes disorders into existence. As long as the majority vote of very large groups is the basis for identifying pathology, the plebiscite's choices *will* express their own average, and psychological normality *will* remain at the unquestioned center.

PSYCHOLOGICAL RESISTANCE TO THE ABANDONMENT OF PSYCHOLOGICAL NORMALITY AS MENTAL HEALTH

What I have proposed, argued, and defended in this book is undeniably a hard pill to swallow, and it would be surprising indeed if there were not very considerable and even unbudging resistance at the very thought of swallowing it: "Psychological normality! —Why it is the expressed aim of parenting, the implied goal of socialization, of public and private education! It is thought to distinguish the innocent man or woman in the street from the sadistic criminal, good citizens from evil perpetrators of atrocities. It is always conveniently on hand to encourage socially approved behavior, and to bring back into line anyone who strays from acceptability, with the exclamation, 'Why that's just not *normal*!' And psychological normality is a defense when your reaction to events is questioned, for then you can claim, 'Why it's what any *normal* person would think/feel/do!' "

And then there is the pride of the average person, who is proud of his or her "ability" to "fit in"; to be "adaptable"; to hold a job, support a family, and come to the defense of country in the name of patriotism; to serve obediently when called upon to serve; to obey, conform, comply, and imitate the models urged upon him or her by family, church, ethnic group, school, professional association, and nation. It is a pride that is continuous with the pride of the mediocre, which, as we saw in the last chapter, caught the attention of Nietzsche, Jung, and Sartre. The pride in being psychologically normal is an even more expansive pride: it expresses the narcissistic self-importance in being *typically human*—a mere short step away from species pride, a preemptive degree of narcissistic arrogance that is immune to challenge and places the human species in a supervening take-whatever-you-want role in relation to other species (Bartlett, 2002, 2007).

But psychological normality has come to mean much more than this since it has been turned into a calcified, skeletal framework upon which psychiatry, much clinical psychology and social work, and the supporting mental health industry hang a rapidly growing collection of artificially constructed diagnostic labels that justify the *business* of providing mental health services. The equation of psychological normality with good mental health is implicit here, explicit there; it surfaces, and it goes below the surface; it is sometimes visible, at other times not; but it is never seriously questioned.

To question it seriously is, first of all, counterintuitive. To think this way runs against what we've been instructed to take for granted and hence believe. It therefore feels absurd even to countenance the possibility that mental health is not captured by the way everyday, average, and simply *normal* people think, feel, and behave.

But to question the established standard of mental health isn't just counterintuitive; we don't *want* to think this way! It would be psychologically unsettling; it would stand prevailing theory and practice on their heads; we wouldn't know which way is up! "Not only does this way of thinking run counter to obvious vested interests," the protestor complains, "it is downright offensive to suggest that psychological normality is fundamentally flawed, and flawed to such a degree that it involves real, nonmetaphorical pathology. This is beyond audacious, it is outlandish, and it probably bespeaks no more than a not very well camouflaged misanthropy on Bartlett's part!"

But "misanthropy" plays no part in the medical science of pathology.[5] When we see a condition that causes harm, suffering, and disability, not merely to one person but to countless people, decade after decade, century after century, there is no alternative but to recognize pathology. And yet there will be many who will object to such recognition.

What we see in their protests and complaints is *resistance*, and it is deeply seated, unyielding, obdurate, and resolute. I began this chapter by listing numerous ways in which human psychology is subject to internal limitation. Such internal psychological limitation is essentially characterized by resistance to change: people who are psychologically constrained in the ways I have described will predictably oppose and defy any attempts to get them to develop beyond those constraints. So much is this the case when we make the attempt to question the standard of psychological normality that it is not clear that there exists a common mental space in which a dialogue might occur. It is, I hazard to think, very much like the conflict between the lover of classical music, on the one hand, and the tone-deaf, primal-rhythm lover of rap and street dance, on the other. To claim, as I have, that different levels of sensibility are involved is already to presuppose what is at issue, but at least this sensibility thesis is honest, and the buck stops there. It is an honest thesis which, I trust Romanes would see immediately, is true and in need of no further evidential support, unless we wish to trace sensibility to another level—perhaps, as is popular now, to the neurological.

I refer to "sensibility" once again because this is where intellectual honesty realizes the matter must rest. Some of us recognize that our grim human history has gone on long enough to warrant strong impatience and frustration, so much so that we're confident in claiming that the psychological average is a sad and sorry thing, which we need, in the interests of humanity and of other species, to outgrow as soon as possible. Others of us, and certainly the great majority of us, do not feel this way at all, but on the contrary see a "nobility" in the struggles of Everyman, and "true tragedy" in what we judge to be humanity's entrapment in a vicious but inescapable cycle of repetition of wars, genocides, persecutions, and the rest. Those of the majority do not perceive the irony, and indeed, in the current sense of this word, the "egregious" nature, of equating psychological normality with mental health. To see that irony requires that we step back from the herd—"egregious" in the old, original sense of the word.

To perceive this fundamental irony is a matter of sensibility, taken in its broad meaning that includes a degree of enlightenment and moral intelligence that is uncommon.

But this claim, however candid it may be, is immediately subject to politically correct ridicule, an expression of the deeply rooted resistance I'm referring to. It takes this form: "To propose a standard of mental health that has its basis in a *rare* capacity to comprehend human psychology—a basis in an uncommon variety of intelligence and sensibility not possessed by, and perhaps not even accessible to, the common man— why that is *elitism personified*! It cannot be tolerated!"

This reaction is understandable. It bears out what this book has been about. It is to be expected. But it is an unfortunate and indeed crippling reaction.

If we are to be realistic, psychological normality is likely to remain pretty much where it is: a presupposed standard by means of which the larger society and its authorized mental health theorists and practitioners will persist in judging that many aberrations from that baseline involve "mental disorders." They will make such judgments in a psychologically normal, often intellectually mediocre, way, sometimes with stubbornly stupid insistence, sometimes with signs of professional meanness that is a sign of barbarity, and often resorting to distorted, projective thinking. Normality will continue to live on in the whispered toasts whenever the cocktail glasses of psychiatrists and insurers clink, for resistance to its open-minded systematic criticism, to its empirically based questioning, is simply too strong.

The predictable psychological obstacles that a paradigm change will encounter has never been a deterrent to the hardy perseverance of anti-establishment thinkers. In writing this book, "tilting at windmills" is a phrase that has sometimes come to mind. I have felt that perhaps the most that can be hoped for such a book is to knock, or at the very least to nudge, the profession of psychiatry out of its *DSM* self-induced complacency. This is what Kant also wanted to accomplish, but in connection with "the dogmatic slumber" of philosophy. It is intellectually healthy to engage in some knocking and nudging of this kind. Antipsychiatrists like Szasz, Laing, and Scheff have protested that mental disorders are artificially created constructs that merely serve socially approved purposes. But none of the antipsychiatrists has yet pointed to *the fact that the standard of mental health assumed and applied by psychiatry is inherently defective.* Psychiatry's reliance upon psychological normality involves recourse to mental health norms that have been derived from a population characterized by pervasive, harmful, and disabling traits. Although in obvious ways the average, majoritarian population is able to function, it is, for all that, severely dysfunctional in psychologically critical ways. It is in our own best interest to recognize this and to make whatever changes in our theory and practice are required by that recognition.

PSYCHOLOGICAL PRIMITIVENESS

People who share traits of internal psychological limitation—characteristics such as acedia, mediocrity, stupidity, barbarity, and projective cognitive distortion—are, as a result of these internal limitations, *comfortably walled in.* Their mental space or horizon is occupied by views that are solidly shallow; their beliefs tend to be held with incredible hardihood even in the face of contrary evidence. They are, furthermore, proud of the tenacity with which they hold to their views and beliefs, and at times most especially proud when they keep faith in their beliefs even when face to face with the fact that they have no empirical evidence for them. Comfortably walled in, they therefore do not willingly reflect on their concerns within a more inclusive frame of reference spanning eons—for example, the reference frame of evolutionary history, or even the much narrower frame of reference of the history of human civilization. But it is healthy to do this, as we shall try briefly to do here.

We've seen in several chapters of this book how levels of human ability, competencies, sensitivities, and sensibilities can be ranked or graded on scales that discriminate "better" or "more advanced" from those that are "inferior" and "less developed." In Chapter 1, I referred to psychologists and psychiatrists who have studied "highly developed people," people who exemplify excellence in their psychological health. We remember that Maslow, for example, focused his research on the "more highly evolved person" (Maslow, 1971, p. 96). Researchers who have focused attention on such extraordinary people have often made use of concepts relating to degree of development or evolution.

Little attention, however, has been directed in the opposite direction, to describe the nature of the *psychologically primitive*. In many obvious ways, the internal psychological limitations that I've described in this book reflect psychological primitiveness. Acedia, an incapacity for higher culture; mediocrity, defined by a varied set of rigidly constraining traits; human stupidity, whose self-imprisoning dynamic dulls awareness and blocks growth; barbarity, which opposes cultivation; and projective thinking, an apparent vestige of animism—all can appropriately be grouped under the general heading of psychological primitiveness.

To classify an individual or group as "primitive" is to call attention to his, her, or its little-evolved qualities that are signs of an early stage of development. We have such concepts as "elementary," "rudimentary," and "immature" to express this. But the notion of "primitive" includes more than this: It is informative by telling us that the level of development in view is still rough; it is unshaped and therefore coarse and crude, not yet refined or polished. To be primitive is to be close to one's animal origins, to be "brutish" or "bestial." Beyond this, primitiveness implies, on a level of taste, manners, and sensibility, the presence of crudeness, incivility, rudeness, and discourtesy (once civilization came to involve royal courts, then it was called "uncourtliness"). Further, in terms of level of cultural development, to be primitive is to be uncultivated, uncultured. And, on a moral level, primitiveness means savagery, cruelty, cold-heartedness, and therefore lack of empathy and compassion. These different meanings that we associate with primitiveness relate directly to the varieties of internal psychological limitation that I've described.

We can think of a "less evolved person" as someone who is primitive in any or all of these ways: coarse, brutish, unmannered, tasteless, uncultured, uncompassionate. To develop beyond the level of the primitive has commonly required natural evolution over long periods of time. On the much shorter—human—time scale, we rely on an individual's natural growth, parental training, and later education and experience to bring about increased maturity, growth in sensibility, advancing knowledge, and improved compassion. But unfortunately, to rely on these is more a matter of optimism than assurance.

The concept of psychological primitiveness allows us to distance ourselves from ourselves and to recognize that the different ranges of ability, sensitivity, moral sensibility, and the other characteristics that I've examined in this book all lend themselves to being placed on a scale of development that ranges from primitive to more highly evolved. When we situate on a comparative developmental scale psychological traits that exemplify greater individual development, and locate on the same scale traits that characterize psychological primitiveness, we can take note of the very large discrepancy, the very large gap, between the two. It is not a radical or unreasonable thing that some members of the human species will, at any stage of the species' development, show signs that they are more fully evolved than others. We identify such individuals as comprising an evolutionary vanguard, whose psychological traits are more highly developed.

From such an evolutionary perspective, it would be unlikely that the majority population of the average, the typical, the psychologically normal should possess characteristics that place them at the forefront of human development. Throughout this work, I have pointed to remarkable individuals, men and women who, in comparison to the psychological normal, are mentally healthier and hence more highly developed in psychologically important ways. I have also pointed to traits shared by the psychological normal that show they are, again in comparison, deficient and psychologically limited in ways that constrain them to their level of deficiency. To observe these facts is, in part, to recognize that a diversity of mental abilities, whether we have in view cognitive, emotional, aesthetic, or moral sensibilities, is a fundamental fact of nature.

Human health, whether we have physical health or mental health in view, should therefore be understood in two conjoined ways: by identifying what excellent health *is* as exemplified by those who show it to a fully functioning degree, and by explicitly excluding from our conception of good health internally limiting traits that prevent people from developing to that fully functioning level. In psychology, approached from a developmental or evolutionary point of view, our task then is to formulate a concept of mental health that embodies both (1) a clear understanding of an excellent level of psychological functioning and (2) an explicit understanding of psychological pathology that informs us how people are prevented from reaching that level of mental health.

Psychological normality should therefore play no role in framing an effective and meaningful concept of mental health. Normality characteristically involves traits of psychological primitiveness, while at the same time it is internally limiting, blocking individual and human advancement. If human development truly concerns us, individually and as a species, it makes no sense to continue to identify human psychological normality with mental health.

IATROGENIC EFFECTS OF PSYCHIATRIC LABELING

> Clinical observations on the concept of normality reveal that to a certain segment of our population the term has meaning as an extension and a derivative of the concept of 'good'.
>
> —Reider (1950, p. 50)

In Chapter 2, I described the extent to which contemporary psychiatry has indulged in an "inflationary ontology," creating and then giving its stamp of approval to an increasingly populous and crowded universe of "mental disorders." A widely recognized effect of such labeling is to stigmatize people upon whom these labels are placed. As Reider remarked in the above quotation more than half a century ago, there is a tendency to equate "normal" with "good," which is another way of expressing the unquestioned thesis this book has opposed, the equation of psychological normality with good mental health. Unfortunately, the authoritative pronouncements of nosology-oriented psychiatry have a pronounced effect on the beliefs of the society. Once our accepted professional authorities elevate normality to serve as a diagnostic standard, society pads along obediently and judges those who don't meet the authorized diagnostic standard to be aberrations from what is "good." Immediately a source of social stigma is created, a stigma that must be borne by those whom psychiatry has labeled "mentally ill."

Reider noted that psychiatric labeling has clear iatrogenic effects: "[T]here are numerous instances of individuals who are worse for their knowledge [of the diagnostic label placed on them by a psychiatrist]" (Reider, 1950, p. 43). Reider's intent, I believe, was to communicate the extent to which a mental disorder label can do inner damage to the patient, leading him or her to internalize the label of sickness derived from psychiatry's unquestioning application of the standard of psychological normality. As we've seen in earlier chapters, the capacity to think critically, to weigh socially and professionally endorsed beliefs in terms of the existence of empirical evidence to support them, is found relatively rarely in the overall population, and so it is not likely to be found in individual patients. Instead, most succumb easily to diagnostic classification, and the way in which they think and feel about themselves can be profoundly influenced by the labels placed on them by those whom they believe to be authoritative and hence trustworthy and hence convincing.

The conviction that one is "mentally ill" can have far-reaching and undesirable consequences. That conviction can itself be disabling— encouraging and sometimes compelling the diagnosed person to conform to the criteria applied to him or her and, as a result, to exhibit in his or her thought, affect, and behavior expectations to which such mental disorder labeling leads.[6] In other words, the application of conventional psychiatric diagnoses can, when internalized by patients, assume the form of yet another handicapping internal psychological limitation of the kind we have studied in this book. Such internal limitation can be the inner result of psychiatric labeling, which can in such people act not in a helpful, therapeutic capacity but as an internalized, harm-producing, iatrogenic pathology.

Beyond this, there is of course the well-known external stigma of mental illness. As we have seen in different contexts, the psychologically normal are "primed" to react negatively to deviations from normality. The psychology of mediocrity contributes to this reaction, as often also does the psychology of stupidity. As a consequence, virtually no efforts are made by the public to question or evaluate psychiatry's rapidly inflating catalogue of mental disorders, which they swallow wholesale. Beyond the public, insurers are not in the business of asking fundamental questions, and so they also passively yield to and process without selective, critical oversight whatever *DSM* diagnostic codes are duly submitted to them. In this process in which ready credulity plays a central part, "concepts of normality have become the morality" (Reider, 1950, p. 43) advocated by the mental health industry.

AFTERWORD

In relation to the concept of mental health described in this book, it would be fallacious logic to reason that if deviation from psychological normality does not identify the mentally ill then deviation from normality should be a sign of mental health. This consequence does not of course follow. Individuals who are "more fully evolved" exhibit traits not typically found among the population of the psychologically normal, but it should go without saying that the population of psychologically nonnormal people, people who are psychologically atypical, includes many who are neither remarkable in Maslow's sense nor characterized by other qualities I've described that typify exceptional people who have reached a more advanced stage of development. Psychological normality is not equivalent to mental health; but neither is psychological abnormality. This point cannot be emphasized enough, since it is an ingrained tendency of human thinking to swing from one excess to its opposite. The truth is usually to be found between extremes.

Vacillating between those extremes, there should come an equilibrium point at which we recognize that psychological problems are not confined to the psychologically abnormal *or* to the psychologically normal. Psychological problems show no preference in whom they afflict.

In Chapter 1, I distinguished between "optimal functioning," which takes into account the limitations of the individual, and "excellence of functioning," which indicates that an individual has reached the highest level of performance, distinction, or development in connection with a given ability. The two concepts of mental health proposed in this chapter correspond to this distinction: Mental health in the sense of excellence of functioning makes use of standards derived from statistically rare groups of individuals who exemplify the highest levels of genuinely good psychological functioning. Mental health in this first meaning is not to be found among those who are average, ordinary, normal.

In comparison, mental health understood in the sense of optimal functioning is altogether relative to an individual's "self-adaptation," to his or her self-acceptance and self-contentment in relation to the person's specific life circumstances, values, abilities, and goals. This individualized, relative level of mental health is by no means restricted to the more fully evolved, but is attainable by an extremely wide and psychological diverse population.

Both degrees of mental health share in the requirement that they be free—*comparatively* free, for this is a matter of degree on a continuum— from the internally limiting pathologies I have identified. To be psychologically healthy as described in this book requires, whether for individuals who have optimal psychological health or for individuals who in the fullest sense have excellent psychological health, that they be comparatively free from the internally limiting mental dysfunctions we have discussed.

As remarked in Chapter 1, mental health is more than a state of not having a mental disorder. To be mentally healthy is to be free from the internally limiting traits that we recognize in the pathologies of normality, mediocrity, acedia, barbarity, and destructive projective thinking, as well as to have reached a level of psychological maturity which is either optimally integrative for the person or reflects a high degree of excellence of development that we find only rarely among similarly remarkable people.

NOTES

1. Even so, behavioral science—in the form, for example, of the many-times-replicated obedience experiments—tells us that the majority (at least two out of three) of psychologically normal men and women will inflict harm on others in simple obedience to the authority of their leaders. The Romanes Principle applied in a casual review of history would lead us at least to this understated figure, without recourse to laboratory experiment.

2. Related to this observation, see the Afterword of this chapter and Appendix III.

3. For a discussion of behavioral scientists who have been exceptions to this rule, see Bartlett (2005).

4. The reflective reader will note immediately that in the two examples I've given reference is made to an "expert group" or an "informed group" whose judgment that pathology exists is subsequently relied upon. There is no way to circumvent the need for a reliable source of diagnostic judgment, and here lies a point potentially subject to theoretical contention: Advocates of the *DSM* plebiscite process will argue that a committee of a thousand should be accepted as well-informed, impartial, and trustworthy. I have argued, in opposition, that we should doubt its impartiality and knowledge, and hence its trustworthiness. As discussed below in the main text, a consensus conception of mental health, derived from such a large group of people, will automatically advocate adherence to a standard of psychological normality. I've argued that such a committee—given the typical or normal psychology that of necessity dominates its numerous members, a psychology that underlies the definitions of its nosology (see Chapter 2 of this book) and that makes mistaken use of normality as a standard of mental health—can be expected to make choices that are conceptually invalid and empirically wrong.

5. See Appendix I.

6. Related to this unfortunate result is "illness of work incapacity," a phrase used by Hadler (2004, p. 141) to mean illness that is made worse by the need to document it for legal or insurance purposes. This is quite different from "malingering": Hadler has in view illnesses that are in fact made worse by the pressure placed on patients to prove that they have them.

PART IV

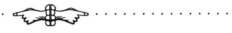

In Retrospect

10

The Reflexive Turn in Psychology

We are most limited by conditions we choose to ignore.

—SJB

Relatively few clinicians have time for theory. Their clinical practice is all-absorbing, so much so that the asking of psychologically fundamental questions is indeed a luxury—if any time at all can be found for it. Theoretically focused psychologists and psychiatrists may have the time, but they are usually busy applying and extending their own research. The incentive to step reflectively back from a habitually employed theoretical standpoint is rare and is probably most often found in philosophers. This is a pity, since as soon as fundamental questions are relegated to *philosophy*, the implication is that asking such questions is likely to be only speculative and obscure, resulting in reflections that are abstract and conceptually complex, multiplying into infinitely debatable and inconclusive conjectures.

Philosophy's generally bad reputation in these respects is, I believe, well-deserved, and I do not propose in this chapter to wax philosophical. On the other hand, I am convinced that psychiatry and clinical psychology suffer from unrecognized theoretical disabilities which a concerted effort in a reflective direction can serve to ameliorate. In this final chapter, I invite readers to gain some distance from the content of the preceding chapters and to look back reflectively, with a sense of perspective and detachment, at the ground we've covered.

THE ECONOMICS OF HUMAN EMOTION

In the course of this book, I've described a variety of internal limitations of human psychology—among these, acedia or the incapacity for culture, traits of barbarity, pathologies of normality, the psychology of mediocrity, and the distorting nature of projective thinking. My purpose in studying these has been to serve a single main purpose, to motivate readers to doubt whether the unquestioned equation of psychological normality with mental health is desirable; to ask whether this equation, in the light of what we know about human behavior, is justifiable; and to consider whether there is not a more theoretically plausible, rationally valid, and empirically convincing alternative model for good mental health.

My approach in the previous chapters has been informally heuristic, descriptive of ways in which men and women throughout history have succumbed to internal psychological limitation, usually without knowing this and virtually always without struggling against it. Each of the varieties of human pathology I've described is associated with forms of psychological gratification that cut off development beyond it. The psychological pattern of forces, the dynamic, that we see in each form of pathology is similar: there is an "emotional profit motive" that is deeply seated in most people, which leads them to remain in a self-limiting and destructive pattern of thought, emotion, or behavior, and to resist abandoning that pattern. If an explicit "economics of human emotion" were to be developed, we should find one of its main objects of study here, in the human unwillingness to give up powerful sources of gratification that attract and bind people to those gratifications and that create in them incredibly strong resistance to relinquish them.

In parallel with economics, we should find a psychological application of the "principle of economic scarcity," which recognizes that investment in one course of action tends to be exclusionary, eliminating consideration of alternative courses of action. We see this in psychology in the all-too-familiar phenomenon in which a person's or group's emotional investment in one alternative excludes all others. Each of the psychological varieties of internal limitation brings people evident kinds of satisfaction that very strongly encourage them to invest their beliefs and efforts in certain directions—and, in accordance with the principle of economic scarcity, to disregard alternatives that may potentially be open to them.

If you, the reader, will put these two "economic" perspectives together, you may be willing to think in the context of a heuristic frame of reference similar to the author's. From that standpoint, we see that a study of the psychology of varieties of psychological internal limitation has not, in any serious measurable, quantitative fashion, even begun. There are, for example, no psychometric tests to show how strongly predisposed a psychologically normal person is to inflict harm on others or to place himself and his fellows in harm's way simply to promote or defend his ideology. Nor do we have any such tests to determine under what circumstances a man or a woman will engage in violence or atrocity, nor do we have any way to anticipate in advance what degree of satisfaction or remorse the person would later feel as a result. The same is generally true in connection with virtually any human patterns of thought, emotion, and behavior typically exhibited by the psychologically normal population, patterns that involve, for example, aggression, destructiveness, envy, rage, laziness, or greed; absence of compassion; a willingness to dehumanize others; species pride and resulting environmental depredation; or, on a more specialized plane, professional jealousy, backstabbing, and the struggle to block new and potentially better ideas.

We see all of these phenomena in great profusion, and still we do not know how to test an individual with any known method in order to disclose the likelihood that he or she will, under specifiable circumstances, think, feel, or act in such ways. Similarly, in terms of the management of society, we have no reliable standards with which to determine in advance how a seemingly mentally healthy leader is liable to think, feel, and behave once placed in a position of power.

Nor do there exist psychological tests that have been designed specifically to measure mediocrity and the extent of its heritability, nor the recalcitrant stubbornness of stupidity, nor the incapacity for culture, nor the predisposition to misrepresent reality through projective thinking.

As a result and on an individual level, quantitative data about these internal limitations are lacking and will continue to be lacking as long as a serious study of the subject is ignored and evaded. We are therefore not yet in a position to know very much at all about such predispositions *when the highly individual, living person is in question.* However, we *do* know a great deal about all of these predispositions *on the level of large groups.* For this purpose, a psychological study of history, as remarked in the last chapter, provides more than adequate evidence that psychologically normal people are, as a group, predisposed to engage in patterns of behavior, thought, and emotion that are internally limiting, blocking individual and species-wide development.

The evidence that shows this is substantial; indeed it is compelling when there is firsthand acquaintance with its strength and breadth. That evidence is not fully communicable within the confines of a single chapter in a book. Perhaps it is in a full-length and detailed study (e.g., Bartlett, 2005), but perhaps not even there—except for those who are already keenly aware of the weight of the evidence and need no reminders. There is a sense in which an unfortunate dilemma besets the researcher who ventures beyond our prevailing internal psychological limitations: either to preach to the choir or to the impenetrable wall erected by the very internal limitations that are in view.

Notwithstanding the inherent pessimism of this meta-remark, the most promising basis on which future research can build given the present stage of our knowledge of forms of internal psychological limitation is to identify and discriminate principal traits that characterize internal psychological limitations. And it is in relation to this task that I've tried to make a first step through detailed description.

THE PSYCHOLOGICAL DYNAMIC OF A DARK AGE

Any application of the phrase "dark age" to the future of course suggests gloom. When the phrase is used, as in Lasch's (1979) *The Culture of Narcissism* or McIntyre's (2006) *Dark Ages: The Case for a Science of Human Behavior*, it is in the context of cultural criticism and not, as here, in connection with specific ways in which human psychology acts to hold people back in cognitive, emotional, moral, and behavioral patterns that are humanly self-destructive. In Chapter 5, I described the way in which a loss of the liberating spirit and liberating content of higher education lays the groundwork for a new Dark Age. Other forces contribute, among them:

- The domination of such an age by acedia, an incapacity for culture;
- The suppressive effect of a system of intellectual prepublication restraint in which an internally limiting psychology of peer review and editorial bias can be expected significantly to block original intellectual work;
- The role of the psychology of mediocrity in impeding individual and collective human development in a multitude of ways; and, of course,
- An uncritical approach in psychiatry and much clinical psychology that is based on an equation of psychological normality with good mental health.

Together, these forces reinforce one another and help to promote and perpetuate an environmentalist-egalitarian, multiculturalist-relativist, anti-elitist, anti-intellectual attitude toward higher education, higher learning, individual attainment, and original thought. These are the psychological ingredients needed for a dark age. We note that technology is able to thrive in such a culturally depleted atmosphere; a dark age in which there is more and more technological progress is not a contradiction in terms.

A dark age is perpetuated by any society's commitment to conformity, conservatism, and conventionalism, all of which make it especially difficult, and sometimes unpopular, for people to question what they have not questioned before and may not have been *willing* to question. In such a period, it is decidedly more difficult but all the more imperative for us to examine our major premises and to be prepared, at least for a time, to put preferred and comfortable beliefs to one side. "Imperative" does not mean, however, that everyone is going to be enthusiastic about doing this, especially when, as we saw in the last chapter, this means facing the challenge of a wholesale revision in established concepts of "mental health" and "mental disorder."

In contemporary psychiatry and much clinical psychology and social work, the prevailing commitments to conformity, conservatism, and conventionalism collaborate to support the belief that "adjusting the young to their environment" is desirable and therefore should be an explicitly urged goal not only by our families and educational system but by establishment mental health services, where the routine therapeutic aim is to *normalize* through the use of psychiatric medication and to encourage and produce normality through the corresponding use of psychotherapy.

This mindset acts as a brake, a constraint, that blocks human advancement. It checks individual development, deters original thought, discourages creative efforts to achieve positive growth, and stands in the way of paradigm change. We've seen this phenomenon in connection with the psychology of definition in psychiatric nosology, in terms of the psychology of the creative artist, the psychology of today's college students and of their liberal arts professors, the psychology of peer review and editorial bias, and of course in discussions of the psychology of normality and mediocrity. Brakes hold back a vehicle, a person, or a group from movement or advancement—which is change. The internal psychological limitations studied in this book are brakes of a certain kind: they impede change, and they preserve and protect a variety of forms of cognitive, affective, and behavioral disability.

As we have seen, there is an in-built brake in the psychologically normal population that holds its members back in typical patterns of pathology. For the mediocre, the majority of whom are psychologically normal, there are in-built impediments that prevent them from becoming more than they are, as there are obstructions ready to hand that they place in the way of those who would become better than they.

But there is more to the dynamic of psychological forces that bring about a dark age. There is, as we've seen in chapters dealing with acedia and barbarism, a growing antipathy toward culture in its liberating, classical meaning; there is also a growing anti-intellectualism, a product of intellectual mediocrity and a politically correct denial of the natural fact of the inequality of individual abilities and sensibilities. There is a passionately rigid opposition to anything that smacks of elitism, and hence an enthusiastic embrace of cultural relativism, multiculturalism, and the rejection of standards that discriminate between higher and lower.

Irony is added to the human tragedy of this drama thanks to the success of psychiatry's nosology that has elevated psychological normality to an unquestioned role as arbiter in distinguishing "mental health" from "mental disorder." In doing this, the psychiatric diagnostic system of classification has evolved into a habitually accepted theory and approach to therapeutic practice that precisely embodies many of the internal limitations that have occupied us in this volume.

We need to perceive the "larger picture" in which a multiplicity of factors—that is, a substantial number of psychological predispositions and traits—interact, reinforce one another, and together contribute to an outcome that is deeply resistant to positive change. If it were the case that only one, or two, or three such factors were at the basis of the major psychological faults of the human species, the undesirable situation and its possible remedy would be greatly simplified. But the contributing factors are complex and they are numerous. They constitute major failings in the psychologically normal constitution as it is at the present time.

It has been my intention in this work (1) to draw attention to certain of these major faults, faults of which people, including mental health theorists and practitioners, are generally oblivious and prefer to be; (2) to remind us of what is most important in life, but what is rapidly being forgotten as liberating higher values recede into shadow and then potentially into oblivion; and (3) to provide a more promising and solid conceptual framework for subsequent work in clinical psychology and psychiatry by eliminating obstacles to clear thinking. To accomplish these things, it is essential that we clarify our fundamental concepts and question the validity of our reasoning by means of them, for they form the basis of theoretical psychology and hence the basis for the approaches to therapy to which it leads.

SUBORDINATING MUNDANE REALITY

[E]ach morning, reality resembles more and more a nightmare.
—Jorge Luis Borges (1940)

In *The Man in the Mirror of the Book: A Life of Jorge Luis Borges*, biographer James Woodall (1996) describes how Borges managed—always, throughout his life—to "subordinate" events of the everyday world in order to guard and cultivate more important things. Those "more important things" are among those things that in this book I've called "higher." This is an expression of an ancient attitude found in Plato's resort to allegory, in his effort to express what is not easily expressed in language, at least not intelligibly to those who do not *already* understand. Here, I believe, is one of the most articulate and intellectually honest expressions of this difficulty, dilemma, and challenge:

> That the world is a prison and our life and hope respectively are servitude and release, is a universal image, powerful enough to be transformed into a myth, and hence, to become imprisoning in its own right if it is nonsense or is false. For then we will be held captive only by the belief in our captivity.
>
> Plato's version is the reverse of this. . . . According to him, our imprisonment consists exclusively of the fact that we are *not* aware of being in our prison. So we cannot (logically) both be in this condition and know that we are in it, and knowledge of our condition is instantly delivering, like a cure for a disease which consists only in not having the cure. But deliverance is complicated by the extraordinary difficulty of explaining to the prisoners, in terms intelligible to them, that prisoners are what they are. For the conditions which make self-understanding possible are incompatible with the conditions they are in, and he who speaks of imprisonment to prisoners must be regarded by them as a madman in his raving. For the bonds which hold them captive are the boundaries of the understanding, and how are we to bring the boundaries *within* themselves to make them understood? The limits of understanding are not part of what is understood. (Danto, 1971, p. ix)

This, as I see it, is far from being a parlor trick in a logician's fable; nor is it simply an epistemological predicament (which it certainly is); but, more importantly here, it describes a *psychological impasse* that owes its existence to the widely varying psychological constitutions of individual people. For some people, the bonds that hold them captive to rigidly habitual patterns of thought, feeling, and behavior are undetectably felt. For others, such as the creative artists described in Chapter 3, *any* shackle, any sense of imprisonment, is felt keenly, sometimes painfully, and is nearly always met with a spirit of defiance and rebellion. In contrast, the majority of people show a pronounced inability to get beyond the impasse hardened by their own internal limitations. For them, that they are internally limited is as imperceptible to them as a self-conscious sensation of water probably is to a fish. The limitations of their understanding are not, as Danto expressed this, part of what they understand.

I've tried to place a description of their main psychologically limiting traits in more distinct relief than our usual acceptance of normality prefers, and in this I've chosen a direct approach to communication rather than allegory. I have tried *not* to mince words in formulating these descriptions, since we gain nothing by vagueness and overcautious qualification. If at times it may seem that I've indulged in overstatement, my rationale is that when stretching the boundaries of understanding, clear assertion that for some may be too bold is sometimes the only effective alternative to allegory—or parable, poetry, or fantasy.

Psychiatric nosology has defined itself into its own sort of Platonic cave, and its authoritative definitions of mental disorders have permeated our society as though from a biblical source. Not only have its diagnostic classifications assumed a reality of their own, but they have persuaded the credibility of their creators, who are, in short, imprisoned within a prison of their own devising.

> The sum of what the prisoners know is shadows and images of things, projected onto the cave's wall. These compose reality for them. The shadows are the touchstone of intelligibility of creatures in their circumstances, for since shadows are all they know, no statement except one about shadows will be meaningful to them. It is this which makes it difficult, which perhaps makes it impossible, that they should know the limits of their world or even that their world has limits, for how is the expression "only shadows" to be made intelligible in terms which refer alone to shadows? This is a statement made about reality from without, and one who understands reality only from within cannot then know that he does so. (Danto, 1971, p. x)

We might be reminded here of the linguistic relativity hypothesis of Whorf (1956/1962) and Sapir (1949/1958). In its strong formulation, it claims that speakers of a given language are internally limited by the perceptual and conceptual discrimination capacities of their language. Whorf and Sapir did not employ the concept I've called "internal psychological limitation"; their concern was rather *linguistic*, suggesting that natural languages have boundaries that potentially circumscribe what its users do or can experience. In contrast, Danto's focus in the two passages I've quoted has to do with the boundaries of human understanding. And in further contrast with Whorf, Sapir, and Danto, my focus has a less broad compass but a more explicit application, for I've had in view specifically the way in which the contemporary psychiatric paradigm of mental health and mental disorder is internally limited.

In part, I've attempted to show readers that such internal limitations are actually operative by pointing to "levels or orders of reality" in comparison with which everyday, mundane reality can be perceived as unreal, artificially constructed, and lanthanic, that is, involving unrecognized pathology. To make this step of meta-analysis, you must step up at least one rung on a ladder of progressive reflection. The last line of Philip Glass's opera "Waiting for the Barbarians" is: "I'm caught in an ugly and stupid dream." The three concepts—"ugly," "stupid," and "dream"—all require that we take a step back from or above the everyday standpoint. To make these judgments, Glass presupposes that his listeners will be able to situate their thinking at least one step removed from ordinary reality. So does Plato's allegory of the cave. So does Borges in many of the themes one finds in his writing, in which the judgment is expressed that what we see is unreal and untrustworthy, so much so that a step into reflective fiction must be relied upon—to establish a level of reality that is higher because only within its borders (daring to speak here for Borges) can we come to know what is true.

In a real and nonliterary, nonmetaphorical fashion, the same is true in connection with our subject, the seemingly heretical proposal that psychological normality is a bad, even monstrous, choice of standard for human mental health. For many people, in order for them genuinely to recognize the truth of this claim, a review of the supporting evidence will *always* be insufficient—except for those who are already convinced or who have a comparatively rare capacity for reflective disengagement from their own habitual commitments. And this assertion, too, is no logician's sleight-of-hand, but it reflects the internally limitative human predicament. Such a recognition requires, as a condition of its very possibility, that a person be able to step beyond or outside the familiar and comfortable constraints of his or her experience. Not many people have the ability, much less the willingness, to do this. Psychiatrists, psychologists, and social workers are no exception.

There are usually alternative routes to the knowledge that something is the case. In this book, I've pointed to two routes. Each requires a reflective turn by psychology, that is, a willingness to assume a reflective metastandpoint toward either or both of two concerns. These two concerns by this point are well-known to readers. The first is the concern that the population of the psychologically normal is far from being mentally healthy, and the second is that much that is of great significance in human life goes unnoticed and remains invisible to the average, typical man and woman. Either recognition—that psychological normality is in many ways dysfunctional and destructive, and that "elevated living" possesses a wealth of meaning in contrast to the poverty of mind of the psychologically normal—either recognition can, for readers with the requisite intellectual receptiveness, provide a psychological foundation that allows them to *subordinate* ordinary reality. But, as Danto has expressed so well, this is a demanding challenge. It is *psychologically demanding* for anyone who is not already among the "converted," for at this juncture most people will run headlong into a face-to-face confrontation with their own internal psychological limitations.

PRACTICAL IMPLICATIONS

You, the reader, have noticed the occasional appearance in this book of such names as Plato, Hesse, and Borges—one man a philosopher, another a novelist, and the third a writer of intellectual fantasy—all, no doubt, idealists! As a result, you may have gotten the mistaken impression that I'm urging a highly idealistic point of view that lacks practical application. The perspective I've described is firmly rooted in a set of ideals, but in fact they have very practical implications.

Having reached the end of this work, we should not hesitate to ask in retrospect, "What, then, is the practical *point* of a descriptive psychology of human pathology?" This is a legitimate question, to which I have these answers: First, and in more general and deceptively simple terms, we need to understand ourselves better if we are to learn how we might become better. We need to take seriously Einstein's observation with which this book began, that if we are to have a better world, "you have to have better people." Second, if it is the case that built into the present psychological constitution of most people are constraints that block their own development and further stand in the way of the development of others, then we need to become fully conscious of those limitations if ever we are to grow beyond them.

Both answers give the initial impression of vagueness and of lacking useful application, so we need to move to the level of the very concrete: the point of studying the psychology of human pathologies is ultimately to provide us with an understanding of people that can be applied on such practical levels as psychological therapy, education, and vocational guidance. Earlier chapters in this book have directed attention to the need to reevaluate the general equation of psychological normality with mental health, to reassess the direction of human education, and to enlarge the scope of values to which we are sensitive. These are practical and concrete ends: Taking them seriously leads to a revisionary approach to mental health and to the treatment of psychological problems, as we have seen in earlier chapters. A serious commitment to these ends also leads directly, as Robert Hutchins (1937, 1952) has shown, to a specific conception of higher education and of specified content to be studied. Further, were we to take these ends seriously, we should be able to develop a map in terms of which to orient how we wish humanity to develop, and then seek practical steps to achieve those goals. In much of this effort, there would be no need to reinvent the wheel, for the work has already been done: it resides on the shelves of libraries, in volumes that would need to be dusted off, expressed in language that could tolerate some refreshening, but little more.

A serious decision to rethink where we should go from here requires that we first understand with uncompromising honesty where we stand at the present time. The phenomenon of mediocrity needs to be taken seriously as a warning, rather than a trivialist's celebration. The psychology of mediocrity is humanity's ball and chain, whose mass and therefore inertia are unappreciated and casually dismissed. A healthy recognition of individual differences needs to be developed in conjunction with an equally healthy affirmation of standards of good mental health in which psychological normality no longer plays a central role. These, too, are specific and concrete goals with applicability that does not require much imaginative effort. There are obvious social and political implications if we affirm the reality of individual differences. Education would need to concern itself foremost with the encouragement and cultivation of exceptional individual merit and attainment, realizing that "no child left behind" is a mistaken mythology that holds children back to a level of mediocrity. We need to make human excellence the explicitly stated goal of education; we should celebrate it: "Excellence exists, and it is time to acknowledge and celebrate the magnificent inequality that has enabled some of our fellow humans to have so enriched the lives of the rest of us" (Murray, 2003, pp. 449–50).

From a clinical point of view, we should see that successful psychological therapy is much more of an art than a science, given that the individual and his or her individual circumstances, abilities, sensibilities, attitudes, values, and goals must together be comprehended and taken into account through the way a therapist responds and offers help to the person who is suffering. Whenever the focus becomes concentrated on the individual, and universal principles of etiology and symptomatology cannot be found, then science must give way to art, for art deals with the individual, science with generalizable and invariant principles. The practice of physical medicine also used to be regarded as an art, and no doubt to some extent it still is, but it has become less so as the many forms of laboratory testing facilitate diagnosis and obviate a large portion of what used to be diagnostic intuition and judgment.

As Norman Sartorius, director of the Division of Mental Health of the World Health Organization, wrote in his preface to the *ICD-10 Classification of Mental and Behavioural Disorders: Clinical Descriptions and Diagnostic Guidelines* (World Health Organization, 1992, p. vii): "A classification is a way of seeing the world as a patient in time." This is eloquent but perhaps too concise for a meaning that needs to be explained. Were clinicians to "see the world as a patient in time," what would this mean? I don't propose to speak for Sartorius, but here are two interpretations: The first is that we consider the world of humanity as a patient in need of therapy; the second is that we consider each individual patient as an expression of the world as experienced by him or her. The first is compatible with

concepts of mental health and psychological pathology that have concerned us in this book, while the second is compatible with the highly
individualized approach that I advocate to help people who experience
psychological distress.

I do not really think Sartorius had these interpretations in mind (unless
he is more than a psychiatrist, but also a poet at heart!), and whether he
did or not isn't relevant here. These two imagined approaches to "seeing
the world as a patient in time" do serve, however, to underscore their stark
contrast with the current attitude of diagnostic psychiatry: As we have seen
in some detail, the way that today's diagnostic psychiatry "sees the world" is
heavily influenced by a projective psychology of reification that systematically misconstrues symptomatology as mental disorder, mistakes stipulative definition in psychiatric nosology for real, scientific definition, and, in
this process, elevates psychological normality to serve as psychological
arbiter of good mental health.

The practical implications of "seeing the world as a patient in time," as
I've no doubt extended and supercharged this phrase, can be as specific as
we choose. They can include, as I've mentioned, a revitalization of
psychological therapy, education, and vocational guidance—all with the
individual's self-adaptation in mind and with a concerted attempt to
remove from the individual's way obstacles that are placed there by the
internal psychological limitations I have identified.

The idealism expressed in this volume is not of the familiar variety that
is impracticable, for it does have clear and definite applications. But its
implementation is so daunting, affecting so much of human reality, as to
be felt impossible, perhaps indeed hopeless, and so it is tempting to judge
it as just so much "pure idealism." This interpretation leads directly to
pessimism, which, very much like optimism, has its shortcomings. Hope
helps us to accommodate to a reality we know is undesirable; pessimism
can tie our hands as we wring them. Either way, our capacity to change a
reality we should no longer be prepared to accept can be disabled.

The fact that the practical implications of this approach are overwhelming should not be confused with the notion that it has none: the
practical implications are legion. They extend to many critical areas of
human life, from the ethics of reproductive choice in a precariously overpopulated world to the values encouraged in children, the treatment of
criminals, the evaluation and appointment of society's leaders, socially
approved attitudes toward violence generally and war in particular, and
the list could be made to go on indefinitely, each item on it reflecting
the need to reappraise values that have too long gone unquestioned.[1]

This, surely, is idealism, but it is not idealism without practical consequences.

IDEALISM THAT IS NOT HOPEFUL

Optimism makes reality more tolerable. When much of psychologically normal reality is unacceptable and no longer to be passively tolerated, optimism about that reality is difficult to summon. *Should* it be summoned at all when we realize that it so often leads us to suffer on with what is no longer bearable? Nietzsche thought poorly of optimism; in an earlier chapter, I quoted his claim that, "morally speaking, [optimism is] a sort of cowardice" (Nietzsche, 1992, p. 18). The sheer scale, the overwhelming magnitude, of internal psychological limitation that one finds in the average human population is cause enough to wring our hands. To face human reality with eyes fully open and yet feel optimism Nietzsche would condemn as cowardly denial. Hope can be a refuge sought out of fear, an escape from an undistorted perception of reality. When human pathology is so widespread as to be normal, the susceptibility of optimists to accept intolerable conditions and so to tolerate them can itself reflect a self-destructive form of pathology. In another work (Bartlett, 2005), I describe "the pathology of hope," which successfully brings about humanity's willingness to tolerate its own worst failings.

The psychologically normal response is to *adjust* to the human environment as best we can, which in the end of course changes nothing. We call this "adaptation"; it is socially desired; it is clinically desired. But adjustment to a world increasingly afflicted by pathologies of normality is not a goal to be wished. To revise an observation made by Robert Hutchins (Mayer, 1993, p. 400): Our purpose is not to adjust to the world, but to make it better; if we become maladjusted in the process, so much may this be better for the world. To adjust to a world in which humanity's internal psychological limitations have reached the present level of conspicuous domination is to become yet another victim of normalization. As we saw in an earlier chapter, creative individuals have often been classified by clinicians as maladapted, as misfits in relation to the world of normal humanity. This has been their strength and their merit, as it has often been their source of suffering, often in large measure thanks, as we've seen, to the way normal society has treated them. (Just as surely, we of course recognize that "maladaptation" is no automatic sign of an elevated mind, nor of high attainment, nor of original capacity.)

The concepts of mental health and mental disorder propounded by psychiatry's consensus-based definition of truth reinforce rather than grind down the blocks that obstruct human psychological development. To urge that it be otherwise, to work toward that end, is—under the psychological circumstances—unalloyed idealism, an idealism which does not encourage tolerance of or adjustment to an unacceptable and disappointing human reality, an idealism which has specific, direct, and—predictably for the psychologically normal human majority—sometimes unattractive and objectionable practical consequences.

Sir Richard Burton (1821–1890) was a rarity among scholars and world explorers, for he combined both in a single man, the author of 43 volumes describing his travels and some 30 volumes of translations, the first European discoverer of Lake Tanganyika, and a linguist fluent in 25 languages which, including dialects, amounted to a knowledge of 40 languages—in short, an unusual man. Ensconced in a heavy scholarly section of notes appended to his long narrative poem *The Kasidah of Haji Abdu* is the following observation:

> To consider the world in its length and breadth, its various history and the many races of men, their starts, their fortunes, their mutual alienation, their conflicts, and then their ways, habits, governments, forms of worship; their enterprises, their aimless courses, their random achievements and acquirements, the impotent conclusion of long-standing facts, the tokens so faint and broken of a superintending design, the blind evolution of what turn out to be great powers or truths, the progress of things as if from unreasoning elements, not towards final causes; the greatness and littleness of man, his far-reaching aims and short duration, the curtain hung over his futurity, the disappointments of life, the defeat of good, the success of evil, physical pain, mental anguish, the prevalence and intensity of sin, the pervading idolatries ... —*all this is a vision to dizzy and appall, and inflicts upon the mind the sense of a profound mystery which is absolutely without human solution.* (Burton, 1894/n.d., pp. 58–59)

By now, we should have a firm grasp of the psychological limitations that dissolve and explain much of this mystery. But whether it is utterly without human solution remains to be seen. Certainly the internal psychological limitations depicted in the present work highlight how difficult any solution would be. The odds seem to be overpoweringly against any solution we might be able reflectively to devise for ourselves; perhaps evolutionary or other natural forces over which we have no control will intervene. But a decline of hope, or the birth of pessimism, is not reason enough to give up the task.

William of Orange is reputed to have courageously uttered in the face of overwhelming odds: "It is not at all necessary to hope in order to endeavor, nor to succeed in order to persevere" (Rüstow, 1980, p. xxix).

NOTE

1. Additional practical implications are suggested in Appendix II.

APPENDIX I

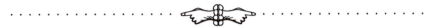

An Apology to Lovers of Humanity?

It is a strange thing that, in studies of medical pathology, authors do not feel called upon to balance their analysis of diseases with praise of good health, whereas the situation is entirely different when it comes to a psychological critique of human psychological normality. Readers who are defensive about "humanity" may feel that a work that studies such things as "pathologies of normality" *owes it* to the humanistic spirit or to species pride to offer a "balanced presentation"—by emphasizing how good many people are, how good much of their behavior is, how much beauty, truth, courage, and heroism humanity is responsible for.

From a psychological standpoint, such a defensive reaction to a study of human pathology that is so widespread as to be *normal* constitutes both an expression of denial and an attempt to take the sting out of a dispassionate assessment of the psychologically normal population's typical destructive predispositions. Complaining that a study of human psychological pathology skips over or does not take the trouble to emphasize human goodness is counterproductive and encourages misplaced emphasis. We do not identify, diagnose, and treat dysfunctional thought, emotion, and behavior by citing counterexamples. The wish for a "balanced presentation" in medical pathology would be seen as irrelevant as it is here.

Yet "irrelevant" is not the entire story: such a wish expresses an attitude that *hinders* the attainment of the goal of pathology, to identify and then treat harmful conditions. We are already ill-disposed to recognize "the enemy within." If we insist upon patting ourselves on the back—*even, and most especially*, in the course of studying our gravest faults—we are likely to miss the point.

There is nothing in a treatise on venereal disease that depreciates human love by virtue of the fact that the treatise omits to mention and praise love; similarly, there is nothing in a study of forms of psychopathology, which

hinder individual and general human development, that should be interpreted as universally depreciating exceptional human attainments,
creations, and exemplary conduct.

But beyond this recognition, there is a compelling need, as I've tried to
show in different contexts in this book, to accept that what is finest about
our species is not captured by the psychological constitution of the majority. My own observations and those of others whose works are mentioned
in this volume suggest that, nearly without exception, extraordinary
achievement comes from an exceedingly small segment of the total human
population, which this book plainly honors. It should make good sense
even to the most ardent lover of humanity to acknowledge the following:
that serious opposition to the equation of psychological normality with
good mental health should not unnecessarily, irrelevantly, and counter-
productively be saddled with the task of praising the very subject in which
deeply seated and largely unrecognized pathology thrives.

APPENDIX II

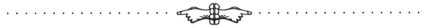

Practical Speculations, or Speculative Practices

A shift in our chosen standard of good mental health, whether we call such a standard a set of criteria, a measure, norm, benchmark, baseline, or arbiter, has potential practical implications. This book, it should be clear, is not a detailed practical engineering manual for social, political, or even psychological reconstruction. Yet, in rereading the text, it struck me that some readers might wish to have a few more *concrete* examples of how the approach that is proposed in this volume can lead to practical application and implementation. In a mere appendix, space for this is clearly limited, but here are a few additional examples, some of greater import than others:

1. The most immediate implication of the shift to a new standard of mental health as proposed in this book would be to undermine the credulity invested by both the public and by mental health clinicians in the plethora of "mental disorders" that are authorized by the *DSM* despite the fact that most have no known organic basis. The majority of the psychological problems that people encounter would then not brand them as "mentally ill," and they would be spared both the internal and the external stigmata that so often result from current diagnostic labeling. As I have proposed, such a change in clinical perspective leads to the recognition that psychological problems are highly individual and require the highly individualized attention and care of clinicians. In addition, I've advocated a thoroughgoing revision in our criteria that are supposed to inform us what constitutes fully functioning mental health. For this purpose we would look not to the population of the psychologically normal but to groups whose psychological traits are exceptions to the rule, whose members express predispositions that, unlike those characterizing

the psychologically normal populace, are free from the pathologies of normality, mediocrity, stupidity, and delusional projective thinking discussed earlier. These two practical implications for psychiatry and clinical psychology have been foremost in my mind in writing this book. But there are other practical implications that one might visualize.

2. The recognition that the world is already greatly overpopulated by our species, coupled with the acceptance that typical, psychologically average people will not curtail their reproductive interests voluntarily, could lead (for instance) to an appropriate politically implemented policy of increased taxation on families in proportion to the number of their children (the very opposite of the prevailing tax exemptions policy in the United States) or to differential taxation so that taxes earmarked for the education and medical care of children are paid only by families that actually *have* children—policies that are clearly unlikely in the absence of crisis conditions. China, of course, has applied a one-child policy, apparently with some success, as well as with attendant problems; selective, directed taxation might in time be more to America's political taste. The looming global problem of "simply too many people" has yet to be faced in any intellectually honest and determined fashion. Once we establish a new center of gravity for good mental health and stop enshrining the norm of normality, we may be more willing to face the manifold problems that are the consequences of excessive population.

3. The psychologically based analysis of higher education that I've given leads directly to the need to elevate educational and disciplinary standards, the reinstituting of liberal arts and foreign language requirements, and an intelligent, self-consciously undertaken publicity campaign that stresses the intellectual and cultural rewards of higher education (and *not* the financial gains to be expected from a vocational degree)—all of these accomplished within a framework that acknowledges, respects, and encourages individual differences among students in their levels of intelligence, sensibility, achievement, and other abilities. A corollary of these policies is the recognition that only a small percentage of students will excel in any given area, and it is upon them that the future largely depends. Other positive and concrete policies relating to education would of course include the permanent removal of sports from the province of higher education and a distinction and separation between higher education and career-oriented vocational training.

4. We recognize that the population of the psychologically normal combined with that of the mediocre comprises a huge group of people

who are predisposed, under suitable circumstances, to think, feel, and behave in well-established, predictable, destructive patterns. This recognition could lead to a deliberate program to encourage benign and productive dispositions in their place. Here, specifically designed education, political, social, and judicial policies are fundamental, as is a fundamentally new approach to the theory and practice of clinical psychology and psychiatry, as already mentioned.

I've given the above concrete examples not only to expand upon the few mentioned in the text. They serve perhaps a more important function. From a psychological standpoint, the reader's reaction to such examples can be enlightening, for he or she will immediately recognize that some, perhaps all, may arouse such dismissive emotions as amusement, scorn, mockery, or outright condemnation. If the reader will take note of his or her reaction, and if it should be of this kind, it may well be symptomatic of the very internal psychological limitations explored in this work. The above list of examples runs afoul of *popularity*, that is, it runs counter to or is abrasive to views supported by *psychological normality*. Such a list can therefore act as a challenge, and therefore literally as an informative affront, to norms that we take for granted. In reading such a list, a negative reaction is very likely a symptom that habitual values have been scratched, causing a tell-tale emotional itch. It is a reaction to which we need to pay reflective attention and not simply scratch and then dismiss what we do not *like* to believe, as we so often are prone to do.

APPENDIX III

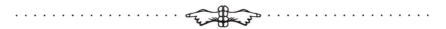

The Distribution of Mental Health

A book that critiques the standard of normality would be incomplete without some mention of the "normal" distribution curve—the so-called bell curve brought to public awareness by Richard J. Hernnstein's and Charles Murray's book of that title, which examined the distribution of intelligence. The normal curve is the quintessential expression of the idea of normality: it presents in graphic form what we mean by average, by a statistical mean, and it shows how the average tapers off into extremes the more distant one gets from the mean. The bell curve for IQ, for example, makes clear that the intelligence of the human majority is centered around a mean IQ of about 100, and that, symmetrically, IQ drops off to the left of that mean, and to the right it rises.

In the past century, human intelligence has been studied in great detail, and numerous tests have been designed to measure it. In comparison, as earlier chapters have shown, positive mental health suffers from lack of precise definition, while definitions of mental disorders have largely been unscientific and highly unstable.

As we've seen, mental health, like intelligence, is a multifaceted thing, consisting of a varied group of individual abilities or skills, sensitivities or sensibilities, attitudes or values, and predispositions to think, feel, and behave. But unlike intelligence, psychometrists have yet to devise a quantitative measure to rank a person's "mental health quotient" (we might call it MHQ) as IQ does with respect to cognitive ability. As this book has argued, genuinely good mental health—in other words, a high MHQ—is not normal, and its distribution in the general population is extremely skewed, as the charts that follow show.

We're accustomed to referring to "positive mental health," but not explicitly to *negative* mental health (although we sometimes speak of a person's "poor mental health"). It can be an aid to clarity for us to think in

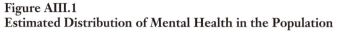

Figure AIII.1
Estimated Distribution of Mental Health in the Population

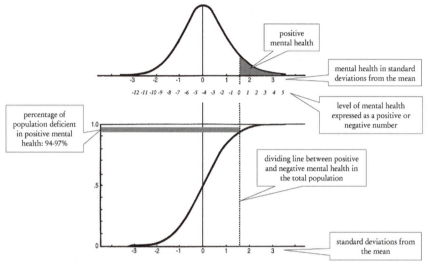

Upper chart: normalized distribution of mental health in the population. Lower chart: associated cumulative distribution curve. Shaded area in the upper chart represents approximately 3-6% of the total population. Positive mental health distribution estimates based on observations by Maslow, Richardson, Johnson, and others; evidence for the negative estimates derived from Milgram, Zimbardo, and other sources (see text).

terms of these two polar opposites (Figure AIII.1). Doing this allows us to represent graphically how mental health, understood in terms of the criteria described in this book, is plausibly distributed in the general population. As a suggestive approximation at this early stage before we can quantify MHQ meaningfully, the two charts below depict curves that show the estimated distribution of mental health in the general population. You will immediately see that although the estimated distribution of mental health is represented in the form of a normal bell-shaped curve, the distribution of positive mental health is confined to the shaded right-hand tail.

For readers unfamiliar with curves like the lower one, a few comments are in order: The lower curve is called a cumulative distribution curve. In relation to the upper bell curve, the lower curve allows us to read off the percentage of the total population that corresponds to any point on the bell curve. For example, the solid vertical line that splits the bell curve symmetrically in two marks the zero standard deviation point, which in both charts represents the mean level of mental health in the total population. The point where this vertical line intersects the lower S-shaped cumulative distribution curve allows us to read off from the left-hand vertical axis of the lower graph that half (.5, or 50%) of the population is at that level of mental health.

Below the horizontal axis of the bell curve is a range of italicized numbers, from −12 to +5, representing arbitrarily chosen equal divisions above and below zero. These numbers are not intended to have special significance, but serve only to divide up a range. What *is* significant, however, is the zero point through which the dotted vertical line has been drawn. It marks the point, somewhere between 1 and 2 standard deviations above the general population's mean, at which an individual's level of mental health is judged to be comparatively neutral, that is, whose mental health is balanced between characteristics that define negative and positive psychological health. (Someone who is one standard deviation above the mean is at the 84th percentile; if two standard deviations above the mean, the individual is at the 98th percentile; if three standard deviations above the mean, the person is in the top thousandth of the population.)

The zero point through which the vertical dotted line is drawn has not been chosen arbitrarily. We have a considerable amount of observational and clinical data that supports a dividing line between positive and negative mental health at that point, between 1 and 2 standard deviations above the mean level of mental health of the total population. Here in an appendix I can only mention some of the sources the charts rely on.

There is strong evidence for the size of both the white and the shaded sides of the top curve. For the size of the shaded righthand side, for example, as quoted in an earlier chapter, Abraham Maslow (1971, p. 92) found that only 1 percent or less of the population has what the upper chart represents as a high level of positive mental health. Lewis Fry Richardson's quantitative, psychologically focused studies of the statistics of war found, as one indication of what I've called "moral intelligence," that fewer than 1 percent of men called to military service in World War I refused on the basis of conscience (Richardson, 1948, I, p. 151; see also Richardson, 1960a, 1960b, and Ashford et al., 1993). Similarly, historian Eric A. Johnson (1999, p. 261) found that only about half of 1 percent of Germans were willing to participate in any kind of resistance against the Nazi regime. (For a fuller discussion of morally intelligent groups see Bartlett, 2005, p. 182). In earlier chapters we found similarly small minorities whenever we looked for fully developed moral intelligence, aesthetic sensibility, commitment to higher values, and behavior consistent with these. But in case the restricted size of these rough estimates may be unduly pessimistic, the percentage of the population in the chart that represents people with high degrees of mental health has been increased severalfold to err on the side of generosity: but whether 1, 2, or 3 percent, or twice that, the group remains a small minority.

There is considerably more evidence for the size of the normal majority population that falls in the negative, unshaded, lefthand region of the upper chart: there are, for the dispassionate mind, the convincing conclusions to be drawn from human history, from Milgram's (1974) and Zimbardo's (2007) studies, from the combined incidence of crime and violent psychotic behavior, and from the evidence of the many normal pathologies of internal limitation discussed in this book and in Bartlett (2005).

The vertical dotted line intersects the lower cumulative distribution curve somewhere between the 94th and the 97th percentiles, as shown by the horizontal shaded band. In other words, 94 to 97 percent of the total population is represented by the white, unshaded area under the bell curve, while only 3 to 6 percent of the population can be characterized, applying the criteria of this book, as possessing genuinely positive levels of mental health. These people are represented by the shaded portion under the righthand tail of the bell curve.

This understanding of the distribution of positive versus negative mental health may appear pessimistic, but it is important to realize that 3 to 6 percent of the world's present population includes 210 to 420 million people with genuinely positive levels of mental health, while in the United States alone there are an estimated 9 to 18 million. Although not common and not normal, positive levels of mental health are to be found in a great many people.

At this stage when we have few ways to measure positive mental health it would be idle to become bogged down in concern over precise percentages. The two charts together place in relief the generally low—that is, negative—level of "normal mental health" of the overall population, in contrast to the relative rarity of genuinely positive mental health in the much smaller population, those who are the exceptions to the rule. If a picture is worth many words, the picture we see underscores the need to question the dictum that to be normal is to have good mental health.

References

Abelson, Raziel (1967). Definition, in *The encyclopedia of philosophy*, vol. 1 (pp. 314–24). New York: Macmillan & The Free Press.

Adler, Alfred (1912/1926). *The neurotic constitution*. New York: Dodd Mead. (First pub. 1912.)

Adler, Alfred (1924). *The practice and theory of individual psychology*. P. Radin (Trans.). New York: Harcourt, Brace.

Adler, Alfred (1929/1964). *Problems of neurosis: A book of case-histories*. New York: Harper. (First pub. 1929.)

Albert, Tim (1997). Why bother with peer review? *The Lancet, 350*, Sept. 13, 822.

Álvarez González, Francisco (1986). *El reto de la mediocridad*. San José, Costa Rica: Universidad Autónoma de Centro América.

American Psychiatric Association (1987). *Diagnostic and statistical manual of mental disorders: DSM-III-R*. Washington, D.C.: American Psychiatric Association.

American Psychiatric Association (1994). *Diagnostic and statistical manual of mental disorders: DSM-IV*. Washington, D.C.: American Psychiatric Association.

American Psychiatric Association (2000). *Diagnostic and statistical manual of mental disorders: DSM-IV-TR*. Washington, D.C.: American Psychiatric Association.

Andreasen, N. C. (1987). Creativity and mental illness: Prevalence rates in writers and their first-degree relatives. *American Journal of Psychiatry, 144*, 1288–92.

Andreasen, Nancy C. (2005). *The creating brain: The neuroscience of genius*. New York: Dana Press.

Ansbacher, Heinz L. & Ansbacher, Rowena (Eds.) (1956). *The individual psychology of Alfred Adler*. New York: Basic Books.

Aquinas, St. Thomas (1265–1273/1912–1925). *Summa Theologiae*. 22 vols. The English Dominican Fathers (Trans.). London: Burns, Oates, & Washbourne. (First pub. 1265–1273.)

Aquinas, St. Thomas (1269–1272/1949). Quaestiones disputatae de malo, in *Quaestiones Disputatae*. 2 vols. Rome: Marietti. (First pub. 1269–1272.)

Arendt, Hannah (1964). *Eichmann in Jerusalem: A report on the banality of evil*. New York: Viking.

Arendt, Hannah (2003). *Responsibility and judgment.* Jerome Kohn (Ed.). New York: Schocken Books.

Armstrong, S. J. (1996). We need to rethink the editorial role of peer reviewers. *The Chronicle of Higher Education, 43*(9), Oct. 25, B3.

Arnett, F. C., Edworthy, S. M., Bloch, D. A., McShane, D. A., Fries, J. F., Cooper, N. S., Healey, L. A., Kaplan, S. R., Liang, N. H., Luthra, H. S., Medsger, T. A., Jr., Mitchell, D. M., Neustadt, D. H., Pinals, S. R., Schaller, J. G., Sharp, J. T., Wilder, R. L., & Hunter, G. G. (1988). The American Rheumatism Association 1987 revised criteria for the classification of rheumatoid arthritis. *Arthritis and Rheumatism, 31*, 315–24.

Ashford, Oliver M., Charnock, H., Drazin, P.D., Hunt, J.C.R., Smoker, P., & Sutherland, Ian (Eds.) (1993). *Collected papers of Lewis Fry Richardson.* Vol. I: Meteorology and Numerical Analysis; Vol. II: Quantitative Psychology and Studies of Conflict. Cambridge: Cambridge Univ. Press.

Asimov, Janet & Isaac (1987). *How to enjoy writing: A book to aid and comfort.* New York: Walker.

Bartlett, Steven James (1971). *A relativistic theory of phenomenological constitution: A self-referential, transcendental approach to conceptual pathology.* 2 vols. (Vol. I: French; Vol. II: English). Ph.D. dissertation, Université de Paris. University Microfilms International #7905583.

Bartlett, Steven James (1975). *Metalogic of reference: A study in the foundations of possibility.* Starnberg, Germany: Max-Planck-Gesellschaft.

Bartlett, Steven James (1976). The idea of a metalogic of reference. *Methodology and Science, 9*(3), 85–92.

Bartlett, Steven James (1980). Self-reference, phenomenology, and philosophy of science. *Methodology and Science, 13*(3), 143–67.

Bartlett, Steven James (1982). Referential consistency as a criterion of meaning. *Synthèse, 52*, 267–82.

Bartlett, Steven James (1983). *Conceptual therapy: An introduction to framework-relative epistemology.* Saint Louis: Studies in Theory and Behavior.

Bartlett, Steven James (1986a). Narcissism and philosophy. *Methodology and Science, 19*(1), 16–26.

Bartlett, Steven James (1986b). Philosophy as ideology. *Metaphilosophy, 17*(1), 1–13.

Bartlett, Steven James (1987). All is not quiet on the Western Front: The not-so-petty crime of noise pollution. *Christian Science Monitor,* July 19, 13.

Bartlett, Steven James (1989). Psychological underpinnings of philosophy. *Metaphilosophy, 20*(3–4), 295–305.

Bartlett, Steven James (1990). *Acedia*: The etiology of work-engendered depression. *New Ideas in Psychology, 8*(3), 389–96.

Bartlett, Steven James (1993a). Barbarians at the door: A psychological and historical profile of today's college students. *Methodology and Science, 26*(1), 18–40. (A concurrent publication in the Netherlands of Bartlett, 1993b.)

Bartlett, Steven James (1993b). Barbarians at the door: A psychological and historical profile of today's college students. *Modern Age, 35*(4), Summer, 296–310. (Readers of this version of the paper are asked to refer to the "Note to Our Readers" printed in this journal in Vol. 36, No. 3, page 303.)

Bartlett, Steven James (1994a). The loss of permanent realities: Demoralization of university faculty in the liberal arts. *Methodology and Science*, 27(1), 25–39.

Bartlett, Steven James (1994b). The psychology of faculty demoralization in the liberal arts: Burnout, *acedia*, and the disintegration of idealism. *New Ideas in Psychology*, 12(3), 277–89.

Bartlett, Steven James (2002). Roots of human resistance to animal rights: Psychological and conceptual blocks. *Animal Law*, 8, 143–76. Electronically republished October 2002 by the Michigan State University's Detroit College of Law, Animal Law Web Center, and maintained on an ongoing basis at http://www.animallaw.info/articles/arussbartlett2002. htm. Translated into German, "Wurzeln menschlichen Widerstands gegen Tierrechte: Psychologische und konceptuelle Blockaden," and electronically published on the following websites in September, 2003: http://www.tierrechts.net/Animal_Law_Roots_ of_Human_Resistance_to_Animal_Rights.pdf; http://www.veganswines.de/Animal_ Law/; and http://animallaw.info/articles/arussbartlett 2002.htm. Accessed February 2006. [For the translation of this paper into Portuguese, see Bartlett (2007).]

Bartlett, Steven James (2005). *The pathology of man: A study of human evil*. Springfield, IL: Charles C. Thomas.

Bartlett, Steven James (2006). The ecological pathology of man. *Mentalities/Mentalités: An Interdisciplinary Journal*, 20(2), 1–18.

Bartlett, Steven James (2007). Raízes da resistência humana aos direitos dos animais: Bloqueios psicológicos e conceituais. *Brazilian Animal Rights Review* (*Revista Brasileira de Direito Animal*), 2(3), July/December, 11–66. [A translation into Portuguese of Bartlett (2002).]

Bartlett, Steven James (2008). The humanistic psychology of human evil: Ernest Becker and Arthur Koestler. *Journal of Humanistic Psychology*, 48(3), 340–63. DOI: 10.1177/ 0022167807305249.

Bartlett, Steven James (2009). From the artist's perspective: The psychopathology of the normal world. *The Humanistic Psychologist*, 37(3), 235–56.

Bartlett, Steven James (Ed.) (1992). *Reflexivity: A source book in self-reference*. Amsterdam: Elsevier Science Publishers.

Bartlett, Steven James & Suber, Peter (Eds.) (1987). *Self-reference: Reflections on reflexivity*. Dordrecht, Holland: Martinus Nijhoff. (Now published by Springer Science.)

Bedeian, A.G. (1996). Improving the journal review process: The question of ghostwriting. *American Psychologist*, 51, 1189.

Beutler, Larry E. & Malik, Mary L. (2002). Diagnosis and treatment guidelines: The example of depression. In Larry E. Beutler & Mary L. Malik (Eds.), *Rethinking the DSM: A psychological perspective* (pp. 251–77). Washington, D.C.: American Psychological Association.

Bierce, Ambrose (1946/1989). *The collected writings of Ambrose Bierce*. New York: Carol Publishing. (First pub. 1946.)

Bisch, Louis E. (1936). *Be glad you're neurotic*. New York: McGraw-Hill.

Blackwell, Richard J. (2006). *Behind the scenes at Galileo's trial*. Notre Dame, IN: University of Notre Dame Press.

Bloom, Allan (1987). *The closing of the American mind: How higher education has failed democracy and impoverished the souls of today's students.* New York: Simon & Schuster.

Bolton, Derek (2008). *What is mental disorder? An essay in philosophy, science, and values.* Oxford: Oxford Univ. Press.

Borges, Jorge Luis (1940). Ellery Queen: The new adventures of Ellery Queen. *Sur, 70,* July.

Bowlby, John (1969–1982). *Attachment and loss.* 3 vols. New York: Basic Books.

Brander, B.G. (1998). *Staring into chaos: Explorations in the decline of Western civilization.* Dallas: Spence Publishing.

Breggin, Peter R. (1994). *Toxic psychiatry.* New York: St. Martin's Press.

Brentano, Franz (1924, 1925, 1928). *Psychologie vom empirishen Standpunkt.* 3 vols. Leipzig: Felix Meiner.

Brown, G. W. & Harris, T. (1978). *The social origins of depression: A study of psychiatric disorder in women.* London: Tavistock Publications.

Browning, Christopher R. (1992). *Ordinary men: Reserve Police Battalion 101 and the Final Solution in Poland.* New York: HarperCollins.

Bruner, J. S. & Tagiuri, R. (1954). The perception of people. In G. Lindzey (Ed.), *Handbook of social psychology* (pp. 634–54). Reading, MA: Addison-Wesley.

Brysbaert, M. (1996). Improving the journal review process and risk of making the poor poorer. *American Psychologist, 51,* 1193.

Buck, Lucien A. (1992). The myth of normality: Consequences for the diagnosis of abnormality and health. *Social Behavior & Personality, 20*(4), 251–62.

Bucknill, John Charles and Tuke, Daniel Hack (1858/1879). *A manual of psychological medicine.* 4th edition. London: J. & A. Churchill. (First pub. 1858.)

Burrow, Trigant (1953/1968). *Science and man's behavior: The contribution of phylobiology.* William E. Galt (Ed.). New York: Greenwood Press. (First pub. 1953.)

Burt, Cyril Lodowic (1940). *The factors of the mind: An introduction to factor-analysis in psychology.* London: Univ. of London Press.

Burton, Sir Richard (1894/n.d.). *The Kasidah of Haji Abdu.* Mt. Vernon: Peter Pauper Press. (Published without a date.) Also available through Project Gutenberg at: http://www.gutenberg.org/cache/epub/6036/pg6036.html. Accessed Feb. 15, 2011. (First pub. 1894.)

Callahan, Raymond E. (1962). *Education and the cult of efficiency.* Chicago: Univ. of Chicago Press.

Campanario, Juan Miguel (1998). Peer review for journals as it stands today— Part 1. *Science Communication,* 19(3), 181–211; Part 2: 19(4), 277–306.

Cannan, Crescy (1972). Social workers: Training and professionalism. In Trevor Pateman (Ed.), *Counter course: A handbook for course criticism* (pp. 245–63). Harmondsworth, U.K.: Penguin.

Cartwright, Samuel A. (1851). Report on the diseases and physical peculiarities of the Negro race. *New Orleans Med. & Surgical Journal,* May, 691–715.

Chevalier, Michael (1838/1961). *Society, manners, and politics in the United States: Letters on North America.* New York: Doubleday. (First pub. 1838.)

Cioran, E. M. (1973/1998). *The trouble with being born.* Richard Howard (Trans.). New York: Arcade. (First pub. in French, *De l'inconvenient d'être né,* 1973; first pub. in English translation, 1976.)

College of American Pathologists Committee on Nomenclature and Classification of Disease (1965). *Systematized nomenclature of pathology*. Chicago: College of American Pathologists.

College of American Pathologists Committee on Nomenclature and Classification of Disease (1979). *Systematized nomenclature of medicine*. Roger A. Côté (Ed.). 2nd edition. 2 vols. Skokie, IL: College of American Pathologists.

Cooper, Rachel (2005). *Classifying madness: A philosophical examination of the* Diagnostic and Statistical Manual of Mental Disorders. Dordrecht: Springer.

Cropsey, Joseph (Ed.) (1964). *Ancients and moderns: Essays on the tradition of political philosophy in honor of Leo Strauss*. New York: Basic Books.

Crosthwaite, Jan (1995). Moral expertise: A problem in the professional ethics of professional ethicists. *Bioethics, 9*, 361–79.

Danto, Arthur C. (1971). *What philosophy is: A guide to the elements*. New York: Harper.

Davidson, William L. (1885). *The logic of definition*. London: Longmans, Green, & Co.

de Gobineau, Arthur (1853–1855). *Essai sur l'inégalité des races humaines*. 4 vols. Paris: Didot.

de Grazia, Sebastian (1962). *Of time, work, and leisure*. New York: Twentieth Century Fund.

de Konig, A. J. J. & Jenner, F. A. (Eds.) (1982). *Phenomenology and psychiatry*. New York: Academic Press.

De Sousa, R. (1987). *The rationality of emotion*. London: MIT Press.

Dewey, John (1949). Democracy and education. In Dewey, John, *Problems of men*. New York: Philosophical Library.

Dobson, K. & Franche, R. L. (1989). A conceptual and empirical review of the depressive realism hypothesis. *Canadian Journal of Behavioural Science, 21*, 419–33.

Dubos, René (1959). *Mirage of health: Utopias, progress, and biological change*. New York: Harper.

Dyson, Freeman (1992). *From Eros to Gaia*. New York: Pantheon.

Ehrlich, Paul R. & Ehrlich, Anne H. (2008). *The dominant animal: Human evolution and the environment*. Washington, D.C.: Island Press.

Eissler, K. R. (1960). The efficient soldier. *The Psychoanalytic Study of Society, I*, 39–97.

Eliade, Mircea (1949). *Traité d'histoire des religions*. Paris: Payot.

Eliade, Mircea (1963). *Aspects du mythe*. Paris: Gallimard.

Ellis, Albert (1973). *Humanistic psychotherapy: The rational-emotive approach*. New York: McGraw-Hill.

Ellis, Albert & Harper, R. A. (1961). *A guide to rational living*. Englewood Cliffs, N.J.: Prentice-Hall.

Ellis, Albert & Harper, R. A. (1975). *A new guide to rational living*. Englewood Cliffs, N.J.: Prentice-Hall.

Elson, Miriam (Ed.) (1987). *The Kohut seminars on self psychology and psychotherapy with adolescents and young adults*. New York: W.W. Norton.

Enserink, Martin (2001). Peer review and quality: a dubious connection? *Science, 293*(5538), Sept. 21, 2187.

Erickson, Milton (1968). The inhumanity of ordinary people. *International Journal of Psychiatry, 6*, 277–79.

Evans, Rowland & Novak, Robert (1988). Bill Bennett: Secretary *for* Education. *Reader's Digest*, March, 106.

Eysenck, H. J. (1967). *The biological basis of personality*. Springfield, IL: Charles C. Thomas.

Eysenck, Hans J. (1972). *Psychology is about people*. New York: Library Press.

Eysenck, H. J. (1990). *Rebel with a cause*. London: W. H. Allen.

Eysenck, Hans J. (1998/1999). *Intelligence: A new look*. New Brunswick: Transaction Publishers. (First pub. 1998.)

Eysenck, Hans J. & Eysenck, Michael W. (1985). *Personality and individual differences: A natural science approach*. New York: Plenum.

Faber, Knud (1923/1930). *Nosography: The evolution of clinical medicine in modern times*. New York: AMS Press. (First pub. 1923.)

Feinstein, A. R. (1967). *Clinical judgment*. Baltimore: Williams & Wilkins.

Fine, M. A. (1996). Reflections on enhancing accountability in the peer review process. *American Psychologist, 51*, 1190–91.

Finkielkraut, Alain (1996/2000). *In the name of humanity: Reflections on the twentieth century*. Judith Friedlander (Trans.). New York: Columbia Univ. Press. (First pub. as *L'Humanité perdue: Essai sur le xxe siècle*, 1996.)

Frankl, Viktor (1955). *The doctor and the soul*. New York: Knopf.

Frankl, Viktor (1959). *Man's search for meaning: An introduction to logotherapy*. New York: Washington Square Press.

Freides, David (1960). Toward the elimination of the concept of normality. *Journal of Consulting Psychology, 24*(2), 128–33.

Freud, Sigmund (1914–1916/1957). On narcissism: An introduction. James Strachey (Trans.). *The standard edition of the complete psychological works of Sigmund Freud*, vol. XIV (pp. 73–102). London: Hogarth Press.

Freud, Sigmund (1930/1952). *Civilization and its discontents*. J. Riviere (Trans.). *Great books of the Western world*, vol. 54 (pp. 767–802). Chicago: Encyclopaedia Britannica. (First pub. 1930.)

Frey, Bruno S. (2003). Publishing as prostitution? Choosing between one's own ideas and academic success. *Public Choice, 116*(1/2), 205–23.

Fromm, Erich (1941). *Escape from freedom*. New York: Rinehart.

Fromm, Erich (1947). *Man for himself*. New York: Rinehart.

Fromm, Erich (1955). *The sane society*. New York: Rinehart.

Galton, Francis (1869/1925). *Hereditary genius: An inquiry into its laws and consequences*. London: Macmillan. (First pub. 1869.)

Gana, K., Alaphilippe, D., & Bailly, N. (2004). Positive illusions and mental and physical health in later life. *Aging & Mental Health, 8*(1), 58–64.

Gans, J. (2000). *Publishing economics: Analyses of the academic journal market in economics*. Northampton, MA: Elgar.

García, J. (1981). Tilting at the paper mills of academe. *American Psychologist, 36*, 149–58.

Gardner, Howard (1983/1993). *Frames of mind: The theory of multiple intelligences*. New York: BasicBooks. (First pub. 1983.)

Gardner, Howard (1993). *Multiple intelligences: The theory in practice*. New York: BasicBooks.

Goleman, Daniel (1985). *Vital lies, simple truths*. New York: Simon & Schuster.

Goleman, Daniel (1995). *Emotional intelligence*. New York: Bantam.

Goodwin, Frederick K. & Jamison, Kay Redfield (1990). *Manic-depressive illness*. New York: Oxford Univ. Press.

Gore, Al (2006). *An inconvenient truth: The planetary emergency of global warming and what we can do about it*. Emmaus, PA: Rodale.

Gould, S.J. & Lewontin, R. C. (1979). The spandrels of San Marco and the Pan-glossian paradigm: A critique of the adaptationist paradigm. *Proceedings of the Royal Society of London. Series B, Biological Sciences, 205*, 581–98.

Greenberg, Daniel S. (1999). Peer review: and the winner is.... *The Lancet, 354*, Dec. 11, 2092.

Greenspan, P. S. (1988). *Emotions and reasons: An inquiry into emotional justification*. London: Routledge.

Grobel, Lawrence (1986). The remarkable Dr. Feynman. *Los Angeles Times Magazine*, Apr. 20, 15–38.

Guilford, J. P. (1936). Unitary traits of personality and factor theory. *American Journal of Psychology, 48*, 673–80.

Guilford, J. P. (1967). *The nature of human intelligence*. New York: McGraw-Hill.

Guilford, J. P. (1975). Factors and factors of personality. *Psychological Bulletin, 82*, 802–814.

Guilford, J.P. & Hoepfner, R. (1971). *The analysis of intelligence*. New York: McGraw-Hill.

Hacker, F.J. (1945). The concept of normality and its practical significance. *American Journal of Orthopsychiatry, 15*, 47–64.

Hadjistavropoulos, Thomas & Bieling, Peter J. (2000). When reviews attack: Ethics, free speech, and the peer review process. *Canadian Psychology, 41*(3), 152–59.

Hadler, Nortin M. (2004). Health hazards in the hateful job, in Hadler, Nortin M., *The last well person: How to stay well despite the health-care system* (pp. 166–76). Montreal: McGill-Queen's Univ. Press.

Hardin, Garrett (1982). *Naked emperors: Essays of a taboo-stalker*. San Francisco: Wm. Kaufmann.

Harlow, H.F. & Harlow, M.K (1962). The mind of man. *Yearbook of science and technology*. New York: McGraw-Hill.

Harnad, Stevan (Ed.) (1982). *Peer commentary on peer review: A case study in scientific quality control*. Cambridge: Cambridge Univ. Press.

Hempton, Gordon & Grossman, John (2009). *One square inch of silence: One man's search for natural silence in a noisy world*. New York: Free Press.

Henderson, Isabella (1960/1963). *A dictionary of scientific terms: Pronunciation, derivation, and definition*. New York: Van Nostrand. (First pub. 1960.)

Herman, Arthur (1997). *The idea of decline in Western history*. New York: Free Press.

Herrnstein, Richard J. & Murray, Charles (1994). *The bell curve: Intelligence and class structure in American life*. New York: Free Press.

Hesse, Hermann (1925/1954). My life: A conjectural biography. In Denver Lindley (Trans.), William Phillips & Philip Rahv (Eds.), *Avon book of modern writing no. 2* (pp. 55–72). New York: Avon Books. (First pub. as "Kurzgefasster Lebenslauf," *Neue Rundschau*, 1925. Also published as "Life story briefly told," in Hermann Hesse, *Autobiographical writings*, Denver Lindley (Trans.), Theodore Ziolkowski (Ed.) (pp. 43–62). New York: Farrar, Straus and Giroux, 1973.)

Hesse, Hermann (1973). *Autobiographical writings*. Denver Lindley (Trans.), Theodore Ziolkowski (Ed.). New York: Farrar, Straus & Giroux.

Hirsch, Eric Donald (1987). *Cultural literary: What every American needs to know*. Boston: Houghton Mifflin.

Hojat, Mohammadreza, Gonnella, Joseph S., & Caelleigh, Addeane S. (2003). Impartial judgment by the "gatekeepers" of science: Fallibility and accountability in the peer review process. *Advances in Health Sciences Education, 8*, 75–96.

Holbrook, Morris B. (1986). A note on sadomasochism in the review process: I hate when that happens. *Journal of Marketing, 50*, July, 104–108.

Horrobin, D. F. (1982). Peer review: A philosophically faulty concept which is proving disastrous for science. *The Behavioral and Brain Sciences, 5*, 217–218; also in Harnad (1982), pp. 33–34.

Horrobin, D. F. (1990). The philosophical basis of peer review and the suppression of innovation. *Journal of the American Medical Association, 263*(10), March 9, 1438–41.

Horwitz, Allan V. & Wakefield, Jerome C. (2007). *The loss of sadness: How psychiatry transformed normal sorrow into depressive disorder*. Oxford: Oxford Univ. Press.

Houts, A. C. (2001). The diagnostic and statistical manual's new white coat and circularity of plausible dysfunctions: Response to Wakefield, Part I. *Behaviour Research and Therapy, 39*, 315–45.

Houts, Arthur C. (2002). Discovery, invention, and the expansion of the modern *Diagnostic and Statistical Manuals of Mental Disorders*, in Larry E. Beutler & Mary L. Malik (Eds.), *Rethinking the* DSM: *A psychological perspective* (pp. 17–65). Washington, D.C.: American Psychological Association.

Houts, A. C. & Follette, W. C. (1998). Mentalism, mechanism, and medical analogues: Reply to Wakefield. *Journal of Consulting and Clinical Psychology, 66*, 853–55.

Hutchins, Robert Maynard (1937). *The higher learning in America*. New Haven, CT: Yale Univ. Press.

Hutchins, Robert Maynard (1952). *The great conversation: The substance of a liberal education. The great books*, vol. 1. Chicago: Encyclopedia Britannica.

Ingenieros, José (1913/1957). *El hombre mediocre*. Mexico, D. F.: Editora Latino Americana. Eighth edition. (First pub. in book form, 1913.)

Jacobs, Tom (2009). Morals authority. *Miller-McCune*, 7(3), May–June, 46–55.

Jahoda, M. (1958). *Current concepts of positive mental health*. New York: Basic Books.

James, William (1904/1958). A world of pure experience. In *Essays in radical empiricism* and *A pluralistic universe* (pp. 39–91). New York: Longmans, Green & Co. (First pub. 1904.)

Jamison, Kay Redfield (1989). Mood disorders and patterns of creativity in 47 British writers and artists. *Psychiatry, 52*, 125–34.

Jamison, Kay Redfield (1993). *Touched with fire: Manic-depressive illness and the artistic temperament.* New York: Free Press.

Jefferson, Tom, Alderson, Philip, Wager, Elizabeth, & Davidoff, Frank (2002a). Effects of editorial peer review: A systematic review. *Journal of the American Medical Association, 287*(21), 2784–86.

Jefferson, Tom, Wager, Elizabeth, & Davidoff, Frank (2002b). Measuring the quality of editorial peer review. *Journal of the American Medical Association, 287*(21), 2786–90.

Jensen, Arthur R. (1972). *Genetics and education.* New York: Harper & Row.

Johnson, Eric A. (1999). *Nazi terror: The Gestapo, Jews, and ordinary Germans.* New York: Basic Books.

Jones, E. (1942). The concept of the normal mind. *The International Journal of Psychoanalysis, 23*, 1–8.

Juda, A. (1949). The relationship between highest mental capacity and psychic abnormalities. *American Journal of Psychiatry, 106*, 296–307.

Jung, C. G. (1916–1917/1967–1983). *Two essays on analytical psychology.* In Jung (1967–1983), vol. 7. (First pub. 1916–1917.)

Jung, C. G. (1946/1967–1983). Epilogue to "Essays on contemporary events." In Jung (1967–1983), vol. 10 (pp. 227–43). (First pub. 1946.)

Jung, C. G. (1958). *Psychology and religion.* In Jung (1967–1983), vol. 2.

Jung, C. G. (1964). Epilogue to "Essays on Contemporary Events." In Jung (1967–1983), *Civilization in transition,* vol. 10 (pp. 227–43). R. F. C. Hull (Trans.). Princeton, N.J.: Princeton Univ. Press.

Jung, C. G. (1967–1983). *The collected works of C. G. Jung.* 20 vols. R. F. C. Hull (Trans.). Princeton, N.J.: Princeton Univ. Press.

Jünger, Ernst (1934). *Blätter und Steine.* Hamburg: Hanseatische Verlagsanstalt.

Kassirer, J. P. & Campion, E. W. (1994). Peer review: Crude and understudied, but indispensable. *Journal of the American Medical Association, 272*, 96–97.

Kelly, George A. (1955). *The psychology of personal constructs.* New York: W.W. Norton.

Kelly, George A. (1956/1978). Man's construction of his alternatives, in Corsini, Raymond J. (Ed.), *Readings in current personality theories* (pp. 107–127). Itaska, IL: F. E. Peacock Publishers. (First published 1956.)

Kernberg, Otto (1975). *Borderline conditions and pathological narcissism.* New York: Jason Aronson.

Kernberg, Otto (1980). *Internal world and external reality.* New York: Jason Aronson.

Kernberg, Otto (1984). *Severe personality disorders.* New Haven, CT: Yale Univ. Press.

Kihlstrom, John F. (2002). To honor Kraepelin . . . : From symptoms to pathology in the diagnosis of mental illness, in Larry E. Beutler & Mary L. Malik (Eds.), *Rethinking the* DSM: *A psychological perspective* (pp. 279–303). Washington, D.C.: American Psychological Association.

Kim, Ha Poong (2006). Confucius's aesthetic concept of the noble man: Beyond moralism. *Asian Philosophy, 16*(2), 111–21.

Kirk, Russell (1978). *Decadence and renewal in the higher learning: An episodic history of the American university and college since 1953.* S. Bend, IN: Gateway.

Klinger, E. (1975). Consequences of commitment to and disengagement from incentives. *Psychological Review, 82,* 1–25.

Klinger, E. (1977). *Meaning and void: Inner experience and the incentives in people's lives.* Minneapolis: Univ. of Minnesota Press.

Knight, R.L. (1948). *Dictionary of genetics, including terms used in cytology, animal breeding and evolution.* Waltham, MA: Chronica Botanica.

Kohut, Heinz (1971). *The analysis of the self: A systematic approach to the psychoanalytic treatment of narcissistic personality disorders.* New York: International Universities Press.

Kohut, Heinz (1977). *The restoration of the self.* Madison, CT: International Universities Press.

Ladrière, Jean (1957). *Les limitations internes des formalismes: Étude sur la signification du théorème de Gödel et des théorèmes apparentés dans la théorie des fondements des mathématiques.* Louvain: E. Nauwelaerts.

Laënnec, René-Théophile-Hyacinthe (1982). Traité d'anatomie pathologique, in L. Boulle, M. D. Grmek, C. Lupovici, & J. Samion-Contet (Eds.), *Laënnec: Catalogue des manuscrits scientifiques* (MS. 2186 (III)). Paris: Maison et Fondation Singer-Polignac.

Laing, R. D. (1960). *The divided self: A study of sanity and madness.* London: Tavistock.

Landau, Jacob (1980). Loneliness and creativity. In Joseph Hartog, J. Ralph Audy, & Yehudi A. Cohen (Eds.), *The anatomy of loneliness* (pp. 486–505). New York: International Universities Press.

Lasch, Christopher (1979). *The culture of narcissism: American life in an age of diminishing expectations.* New York: W.W. Norton.

Lee, Vernon (1920). *Satan, the waster: A philosophic war trilogy.* New York: John Lane. [Vernon Lee was the pseudonym of Violet Paget, 1856–1935.]

Levenson, R. L. (1996). Enhance the journals, not the review process. *American Psychologist, 51,* 1191–93.

Lock, S. (1985). *A difficult balance: Editorial peer review in medicine.* Philadelphia: ISI Press.

Lorenz, Konrad (1940). Durch Domestikation verursachte Störungen arteigenen Verhaltens. [Disorders caused by the domestication of species-specific behavior.] *Zeitschrift für angewandte Psychologie und Charackterkunde, 59,* 2–81.

Ludwig, A. M. (1992). Creative achievement and psychopathology: Comparisons among professions. *American Journal of Psychotherapy, 46,* 330–56.

Maddi, Salvador R. (1967). The existential neurosis. *Journal of Abnormal Psychology, 72*(4), 311–25.

Mahoney, M. J. (1977). Publication prejudices: An experimental study of confirmatory bias in the peer review system. *Cognitive Therapy & Research, 1,* 161–75.

Mahoney, M. J. (1979). Psychology of the scientist: An evaluative review. *Social Studies of Science, 9*(3), 349–75.

Mahoney, M. J. (1990). Bias, controversy, and abuse in the study of the scientific publication system. *Science, Technology, & Human Values, 15*(1), Winter, 50–55.

Mahoney, M. J., Kazdin, A. E., & Kenigsberg, M. (1978). Getting published. *Cognitive Therapy & Research*, *2*, 69–70.

Malik, Mary L. & Beutler, Larry E. (2002). The emergence of dissatisfaction with the DSM, in Larry E. Beutler & Mary L. Malik (Eds.), *Rethinking the* DSM: *A psychological perspective* (pp. 3–15). Washington, D.C.: American Psychological Association.

Marsh, Herbert W., Bond, Nigel W., & Jayasinghe, Upali W. (2007). The peer review process: Assessments by applicant-nominated referees are biased, inflated, unreliable and invalid. *Australian Psychologist*, *42*, March, 33–38.

Martin, Brian, Baker, C. M. Ann, Manwell, Clyde, & Pugh, Cedric (1986). *Intellectual suppression: Australian case histories, analysis and responses*. North Ryde, NSW, Australia: Angus & Robertson.

Maryland Judicial Task Force on Professionalism (2003). Dated November 10. Accessed at: http://www.courts.state.md.us/publications/professionalism 2003.pdf.

Maslow, Abraham H. (1964). The superior person. *Trans-action*, *1*, 10–13.

Maslow, Abraham H. (1970). *Motivation and personality*. New York: Harper & Row.

Maslow, Abraham H. (1971). *The farther reaches of human nature*. New York: Viking Press.

Mayer, Milton (1993). *Robert Maynard Hutchins, A memoir*. John H. Hicks (Ed.). Berkeley: Univ. of California Press.

McCarthy, Nancy (1994). Pessimism for the future. *California Bar Journal*, November. Accessed at: http://www.calbar.ca.gov/calbar/pdfs/members/ 1994-Futures-CBJ.pdf.

McIntyre, Lee (2006). *Dark ages: The case for a science of human behavior*. Cambridge, MA: MIT Press.

Melville, Herman (1852/1995). *Pierre: Or the ambiguities*. Hershel Parker (Ed.). New York: HarperCollins. (First pub. 1852.)

Menninger, Karl, Mayman, Martin, & Pruyser, Paul (1963/1967). *The vital balance: The life process in mental health and illness*. New York: Viking.

Menuhin, Yehudi (1977). *Unfinished journey*. New York: Alfred A. Knopf.

Milgram, Stanley (1974). *Obedience to authority: An experimental view*. New York: Harper & Row.

Miller, Arthur G. (1986). *The obedience experiments: A case study of controversy in social science*. New York: Praeger.

Millon, Theodore (1989). Normality: What may we learn from evolutionary theory? In Daniel Offer & Melvin Sabshin (Eds.), *The diversity of normal behavior: Further contributions to normatology* (pp. 356–404). New York: BasicBooks.

Morris, Kelly (1997). Swedish researchers reveal systematic bias in peer-review. *The Lancet*, *349*, May 31, 1611.

Murphy, Edmond A. (1979). The epistemology of normality. *Psychological Medicine*, *9*, 409–415.

Murray, Charles (2003). *Human accomplishment: The pursuit of excellence in the arts and sciences, 800 B.C. to 1950*. New York: HarperCollins.

Naftulin, D. H., Ware, Jr., J. E., & Donnelly, F. A. (1973). The Doctor Fox lecture: A paradigm of educational seduction. *Journal of Medical Education*, *48*, 630–35.

Naranjo, Luis Ángel Camacho (1992). *Ensayo sobre la mediocridad*. San José, Costa Rica: Editorial de la Universidad de Costa Rica.

Nesse, Randolph M. (2000). Is depression adaptation? *Archives of General Psychiatry*, 57, 14–20.

Newman, John Henry (1852/1960). *The idea of a university*. San Francisco: Rinehart Press. (Based on lectures Newman delivered in 1852.)

Nicholls, Robert D. (1999). Peer review under review. *Science, 286*(5446), Dec. 3, 1853.

Nietzsche, Friedrich (1954). *The portable Nietzsche*. Walter Kaufmann (Trans.). New York: Viking Press.

Nietzsche, Friedrich (1956). *The genealogy of morals*. F. Golffing (Trans.). New York: Doubleday.

Nietzsche, Friedrich (1968). *The will to power*. W. Kaufmann & R. J. Hollingdale (Trans.). New York: Vintage.

Nietzsche, Friedrich (1972). *Beyond good and evil*. R. J. Hollingdale (Trans.). Harmondsworth, U.K.: Penguin.

Nietzsche, Friedrich (1974). *The gay science*. W. Kaufmann (Trans.). New York: Vintage.

Nietzsche, Friedrich (1982). *Daybreak*. R. J. Hollingdale (Trans.). Cambridge: Cambridge Univ. Press.

Nietzsche, Friedrich (1989). *Human, all too human*. R. J. Hollingdale (Trans.). Cambridge: Cambridge Univ. Press.

Nietzsche, Friedrich (1992). Walter Kaufmann (Ed. & Trans.). *Basic writings of Nietzsche*. New York: Modern Library.

Offer, Daniel & Sabshin, Melvin (1966/1974). *Normality: Theoretical and clinical concepts of mental health*. New York: Basic Books. (First pub. 1966.)

Offer, Daniel & Sabshin, Melvin (Eds.) (1984). *Normality and the life cycle: A critical integration*. New York: Basic Books.

Offer, Daniel & Sabshin, Melvin (Eds.) (1989). *The diversity of normal behavior: Further contributions to normatology*. New York: BasicBooks.

Olson, C. M. (1990). Peer review of biomedical literature. *American Journal of Emergency Medicine, 8*, 356–58.

Ortega y Gasset, José (1957/1982). *¿Qué es filosofía?* Madrid: Revista de Occidente en Alianza Editorial. (First pub. 1957.)

Peter, J. P. & Olson, J. C. (1983). Is science marketing? *Journal of Marketing, 47*, Fall, 111–25.

Peters, D. P. & Ceci, S. J. (1982). Peer review practices of psychological journals: The fate of published articles, submitted again. *The Behavioral and Brain Sciences, 5*, 187–95.

Pieper, Josef (1948/1963). *Leisure, the basis of culture*. Alexander Dru (Trans.). New York: New American Library. (First pub. as *Musse und Kult* and *Was heisst Philosophieren?* München: Käsel-Verlag, 1948.)

Pieper, Josef (1977/1986). *On hope*. Mary Frances McCarthy (Trans.). San Francisco: Ignatius Press. (First pub. as *Über die Hoffnung*. München: Käsel-Verlag, 1977.)

Pines, Ayala & Aronson, Elliot (1988). *Career burnout: Causes and cures*. New York: Free Press.

Pitkin, Walter B. (1932). *A short introduction to the history of human stupidity*. New York: Simon & Schuster.

Proust, Marcel (1913–1927/1981). *Remembrance of things past*. C. K. Scott Moncrieff, T. Kilmartin, & A. Mayor (Trans.). 3 vols. New York: Random House. (First pub. 1913–1927.)

Rabinovich, B. A. (1996). A perspective on the journal review process. *American Psychologist, 51*, 1190.

Radbert, St. Pachasius (1857–1866). De fide, spe et charitate, in J. P. Migne (Ed.), *Opera omnia, patrologiae cursus completus*, series graeca. 161 vols. (vol. 120, cols. 1387–1490). Paris [publisher not given].

Redlich, F. C. (1952). The concept of normality. *American Journal of Psychotherapy, 6*, 551–69.

Reichenbach, Hans (1965). *The theory of relativity and a priori knowledge*. Maria Reichenbach (Trans. & Ed.). Berkeley: Univ. of Calif. Press.

Reider, Norman (1950). The concept of normality. *The Psychoanalytic Quarterly, 19*, 43–51.

Rescher, Nicholas (2006). *Epistemetrics*. New York: Cambridge Univ. Press.

Reznek, Lawrie (1987). *The nature of disease*. London: Routledge & Kegan Paul.

Richardson, Lewis Fry (1948). War-moods. Part I: *Psychometrika, 13*(3), 147–74; Part II: *Psychometrika, 13*(4), 197–232.

Richardson, Lewis Fry (1960a). *Arms and insecurity: A mathematical study of the causes and origins of war*. Nicolas Rashevsky & Ernesto Trucco (Eds.). Pittsburgh & Chicago: Boxwood Press & Quadrangle Books.

Richardson, Lewis Fry (1960b). *Statistics of deadly quarrels*. Quincy Wright & C. C. Lienau (Eds.). Pittsburgh & Chicago: Boxwood Press & Quadrangle Books.

Richet, Charles (1919/c. 1925). *Idiot man or the follies of mankind ("L'Homme Stupide")*. Norah Forsythe & Lloyd Harvey (Trans.). New York: Brentano's. (Published without a date; estimated c. 1925. Originally published 1919.)

Roberts, Sam (2009). Big birthday for a powerful little book. *New York Times*, April 22, C3.

Roberts, Siobhan (2006). *King of infinite space: Donald Coxeter, the man who saved geometry*. New York: Walker & Co.

Robinson, Richard (1950/1962). *Definition*. Oxford: Oxford Univ. Press. (First pub. 1950.)

Rogers, Carl R. (1961). *On becoming a person*. Boston: Houghton Mifflin.

Rogers, C. R. (1965). *Client-centered therapy*. New York: Houghton Mifflin.

Rohrlich, Jay B. (1980). *Work and love: A crucial balance*. New York: Summit Books.

Romanes, George John (1883). *Animal intelligence*. New York: Appleton.

Romanes, George John (1888). *Mental evolution in man: Origin of human faculty*. New York: Appleton.

Romanes, George John (1895). *Mental evolution in animals*. New York: Appleton.

Rowland, Fytton (2002). The peer review process: A report to the JISC Scholarly Communications Group. Accessed at http://www.ra-review.ac.uk/invite/responses/stake/21.doc.

Roy, Rustum & Ashburn, James R. (2001). The perils of peer review. *Nature, 414*, Nov. 22, 393–94.

Russell, Bertrand (1957). A free man's worship, in Bertrand Russell, *Why I am not a Christian* (pp. 104–116). New York: Simon and Schuster.

Rüstow, Alexander (1980). *Freedom and domination: A historical critique of civilization*. S. Attanasio (Trans.). Princeton, NJ: Princeton Univ. Press.

Sabshin, Melvin (1967). Psychiatric perspectives on normality. *Archives of General Psychiatry, 17*, 258–64.

Sackheim, H. A. (1983). Self-deception, self-esteem, and depression: The adaptive value of lying to oneself, in J. Masling (Ed.), *Empirical Studies of Psychoanalytic Theories*, vol. 1 (pp. 101–157). Hillsdale, NJ: Analytic Press.

Sadler, John Z. (2005). *Values and psychiatric diagnosis*. Oxford: Oxford Univ. Press.

Sadler, John Z. (Ed.) (2002). *Descriptions and prescriptions: Values, mental disorders, and the DSMs*. Baltimore: Johns Hopkins Univ. Press.

Salovey, Peter & Mayer, John D. (1990). Emotional intelligence. *Imagination, Cognition, and Personality, 9*(3), 185–211.

Santayana, George (1920). The unhappiness of artists. In Logan Pearsall Smith (Ed.), *Little essays drawn from the writings of George Santayana* (pp. 184–86). New York: Charles Scribner's Sons.

Sapir, Edward (1949/1958). *Selected writings of Edward Sapir in language, culture and personality*. David G. Mandelbaum (Ed.). Berkeley: Univ. of California Press. (First pub. 1949.)

Sartre, Jean-Paul (1946/1948). *Anti-Semite and Jew*. New York: Schocken. (First pub. as *Refléxions sur la question Juive*, 1946.)

Sax, Linda J., Astin, Alexander W., Korn, William S., Mahoney, Kathryn M., & Higher Education Research Inst. (1998). *The American freshman: National norms for Fall 1998*. Los Angeles: Higher Education Research Institute, UCLA Graduate School of Education & Information Studies.

Scadding, J. G. (1990). The semantic problems of psychiatry. *Psychological Medicine, 20*, 243–48.

Scadding, J. G. (1996). Essentialism and nominalism in medicine: Logic of diagnosis in disease terminology. *Lancet, 348*, 594–96.

Scheff, Thomas J. (1966/1984). *Being mentally ill: A sociological theory*. New York: Aldine de Gruyter. (First pub. 1966.)

Schiappa, Edward (2003). *Defining reality: Definitions and the politics of meaning*. Carbondale: Southern Illinois Univ. Press.

Sechrest, Lee (1977). Personal constructs theory. In Raymond J Corsini (Ed.), *Current personality theories* (pp. 203–241). Itasca, IL: F.E. Peacock Publishers.

Sedgwick, Peter (1973). Illness—mental and otherwise. *Hastings Center Studies, I*(3), 19–40.

Sharp, D. W. (1990). What can and should be done to reduce publication bias? *Journal of the American Medical Association, 263*, 1390–91.

Shaw, George Bernard (1934). *Too true to be good, Village wooing & On the rocks*. Three plays. London: Constable.

Shostrom, E. (1963). *Personal orientation inventory (POI)*. Educational and Industrial Testing Service.

Simonton, Dean Keith (1994). *Greatness: Who makes history and why*. New York: Guilford Press.

Spearman, Charles E. (1927). *The abilities of man*. New York: Macmillan.

Spitzer, R. L. (1991). An outsider-insider's views about revising the *DSMs*. *Journal of Abnormal Psychology*, *100*, 294–96.

Stang, Ragna (1979). *Edvard Munch: The man and his art*. Geoffrey Culverwell (Trans.). New York: Abbeville Press.

Starbuck, William H. (2003). Turning lemons into lemonade: Where is the value in peer reviews? *Journal of Management Inquiry*, *12*, 344–51.

Stempsey, William E. (1999). *Disease and diagnosis: Value-dependent realism*. Dordrecht: Kluwer Academic Publishers.

Strauss, Leo (1988). *Persecution and the art of writing*. Chicago: Univ. of Chicago Press.

Svitil, Kathy A. (2007). Mind-control microbe. *Discover*, Feb., 14.

Szasz, Thomas Stephen (1957/1961). *The myth of mental illness: Foundations of a theory of personal conduct*. New York: Hoeber-Harper. (First pub. 1957.)

Szasz, Thomas S. (1970/1997). *The manufacture of madness: A comparative study of the Inquisition and the mental health movement*. New York: Syracuse University Press. (First pub. 1970.)

Taft, R. (1956). Some characteristics of good judges of others. *British Journal of Psychology*, *47*, 19–29.

Taylor, Shelly E. (1989). *Positive illusions: Creative self-deception and the healthy mind*. New York: Basic Books.

Taylor, Shelley E. & Brown, Jonathon D. (1988). Illusion and well-being: A social psychological perspective on mental health. *Psychological Bulletin*, *103*(2), 193–210.

Thomson, Godfrey (1939). *The factorial analysis of human ability*. New York: Houghton Mifflin.

Thorndike, E. L. (1920). Intelligence and its uses. *Harper's Magazine*, *140*, 227–35.

Tolkien, J. R. R. (1965). *Tree and leaf*. Boston: Houghton Mifflin.

Tolstoy, Leo (1869/1952). *War and peace*. Louise & Aylmer Maude (Trans.). In *Great books of the Western world*, vol. 51. Chicago: Encyclopedia Britannica.

van den Berg, J. H. (1955). *The phenomenological approach to psychiatry: An introduction to recent phenomenological psychopathology*. Springfield, IL: Charles C. Thomas.

van den Berg, J. H. (1972). *A different existence: Principles of phenomenological psychopathology*. Pittsburgh, PA: Duquesne Univ. Press.

van den Berg, J. H. (1980). Phenomenology and psychotherapy. *Journal of Phenomenological Psychology*, *10*(2), 21–49.

van den Haag, Ernest (1974). Gresham's Law in education. In Sidney Hook, Paul Kurtz, & Miro Todorovich (Eds.), *The idea of a modern university* (pp. 45–49). Buffalo, NY: Prometheus Books.

Wakefield, Jerome C. (1992). The concept of mental disorder: On the boundary between biological facts and social values. *American Psychologist*, *47*, 373–88.

Walsh, Roger & Shapiro, Deane H. (Eds.) (1983). *Beyond health and normality: Explorations of exceptional psychological well-being*. New York: Van Nostrand.

Ware, J. E. & Williams, R. G. (1975). The Dr. Fox effect: A study of lecturer effectiveness and ratings of instruction. *Journal of Medical Education*, *50*, 19–156.

Whitehead, Alfred North (1925). Science and the modern world. Cambridge: Cambridge Univ. Press.

Whorf, Benjamin Lee (1956/1962). *Language, thought, and reality.* John B. Carroll
    (Ed.). Cambridge, MA: Technology Press of MIT. (First pub. 1956.)
Wile, Ira S. (1940). What constitutes abnormality? *American Journal of Ortho-
    psychiatry, 10,* 216–28.
Wood, Dustin, Gosling, Samuel D., & Potter, Jeff (2007). Normality evaluations
    and their relation to personality traits and well-being. *Journal of Personality
    & Social Psychology, 93*(5), 861–79.
Woodall, James (1996). *The man in the mirror of the book: A life of Jorge Luis Borges.*
    London: Hodder & Stoughton.
Woolf, Virginia (1929). *A room of one's own.* New York: Harcourt, Brace & Co.
World Health Organization (1994). *The ICD-10 classification of mental and behav-
    ioural disorders: Clinical descriptions and diagnostic guidelines.* Geneva: World
    Health Organization.
Wulff, Henrik R. (1976). *Rational diagnosis and treatment.* Oxford: Blackwell Sci-
    entific Publishers.
Wynne-Tyson, Jon (Ed.) (1985/1989). *The extended circle: A commonplace book of
    animal rights.* New York: Paragon House. (First pub. 1985.)
Yalow, Rosalyn S. (1982). Competency testing for reviewers and editors. In Harnad
    (1982), 60–61.
Zillmer, Eric A., Harrower, Molly, Ritzler, Barry A., & Archer, Robert P. (1995).
    *The quest for the Nazi personality: A psychological investigation of Nazi war
    criminals.* Hillsdale, NJ: Lawrence Erlbaum.
Ziman, John (1982). Bias, incompetence, or bad management? In Harnad (1982),
    61–62.
Zimbardo, Philip (2007). *The Lucifer effect: Understanding how good people turn evil.*
    New York: Random House.

Index

About the Author

STEVEN JAMES BARTLETT was born in Mexico City and educated in Mexico, the United States, and France. He received his undergraduate degree from Raymond College, an Oxford-style honors college of the University of the Pacific; his master's degree from the University of California, Santa Barbara; his doctorate from the Université de Paris, where his research was directed by Paul Ricoeur; and has done postdoctoral study in clinical psychology. He has been the recipient of many honors, awards, grants, scholarships, and fellowships. His research has been supported under contract or grant by the Alliance Française, the American Association for the Advancement of Science, the Center for the Study of Democratic Institutions, the Lilly Endowment, the Max-Planck-Gesellschaft, the National Science Foundation, the RAND Corporation, and others.

Bartlett brings to the present work an unusual background consisting of training in pathology, psychology, and epistemology. He has published 15 books and monographs and many papers and research studies in the fields of psychology, epistemology, and philosophy of science. He has taught at Saint Louis University and the University of Florida and has held research positions at the Max-Planck-Institut in Starnberg, Germany, and at the Center for the Study of Democratic Institutions in Santa Barbara. He is currently visiting scholar in psychology at Willamette University and senior research professor at Oregon State University.